Methods in Mammary Gland Biology and Breast Cancer Research

Committee on Mammary Gland Biology

Sandra A. Haslam, Chair
Margaret C. Neville, Executive Secretary

Carlos Arteaga

Bonnie B. Asch

Dale E. Bauman

Kermit Carraway

Robert Clarke

Joanne T. Emerman

Armond Goldman

Bernd Groner

Howard Hosick

Nancy E. Hynes

Margot M. Ip

Edison Liu

Ian Mather

Daniel Medina

Malcolm Peaker

Jeffrey Rosen

David Salomon

Floyd Schanbacher

Charles Streuli

Barbara K. Vonderhaar

Methods in Mammary Gland Biology and Breast Cancer Research

Edited by

Margot M. Ip

and

Bonnie B. Asch

Roswell Park Cancer Research Institute
Buffalo, New York

Kluwer Academic / Plenum Publishers
New York, Boston, Dordrecht, London, Moscow

Library of Congress Cataloging-in-Publication Data

Methods in mammary gland biology and breast cancer research/edited by Margot M. Ip
and Bonnie B. Asch.
    p. cm.
    Result of a meeting held in 1997 entitled: "Gordon Conference on Mammary Gland Biology".
    Includes bibliographical references and index.
    ISBN 0-306-46397-0
    1. Breast—Cancer—Laboratory manuals. 2. Breast—Physiology—Laboratory manuals. I.
Ip, Margot M. II. Asch, Bonnie B. III. Gordon Conference on Mammary Gland Biology
(1997)

RC280.B8 M48 2000
616.99′449—dc21

00-025889

A publication of the Committee on Mammary Gland Biology

ISBN: 0-306-46397-0

©2000 Kluwer Academic/Plenum Publishers
233 Spring Street, New York, N.Y. 10013

http://www.wkap.nl/

10 9 8 7 6 5 4 3 2 1

A C.I.P. record for this book is available from the Library of Congress

Printed in the United States of America

Contributors

Domenico Accili   Endocrinology Branch, National Institute of Child Health and Human Development, National Institutes of Health, Bethesda, Maryland 20892

Cheryl A. Ammerman   Department of Radiation Oncology, University of Michigan, Ann Arbor, Michigan 48109-0984

Neal Beeman   Department of Physiology, University of Colorado Health Sciences Center, Denver, Colorado 80262

Joel Brody   Department of Anatomy, University of California, San Francisco, California 94143

Gerald R. Cunha   Department of Anatomy, University of California, San Francisco, California 94143

Trevor Dale   Institute of Cancer Research, The Breakthrough Toby Robins Breast Cancer Centre, London, SW3 6JB England

Charles W. Daniel   Department of Biology, University of California, Santa Cruz, California 95065

Kathleen M. Darcy   GOG Statistical and Data Office, Roswell Park Cancer Institute, Buffalo, New York 14263

Michele L. Dziubinski   Department of Radiation Oncology, University of Michigan, Ann Arbor, Michigan 48109-0984

Connie J. Eaves   Department of Medical Genetics, University of British Columbia, Terry Fox Laboratory, British Columbia Cancer Agency, Vancouver, British Columbia, Canada

Stephen B. Edge   Department of Surgical Oncology, Roswell Park Cancer Institute, Buffalo, New York 14263

Joanne T. Emerman   Department of Anatomy, University of British Columbia, Vancouver, British Columbia V6T 1Z3 Canada

Stephen P. Ethier   Department of Radiation Oncology, University of Michigan, Ann Arbor, Michigan 48109-0984

Priscilla A. Furth   Institute of Human Virology and Division of Infectious Diseases, Department of Medicine and Department of Physiology, University of Maryland Medical School, Baltimore, Maryland 21201

Erika Ginsburg   Laboratory of Tumor Immunology and Biology, National Cancer Institute, National Institutes of Health, Bethesda, Maryland 20892

Michael N. Gould   University of Wisconsin Comprehensive Cancer Center and McArdle Laboratory for Cancer Research, University of Wisconsin-Madison, Madison, Wisconsin 53792

Raphael C. Guzman   Department of Molecular and Cell Biology, Cancer Research Laboratory, University of California, Berkeley, California 94720

Lothar Hennighausen   Laboratory of Genetics and Physiology, National Institute of Diabetes, Digestive, and Kidney Diseases, National Institutes of Health, Bethesda, Maryland 20892

Gloria H. Heppner   Karmanos Cancer Institute and School of Medicine, Detroit, Michigan 48201

Yun Kit Hom   Department of Anatomy, University of California, San Francisco, California 94143

Russell C. Hovey   Laboratory of Tumor Immunology and Biology, National Cancer Institute, National Institutes of Health, Bethesda, Maryland 20892

Thelma C. Hurd   Department of Surgical Oncology, Roswell Park Cancer Institute, Buffalo, New York 14263

Walter Imagawa   Department of Molecular and Integrative Physiology, University of Kansas Medical Center, Kansas City, Kansas 66160

Margot M. Ip   Department of Pharmacology and Therapeutics, Roswell Park Cancer Institute, Buffalo, New York 14263

Frances Kittrell   Department of Molecular and Cell Biology, Baylor College of Medicine, Houston, Texas 77030

Ping-Ping H. Lee   Department of Pharmacology and Therapeutics, Roswell Park Cancer Institute, Buffalo, New York 14263

Michael Lewis   Department of Physiology, University of Colorado Health Sciences Center, Denver, Colorado 80262

Minglin Li   Institute of Human Virology and Division of Infectious Diseases, Department of Medicine, University of Maryland Medical School, Baltimore, Maryland 21201

Daniel Medina   Department of Molecular and Cell Biology, Baylor College of Medicine, Houston, Texas 77030

Fred R. Miller   Karmanos Cancer Institute and School of Medicine, Wayne State University, Detroit, Michigan 48201

Shigeki Miyamoto   Department of Pharmacology, University of Wisconsin Clinical Science Center, Madison, Wisconsin 53792

Satyabrata Nandi   Department of Molecular and Cell Biology, Cancer Research Laboratory, University of California, Berkeley, California 94720

Margaret C. Neville   Department of Physiology, University of Colorado Health Sciences Center, Denver, Colorado 80262

Duy-Ai Nguyen   Department of Physiology, University of Colorado Health Sciences Center, Denver, Colorado 80262

Susan B. Rasmussen   Laboratory of Tumor Immunology and Biology, National Cancer Institute, National Institutes of Health, Bethesda, Maryland 20892

Elizabeth A. Repasky   Department of Immunology, Roswell Park Cancer Institute, Buffalo, New York 14263

Gertraud W. Robinson   Laboratory of Genetics and Physiology, National Institute of Diabetes, Digestive, and Kidney Diseases, National Institutes of Health, Bethesda, Maryland 20892

Edmund B. Rucker III   Laboratory of Genetics and Physiology, National Institute of Diabetes, Digestive, and Kidney Diseases, National Institutes of Health, Bethesda, Maryland 20892

Jerome Schaack   Department of Physiology, University of Colorado Health Sciences Center, Denver, Colorado 80262

Gary B. Silberstein   Department of Biology, University of California, Santa Cruz, California 95065

Harry K. Slocum   Tissue Procurement Facility, Department of Pathology, Roswell Park Cancer Institute, Buffalo, New York 14263

Gilbert H. Smith   Laboratory of Tumor Immunology and Biology, National Cancer Institute, National Institutes of Health, Bethesda, Maryland 20892

John Stingl   Department of Anatomy, University of British Columbia, Vancouver, British Columbia V6T 1Z3 Canada

Henry J. Thompson   Center for Nutrition in the Prevention of Disease, AMC Cancer Research Center, Lakewood, Colorado 80214

Todd A. Thompson   University of Wisconsin Comprehensive Cancer Center and McArdle Laboratory for Cancer Research, University of Wisconsin-Madison, Madison, Wisconsin 53792

Barbara K. Vonderhaar   Laboratory of Tumor Immunology and Biology, National Cancer Institute, National Institutes of Health, Bethesda, Maryland 20892

Kay-Uwe Wagner   Laboratory of Genetics and Physiology, National Institute of Diabetes, Digestive, and Kidney Diseases, National Institutes of Health, Bethesda, Maryland 20892; *Current address*: Eppley Institute for Research in Cancer and Allied Diseases, University of Nebraska Medical Center, Omaha, Nebraska 68198-6805

Steven Weber-Hall   Institute of Cancer Research, The Breakthrough Toby Robins Breast Cancer Centre, London, SW3 6JB England

Yan Xu   Department of Immunology, Roswell Park Cancer Institute, Buffalo, New York 14263

Jason Yang   Department of Molecular and Cell Biology, Cancer Research Laboratory, University of California, Berkeley, California 94720

Lawrence J. T. Young   Center for Comparative Medicine, University of California-Davis, Davis, California 95616

Peter Young   Department of Anatomy, University of California, San Francisco, California 94143

Danilo Zangani   Department of Pharmacology and Therapeutics, Roswell Park Cancer Institute, Buffalo, New York 14263

Foreword from the Committee on Mammary Gland Biology

The Committee on Mammary Gland Biology was formed in the 1980s to promote research and communication among scientists in all the varied specialities necessary to understand the development, function, and diseases of the mammary gland. It has met regularly since that time, with a constantly shifting membership, mainly in conjunction with the Gordon Conference on Mammary Gland Biology. In 1987 the Committee sponsored the publication of a book *The Mammary Gland*, edited by Charles Daniel and Margaret Neville. In 1993 the Committee recognized the need for more extensive communication among members of the community of mammary gland biologists and founded the *Journal of Mammary Gland Biology and Neoplasia*, a review journal currently in its fifth year of publication.

The present book grew out of a meeting of the Editorial Board of *The Journal of Mammary Gland Biology and Neoplasia* at the 1997 Gordon Conference on Mammary Gland Biology, at which a number of members expressed their frustration with the lack of a generally available source for methods for investigation of the mammary gland and breast cancer. The advantages of such an organ for studies of the development and for modeling of mammary tumorigenesis *in vitro* and *in vivo*, if we are to develop a rational approach to breast cancer, were universally clear. What was not clear were the technical details involved in the use of this marvelous organ to advance our understanding of both development and carcinogenesis. This need was reaffirmed at a second meeting of the Editorial Board held in Bethesda two weeks later. Soon thereafter Margot Ip and Bonnie Asch agreed to edit this volume, and they began what seemed like an endless task of recruiting authors, reviewing and editing submitted chapters for consistency and clarity, collecting diskettes and permission forms, and, finally, making sure that every article provided meaningful and up-to-date information.

The Committee on Mammary Gland Biology is now happy to present this long overdue compilation of methods in the field. Some, like transplantation into the cleared fat pad, are old enough to earn the appellation *classic*. Others, like the use of viral transduction, are still under development. Some are quite difficult and require considerable experience. Others are almost a matter of common sense, once the details of the approach are presented. This book is intended as a bench manual, so materials are carefully described and each step of the procedure carefully laid out in a volume that will lie flat on the laboratory bench. Where pitfalls and limitations are present, they are outlined. Where a technique shows promise that has not yet been realized, potential uses are illustrated. We feel sure that the techniques presented here will promote outstanding research, as well as the development of new approaches to the experimental problems that still face us in understanding this most fascinating of organs.

Too many people contributed to the completion of this volume to allow acknowledgment of all the individual efforts, but we particularly thank the reviewers whose input into the editorial process was invaluable and the authors of these chapters who revised their text, sometimes more than once, to bring it to the high standards set by the Editors. The Committee gratefully acknowledges the support of Vysis, Inc., in the publication of a color figure in Chapter 19, by S. Weber-Hall and Trevor Dale. Finally, we wish to express our heartfelt appreciation to Margot Ip and Bonnie Asch, who worked long and hard to bring this volume to fruition.

Margaret C. Neville
for the Committee on Mammary Gland Biology

Preface

One of the most exciting and beneficial developments in research on mammary gland biology and breast cancer has been the influx of increased funding to support this work. This influx, which has been due primarily to the tireless efforts of breast cancer activists to garner additional money from various federal and state sources, has led to a rapid expansion of research efforts by attracting numerous new investigators into the field. These new investigators include students, postdoctoral fellows, and scientists from other fields. Most of these individuals are not familiar with the myriad considerations and factors that are critical for conducting meaningful research on mammary cells and tissues. In addition, scientists who have been working on the mammary gland for many years may need to use a method or procedure that they have not previously used. Until now, however, the important and, in many cases, unique techniques necessary to studies on mammary gland biology and breast cancer have not been available in one place, in a volume convenient for lab use, and containing as many details as possible. Another consideration in producing this volume was that some of the pioneering scientists who developed the special methods and procedures for research on the mammary gland are retiring to follow other pursuits, and we wanted them to provide an accurate description of their protocols before departing. We have tried to include as many critical techniques as possible. The chapters are written by experts in each area with an emphasis on "nitty-gritty" details that are key points for successful use of a method. Techniques included range from the classic clearing of the mammary gland fat pad, with subsequent transplantation of mammary epithelial cells and analysis of the mammary whole mount, a technique now undergoing a rebirth in the evaluation of the consequences of gene deletion, to the technically challenging and still-evolving methodology for conditional deletion of genes in the mammary gland.

The original plan for this volume was to include an atlas of normal and cancer-related histology of the mammary gland in mice, rats, and humans. However, the final number of chapters proved to be too many for one volume. Consequently, the atlas articles will appear in an addendum to the April 2000 issue of *The Journal of Mammary Gland Biology and Neoplasia*. These articles provide a requisite complement to the chapters in this book because the methods described assume the reader has a reasonable understanding of mammary gland architecture in females of different ages and physiological stages. We therefore strongly recommend that anyone who is unfamiliar with the structure of the gland read the appropriate atlas articles to facilitate understanding of the methods given here.

We are most grateful to the editors of *The Journal of Mammary Gland Biology and Neoplasia* for inviting us to serve as editors of this book. We especially want to thank the many contributors for their patient cooperation. They were very responsive to our requests for changes and corrections. We want to emphasize that for certain topics other scientists were equally qualified to describe the technique. However, because of space considerations, it was necessary to limit the number of contributors. The issue is organized into four parts: *In Vivo* Model Systems, Special Techniques for *In Vivo* Studies, *In Vitro* Model Systems, and Molecular Analysis and Gene Transfer Techniques.

Our hope is for copies of this book to become well-worn from extensive laboratory use and for its contents to promote and facilitate high-quality research to help fill the vast gaps in our knowledge about mammary development and carcinogenesis.

Margot M. Ip and Bonnie B. Asch
Roswell Park Cancer Institute

Contents

Part II. Special Techniques for *In Vivo* Studies

Part III. *In Vitro* Model Systems

Part I

In Vivo **Model Systems***

*A useful adjunct to the techniques presented in this part is *The Mouse Mammary Video*. This video, put together by Charles Daniel, presents surgical procedures, small-animal handling, and a general description of mammary development. Further information about this video and how it can be purchased can be found at the website http://www.biology.ucsc.edu/mamvid.

Chapter 1

Mouse Models for Mammary Cancer

Daniel Medina

Abstract. This chapter provides an overview of of the major types of mouse models that are used in the study of breast cancer. The major strengths and limitations with specific caveats for each type of model are provided to guide the reader in the appropriate choice of model to examine questions pertinent to breast cancer research. It is the intent of this overview to help clarify the contributions of traditional models of breast cancer and provide a rationale for the continued development of new models that more closely reflect the human disease.

Abbreviations. loss of heterozygosity (LOH); transforming growth factor α (TGFα); transforming growth factor β (TGFβ); 4-hydroxyphenylretinamide (4-HPR); dimethylbenzanthracene (DMBA); polycyclic aromatic hydrocarbons (PAH).

INTRODUCTION

The mouse has played an historic role in the development of models for breast cancer. Three eras in model building for breast cancer can be defined. The first era, roughly from 1920 to 1960, represented a time when inbred mice were recognized and developed as unique models for susceptibility to specific cancers, including breast cancers. Studies on inbred mice, such as C3H, RIII, GR, A, BALB/c, and C57BL6, led to the hypothesis that specific genetic, hormonal, and viral factors were important for susceptibility to breast cancer (1). These studies resulted in the recognition that MMTV-induced mammary tumorigenesis was a consequence of insertional activation of specific genes of the *wnt* and *fgf* families. The examination of chemical carcinogens and hormones demonstrated the synergistic interactions of these two factors in mammary tumorigenesis and provided additional model systems to assay for prevention modalities (2). The second era, roughly from 1980 to 1995, resulted from the recognition that specific oncogenes and tumor suppressor genes played pivotal roles in mammary carcinogenesis and that constitutive overexpression of specific oncogenes targeted to the mammary gland (e.g., *c-myc, p53mut, v-ras, TGFα, wnt-1, cyclin D1,* polyoma *mt*) resulted in markedly enhanced tumorigenesis (3). The chemical carcinogen models identified specific molecular alterations (e.g., *ras*) and dietary factors (e.g., selenium, retinoids, lipids) that play pivotal roles in tumorigenesis. The constitutively overexpressed gene models are still being constructed or used in bigenic models. The value of constitutively overexpressed gene models lies

Daniel Medina   **Department of Molecular and Cell Biology, Baylor College of Medicine, Houston, Texas 77030.**

Methods in Mammary Gland Biology and Breast Cancer Research, edited by Ip and Asch. Kluwer Academic/Plenum Publishers, New York, 2000.

in the ability to examine the effects of a single gene; however, these models are also limited by the leakiness and multitissue expression of the promoter (i.e., MMTV) that may interfere with the study of mammary specific effects. Additionally, the extent of overexpression is difficult to control as multiple gene copies are integrated into the host genome. Comparable studies using gene deletion models have been restricted to total gene deletion and not mammary-gland-specific deletion and, thus, have not been particularly useful in understanding the role of specific genes in mammary tumorigenesis (4, 5). The third era of model building, which started roughly in 1997, is upon us and takes advantage of tissue-specific gene deletion and activation. The ability to delete a specific gene (i.e., *Brca2, Rb*) restricted to the mammary gland or inducibly activate an oncogene only in the mammary gland provides the opportunity to model the human disease as closely as possible. The development and characterization of such models at the morphological, chromosomal, genetic, and biological levels will identify new molecular targets for therapeutic or prevention treatment modalities.

It is not the intent of this chapter to review each of these models but to provide an overview of the main features of the different models and some of their strengths and weaknesses for understanding breast cancer. A summary of the main characteristics of mouse mammary tumors is provided in Table 1-1.

VIRUSES

Two types of viruses are known to induce mammary tumors in mice: the mouse mammary tumor virus (MMTV) is a retrovirus, and polyoma is a DNA virus. The analysis of different inbred mouse strains led to the elucidation and dominant role of MMTV in mouse mammary tumorigenesis. The classical mouse mammary tumor virus represents a family of closely related retroviruses that are transmitted either via the milk (exogenous virus) from mother to offspring or via the germ cells (endogenous virus). The exogenously transmitted MMTV is associated with a high mammary tumor incidence and a short tumor latency period and is responsible for the strains of mice with a high "spontaneous" mammary tumor incidence, such as C3H, RIII, GR, A, and DBA/2. Elimination of exposure to virus by foster-nursing newborn pups on MMTV-free dams reduces or eliminates mammary tumors. For example, BALB/cV fostered on BALB/c results in a strain (BALB/cVf) with a zero incidence of mammary tumors at 15 months of age. C3H mice fostered on C57BL mice results in a strain (C3Hf) with a reduced mammary tumor incidence and long tumor latency period. The differences in mammary tumor incidence between the BALB/cVf and C3Hf strains reflects the fact that the C3H strain also carries a fully functional, transcriptional active endogenous provirus, whereas the BALB/c strain only carries nonfunctional endogenous proviruses.

The mechanism of exogenous MMTV-induced mammary tumorigenesis is understood in its broad outlines. Tumorigenesis is the result of random insertion of the viral genome into mammary cell DNA (6). Multiple insertion sites have been found and the most common ones in tumors have been mapped and well defined. These sites are *wnt*-1, *wnt*-3, *fgf*3, *fgf*4, *fgf*8, *int*-3, and *int*-6 (6–8). The *wnt* genes are part of a family of developmental genes that act through the β-catenin pathway. The *fgf* genes are growth factors, normally produced by stromal cells in the gland, which are important for growth of normal mammary epithelium. As predicted from these observations, transgenic mice with *wnt*-1 or *fgf*3 targeted to the mammary gland have glandular hyperplasia and elevated mammary tumor incidence. *Wnt*-1/*fgf*3 and *wnt*-1/*fgf*8 bigenic mice have higher mammary tumor rates than single transgenic mice (9). The *int* genes are activated as a consequence of MMTV insertion that results

Table 1-1. Characteristics of the Major Types of Mouse Mammary Tumors

Oncogene	Transmission	Mouse strain	Tumor type	Tumor incidence	Mean latency period	Hormone responsiveness	Metastases
MMTV	Milk	C3H, A, DBA, BALB/cfC3H	Adenocarcinoma types A and B	70–100% (breeders)	<1 year	Ovary, pituitary, hormone independent	Frequent to lung
MMTV	Germ cells	C3Hf	Adenocarcinoma types A and B	<40% (breeders)	>1 year	Ovary hormone independent	Unknown
MMTV	Germ cells, milk	GR	Adenocarcinoma type P	>80% (breeders)	<1 year	Pregnancy dependent	Unknown
MMTV	Milk	DD, RIII, DDD	Adenocarcinoma type P, pale cell carcinoma	>80%	<1 year	Ovary dependent	Frequent to lung
Chemical carcinogens	—	BALB/c, DBA2/f, Sencar, FVB, C57BL, (C57BL × DBA/2f)F$_1$	Adenocarcinoma type B, papillary adenocarcinoma, adenosquamous carcinoma, pale cell carcinoma	20–70%	≤1 year	Ovary dependent (C57BL × DBA/2f)F$_1$, ovarian independent (BALB/c)	Occasional to lung
Radiation	—	BALB/c	Adenocarcinoma type B	25%	>1 year	Ovary independent	Frequent to lung

in truncated gene products. Both of the *int* genes were found in Czech mice, a strain that lacks endogenous MMTV genes and transmits MMTV only via the milk. *Int-3* is related to the *notch* family of developmental genes. The consequence of MMTV insertion is inappropriate activation of the genes, which then function as oncogenes.

Mammary tumors arise from hyperplastic alveolar nodules (HAN) induced by MMTV infection (2). Transplantation experiments into syngeneic mice demonstrate in a direct fashion that HAN are precursors to mammary adenocarcinomas. The targeted overexpression of MMTV-activated *wnt* genes results in mammary hyperplasia prior to tumor formation. Finally, the presence of HAN has been used as an assay endpoint for carcinogenesis and chemoprevention studies (10).

Mammary tumors arising in MMTV-infected mice are highly metastatic and are strain dependent (reviewed in 2). Spontaneous mammary tumors in mice metastasized with a high frequency that depended on the strain, type of MMTV, and the tumor–host relationship. Mammary tumor metastases, primarily to the lung, have been reported in strains RIII, BALB/c, C3H, A, DBA, BALB/cfC3H, BALB/cf RIII, and (BALB/c × DBA/8)F$_1$. C3H mice have a 49% incidence of metastasis in retired breeders, whereas RIII have a 17% incidence. Interestingly, BALB/cfC3H mice have a higher incidence of metastases (63%) than BALB/cf RIII mice (17%). In (BALB/c × DBA/8F$_1$) mice, 67% of spontaneous tumors metastasized within 7 to 63 days after initial observation of the primary tumor. The incidence of metastases was proportional to the size of the primary tumor but was not correlated with the growth rate of the tumor when implanted subcutaneously. In a large study using several different strains, metastases were increased by breeding, administration of estrogen, pituitary isografts, and tumorectomy, but were not related to size or location of tumor, histological type, or latent period of tumor growth. A conscientious effort is required to detect distal metastases, as several investigators have demonstrated a high frequency of metastases to lungs and liver 6–9 weeks after removal of the primary tumor. The frequently stated opinion that mouse mammary tumors are not highly metastatic is a misconception that has not been effectively laid to rest, although the data argue convincingly against it.

An appreciable number of mammary tumors in mice are hormone dependent. The term *hormone dependent* is used to designate tumors that depend on reproductive hormones for tumor growth. In most experiments the exact set of hormones that influence the growth of tumors has not been defined; however, the organ (i.e., ovary) or condition (i.e., pregnancy) has been determined. Although mammary tumors appearing in the conventional American-derived strains of C3H, C3Hf, DBA, A, BALB/cfC3H, and BALB/c are ovary independent, several investigators have shown that MMTV-induced tumors in the European-derived strains GR, BR6, RIII, and DDD mice are pregnancy dependent (2).

There is very little convincing evidence that mammary tumor viruses play an etiologic role in human breast cancer. Nonetheless, the MMTV mouse models have led to the identification of mammary cellular oncogenes that may play a role in human breast cancer. At least three *wnt* genes (*wnt* 2, 5a, and 7b) have been reported to be overexpressed in human breast cancers compared to normal tissues (11, 12); however, functional data for the oncogenic potential of these genes is still missing. The *fgf* genes play a role in ductal branching, although their role as human mammary oncogenes remains poorly described. The utility of the MMTV mouse models currently lies in the elucidation of the roles of the activated genes, and for this reason there has been a shift from using the traditional inbred strains carrying exogenous MMTV to developing and studying transgenic models in which specific *wnt* or *fgf* genes are overexpressed in the mammary gland. Furthermore, it has been recently argued that transgenic mice provide a more useful tool for mechanism-based cancer prevention research (13).

   The second virus model of mammary tumorigenesis is the polyoma virus, which is a DNA virus. The limited number of investigations of the oncogenicity of this virus convincingly demonstrate that infection of newborn BALB/c mice with polyoma virus results in a rapid and high incidence of mammary tumors (14). The infection results in ductal hyperplasias prior to mammary tumor formation. Transgenic mice with polyoma middle T(*mt*) targeted to the gland recapitulate the high mammary tumor incidence and demonstrate the metastatic properties of these tumors (15). The advantage of the transgenic polyoma model lies in the constitutive overexpression of the gene in the mammary gland of an inbred strain (FVB) instead of having to continually infect young mice with viral preparations each generation. The model is also useful for dissecting mechanisms of DNA-virus-induced mammary oncogenesis. Although DNA viruses are not known oncogenic agents for the human breast, the molecular targets of the oncogene, polyoma *mt*, involve signaling pathways of both phosphatidylinositol 3′ kinase and the Shc adapter protein. The ability to engineer mutants of the middle T gene, which lack either of these two activities, and examine the consequences for early pathogenesis (e.g., hyperplasia), primary tumor formation, or metastases presents a powerful and useful approach (15).

   In summary, the traditional mammary tumor virus models, both RNA and DNA viruses, have been effectively replaced by transgenic models that focus on the functional activities of the relevant oncogenes. One might argue that the C3H, GR, and Czech mice might still be useful for the discovery of additional oncogenes that may play a role in human breast cancer, but the transgenic mice are the best models to use for dissecting out functional activities of these genes and for serving as appropriate test mice in studies of mechanism-based cancer prevention.

CHEMICAL CARCINOGENESIS

Strain Differences in Susceptibility

   Chemical carcinogenesis in the mouse mammary gland has been studied since 1940. Early studies demonstrated that numerous strains of MMTV-free mice are susceptible to polycylic-hydrocarbon-induced mammary tumorigenesis and that hormonal stimulation facilitated the tumorigenic effects of carcinogens. The relative susceptibility of different mouse strains to specific carcinogenic-induced mammary tumorigenesis can be gleaned from different experiments. In response to polycyclic hydrocarbons (e.g., 3-methylcholanthrene), the relative susceptibility from highest to lowest was DBA/2f, BALB/c, C3Hf, and C57BL (16) (Table 1-2). The F1 hybrid between DBA/2f and C57BL is highly susceptible even in virgin mice (17). Two recent strains of interest are FVB and Sencar. The FVB strain is widely used in transgenic models (18). Compared to BALB/c mice, FVB mice are slightly less susceptible when treated as virgin mice (37% vs. 24%) but are equally highly sensitive if hormonally stimulated (Table 1-2). The typical tumorigenic response to 4 mg DMBA in the presence of hormone stimulation is shown here for FVB (Figure 1-1). At high doses close to 100% tumors were produced 8–13 weeks after the first dose. Reducing the dose from 4 to 1 mg increases the mean tumor latency as shown here from 9 to 32 weeks (Figure 1-1). The Sencar mouse seems to be the most sensitive of all mouse strains because it develops a high frequency (65%) of mammary tumors relatively rapidly (4.5 months) in virgin (not hormonally stimulated) mice (19).

   Mice treated with chemical carcinogens frequently die of cancers other than mammary tumors. The most frequent causes of death (other than mammary cancer) are lymphomas,

Table 1-2. Relative Susceptibility of Mouse Strains to Chemical Carcinogen-Induced Mammary Tumors

Strain	Virgin[a]	Hormone-stimulated[a]
DBA/2f	57 (13)[b]	90 (11)[b,c]
BALB/c	67 (18)[b]	90 (12)[b,c]
C3Hf	27 (14)[b]	46 (12)[b,c]
C57BL	3 (18)[b]	30 (18)[b,c]
Sencar	65 (4.5)[d]	N.D.
BALB/c	37 (10)[d]	90 (4)[e]
FVB	24 (10)[d]	90 (3)[e]

[a]Percent mammary tumors with mean age of mice (in months) given in parentheses.
[b]9 mg 3-methylcholanthrene administered orally, 1 mg weekly.
[c]Mice were forced breeders.
[d]4 to 5 mg DMBA administered orally.
[e]4 mg DMBA administered orally in mice with a pituitary isograft.
ND = not determined.

ovarian cancer, and gastric cancer. These cancers can complicate the usefulness and interpretation of any carcinogenic treatment. For example, in the progesterone receptor knockout (PRKO) mouse, which has a (129/Sv × C57BL) genetic background, the ovarian cancer incidence was 70% in virgin mice and exceeded the mammary tumor incidence. Similarly, Sencar mice treated with a total dose of 1.8 mg DMBA had a 75% incidence of lymphoma and a 30% incidence of mammary tumors. Lowering the total dose to 600 μg (20 μg/day × 6 weeks) resulted in 65% mammary tumors by 47 weeks and only 25% lymphomas (20).

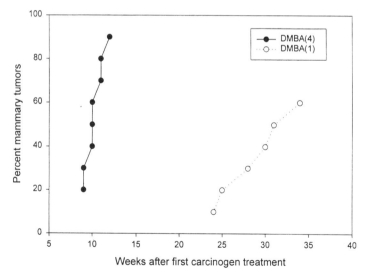

Figure 1-1. DMBA-induced mammary tumorigenesis in FVB mice. The response of pituitary-isograft-bearing FVB female mice to a high dose of 7,12-dimethylbenzanthracene (1 mg per week for 4 weeks;) is compared to mice receiving a low dose (0.5 mg per week for 2 weeks;). In both cases the carcinogen was first administered to 8-week-old mice.

Co-carcinogenesis

Chemical carcinogens can be utilized in multiple protocols. They can be administered as subthreshold initiating agents where a phenotypic effect is not detected until a promoting stimulus is applied subsequently. They can be administered as one or multiple doses sufficient to induce a phenotypic effect (e.g., hyperplasia or neoplasia), as discussed in the preceding sections. Finally, they can be administered to existing preneoplastic mammary cell populations to trigger or enhance tumor development. The latter protocol has been extensively utilized (21). The susceptibility of existing preneoplastic cell populations to chemical carcinogens, such as DMBA and urethane, is very high. For instance, whereas a total dose of 6 mg DMBA is required to neoplastically transform normal virgin ductal epithelium in BALB/c mice, only 0.5 mg is required to induce tumors in BALB/c preneoplastic mammary cell populations (21). As in normal mammary glands, *ras* is frequently activated. The increased susceptibility of mammary preneoplastic cell populations to DMBA is also observed in mammary cells of transgenic mice. Both TGFα transgenic mice (22) and p53[172Arg-His] transgenic mice (23) exhibited increased susceptibility to DMBA-induced transformation. The response of the mammary cell to a chemical carcinogen is a useful approach to determine if genetic alterations that do not convey an obvious phenotypic property can alter susceptibility of the mammary epithelium to tumorigenesis.

Role of Hormones

The importance of hormone stimulation in mammary tumorigenesis was documented by the earliest investigators. As shown in Table 1-2, concomitant hormone stimulation of the carcinogen-treated gland markedly enhanced tumorigenesis. Several methods of hormonal stimulation have been used, including pregnancy, estrogen plus progesterone treatment, medroxyprogesterone, or a pituitary isograft. The latter results in elevated circulating blood levels of estrogen, progesterone, and prolactin. Experiments have demonstrated that concomitant hormone stimulation is necessary for initiation and promotion of carcinogen-altered cells (24). In the experiment illustrated in Figure 1-2, a high incidence of mammary tumors was induced if a pituitary isograft was in place prior to, during, and for 8 weeks after carcinogen treatment. If the pituitary isograft was removed immediately after the last dose of carcinogen, mammary tumor incidence decreased by 50%. If the pituitary isograft was implanted 8 weeks after the initial carcinogen treatment, there was no increase in mammary tumors above the incidence in mice exposed only to carcinogen. Mammary tumors that develop in the presence of a pituitary isograft are not hormone dependent. Progesterone is the critical hormone as shown by the observation that mammary tumorigenesis in the chemical-carcinogen-treated, ovariectomized female mouse required progesterone (25). Estrogen and progesterone, but not estrogen alone, were both necessary for mammary tumorigenesis in ovariectomized mice exposed to chemical carcinogen. Similarly, mammary tumorigenesis was significantly decreased in the carcinogen-treated PRKO mouse compared to the wild-type mouse (25% vs. 75%, respectively) (Lydon and Medina, unpublished data).

Types of Carcinogens

The types of carcinogens used in these studies have not been extensive. Polycyclic hydrocarbons, such as methylcholanthrene, dibenzanthracene, and dimethylbenzanthracene are frequently used (2). The alkylating agents methylnitrosourea, ethylnitrosourea, and

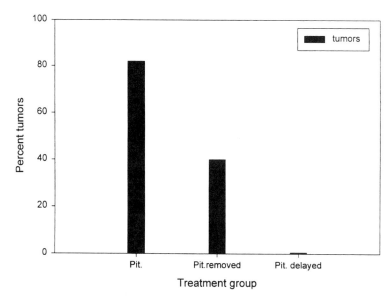

Figure 1-2. Effect of hormone stimulation on carcinogen-induced mammary tumors. The effect of hormone stimulation of the mammary gland provided by a pituitary isograft on 3-methylcholanthrene-induced mammary tumorigenesis in BALB/c mice is shown. The carcinogen (1.5 mg) was given in doses of 0.5 mg once a week for 3 weeks starting at 8 weeks of age. In one group (pit.), the pituitary isograft was in place for 12 weeks starting at 4 weeks of age. In a second group (pit. removed), the pituitary isograft was in place for 6 weeks starting at 4 weeks of age. In a third group (pit. delayed), the pituitary was in place for 12 weeks starting at 16 weeks of age. The ordinate indicates the percent mice bearing mammary tumors.

urethane also induce mammary tumors (2, 26), and 1,3-butadiene given chronically induces mammary tumors at a modest frequency (27). Although both major classes of chemicals are effective carcinogens for the mouse mammary gland, there are subtle differences (Table 1-3). The optimal agent may well be ethylnitrosourea because it can be given as a single dose and induces only adenocarcinomas. The polycyclic hydrocarbons urethane and methylnitrosourea induce adenocarcinomas and adenosquamous carcinomas. Because the latter tumor is not

Table 1-3. Comparison of Polycyclic Aromatic Hydrocarbons and Nitrosoureas as Mammary Carcinogens

Property	PAH	NU
Virgin host	+	−
Hormone stimulation	+	+
Single dose	−	+
Mammary adenocarcinoma	+	+
Adenosquamous carcinoma	+	±
Hormone responsiveness	35%	12%

PAH = polycyclic aromatic hydrocarbons; NU = nitrosourea.
MNU induces both mammary adenocarcinomas and adenosquamous carcinomas, whereas ENU induces only mammary adenocarcinomas in BALB/c mice (26).

frequently encountered in human breast cancer, the presence of this histological class of tumor confounds mechanistic approaches to determining the molecular basis for chemical-carcinogen-induced mammary tumorigenesis in the mouse.

The transforming activity of additional chemicals for the mouse mammary gland has also been investigated using the *in vitro* whole organ assay (28, 29). This assay utilizes hormone-dependent nodule-like alveolar lesions (NLAL) as an endpoint for carcinogen treatment. The assay is short (one month), relatively easy to perform, and yields quantitative data. The assay has been used to examine chemicals that may have carcinogenic potential as well as factors with possible chemopreventive activity. Using this assay, researchers demonstrated that nitrosamines (e.g., *N*-nitrosodiethylamine, *N*-methyl-*N'*-nitro-*N*-nitrosoguanidine), fluorenylacetamides and their activated derivatives, and naphthylamines (both 1- and 2-NA), in addition to PAH and nitrosoureas, are effective carcinogens for the mammary gland.

Pathogenesis

Pathogenesis with both major classes of chemical carcinogens is similar. Alveolar hyperplasias and ductal hyperplasias are induced by chemical carcinogens. In virgin BALB/c and (C57BL × DBA/2f)F_1 mice, ductal hyperplasias are frequent and appear prior to palpable tumors (2). These hyperplastic lesions exhibit extensive intraluminal epithelial proliferation, and transplantation of the ductal hyperplasias into mammary-gland-free fat pads of syngeneic mice directly demonstrated the tumorigenic capability of these lesions. There are multiple (4–5) lesions per animal.

A minority of the tumors (about 35%) derived from these lesions are responsive to hormonal regulation of their growth, either as hormone-dependent or hormone-sensitive cell populations (growth repressed by ovarian hormones). Urethane-induced mammary tumors in BALB/c mice and BD2fF_1 mice, and DMBA-induced tumors in BD2f/F_1 mice, are ovary dependent for growth (2). Interestingly, assessment of the hormone dependency of BD2fF_1 tumors by transplantation into ovariectomized mice demonstrated that 65% grew equally well in ovariectomized versus control mice, 18% required ovarian hormones for growth, and 17% grew better in the ovariectomized mice than in intact mice. The last phenotype was stable for several transplant generations. Ovarian hormone-dependent tumors arising in chemical-carcinogen-treated mice are positive for estrogen and progesterone receptors (30) and have been used as model systems to examine antiestrogen function and tumor progression (31, 32).

The metastatic potential of chemical-carcinogen-induced mammary tumors has not been adequately studied, but metastases to the lung have been noted (2). There is no reason to assume that these tumors are not frequently metastatic, since MMTV-induced mammary tumors, as noted earlier, and spontaneous BALB/c mammary tumors are highly metastatic; that is, the TM set of BALB/c tumors has a metastatic frequency of 29% (33).

Molecular Alterations

The molecular changes in chemically induced mouse mammary tumors have not been systematically investigated for any model. In BALB/c and Sencar mice, DMBA and MNU treatments result in Ha-*ras* and Ki-*ras* activation, respectively; however,

ENU-induced tumors in the same strain (BALB/c) do not result in Ki-*ras* activation. This result shows that similar chemicals have different spectra of genetic lesions *in vivo* as well as *in vitro*.

The tumor suppressor gene p53 is infrequently mutated in DMBA-induced BALB/c mammary tumors (34). This finding contrasts with an abstract in which frequent p53 mutations in DMBA-induced mammary tumors were reported in Sencar mice (35). However, p53 mutations are frequent in spontaneous mammary tumors in BALB/c mice (36).

Cytogenetic analysis of MMTV-induced mouse mammary tumors shows a diploid karyotype (2). Recently, Aldaz and co-workers examined DMBA-induced mammary tumors in (BALB/c × DBA/2)F$_1$ mice and demonstrated that early arising tumors were essentially diploid (37). However, a higher frequency of loss of heterozygosity (LOH) was detected in tumors arising with a long latency and in transplanted tumors. The authors implicated chromosomes 4, 8, 11, and 14 as frequently exhibiting LOH. Mice chronically exposed to 1,3-butadiene develop mammary tumors with a high frequency of aneuploidy and show a high frequency of LOH in chromosomes 11 and 14 (27).

Dietary Modulation

The BALB/c and Sencar strains have been used in studies of dietary modulation of DMBA-induced mammary tumors. Studies have shown that dietary fat can enhance mammary tumorigenesis (38), whereas specific agents, such as selenium compounds (10) and dibenzoylmethane (39), can inhibit mammary tumorigenesis. Retinoids as a class have little inhibitory effect on DMBA-induced mammary tumors, and some retinoids, such as 4-HPR, slightly enhance mammary tumorigenesis (40). The presence of tumors in secondary sites can even be an advantage in these studies, because some agents, such as curcumin (an antioxidant and free-radical scavenger), inhibit lymphomas but not mammary tumors in Sencar mice (39). Although chemical-carcinogen-induced mammary tumorigenesis in mice is not used as frequently as the similar rat mammary tumor system, it has been a useful second model system to examine the efficacy of any chemopreventive modality. With the advent of transgenic mice with specific molecular alterations, it is likely that the transgenic mouse will be the assay system of the future.

RADIATION

Radiation-induced mammary cancer has not been extensively investigated in the mouse primarily due to the low incidence and long latency of the induced mammary tumors [reviewed in (2)]. Radiation-induced mammary tumors are dose dependent over a dose of 0.25 Gy to 2 Gy. Radiation (4 Gy) increased mammary tumor incidence slightly (20% vs. 10% controls) in WHC mice. In BALB/c mice exposed to 2 Gy of γ-radiation or acute neutron radiation, mammary tumor incidence increased from 7% to 20%. If radiation is provided chronically (0.01 Gy/day, 1.9 Gy total), a 45% incidence was induced in BALB/c mice. The irradiated BALB/c mouse model has been extensively studied by Ullrich and co-workers, who have shown that BALB/c mice are more sensitive than C57BL mice to γ-irradiation (41) and that the initial genetic damage is expressed as increased chromosomal instability at the molecular level (42) and as ductal hyperplasias at the cell level (43). The ability to assess irradiation-induced damage at both levels provides a unique model system to examine and detect specific molecular alterations that occur at the earliest stages of neoplastic development (e.g., ductal hyperplasias). The ductal hyperplasias can be detected in out-growths resulting from cells isolated 24 h after 1 Gy irradiation and transplanted into syn-geneic hosts. The frequency of the ductal hyperplasias was equal to that induced by a low dose of DMBA. Irradiation-induced mammary tumors are classical type A and type B mammary adenocarcinomas, ovarian-hormone independent, yet highly metastatic to lung (2). Since irradiation is the only firmly established human breast carcinogen, this model system deserves more attention. γ-Irradiation also significantly enhances the neoplastic transforma-tion of mammary preneoplastic outgrowth lines, an effect that is apparently independent of the p53 status of the mammary cells (44).

TRANSGENIC MICE

The development of mammary epithelial-targeted gene expression of oncogenes has provided an entirely new set of animal models for mammary cancer (3). The pioneering studies of Leder and co-workers (45) have led to new approaches for examining gene inter-actions and the interactions of genes and environmental carcinogens. These models are pro-viding new approaches for examining mechanistic-based chemoprevention agents (13). It is not our intent to discuss the characteristics of the numerous transgenic models currently available. This information is available in recent reviews (5) and on websites, such as www-mp.ucdavis.edu/tgmice/firststop.html and mammary.nih.gov. In this chapter I will discuss the relative strengths and weaknesses of the transgenic mouse as a model for breast cancer. As mentioned, transgenic mice provide a functional analysis of the mammary onco-genicity of a given gene and sets of genes. These results have reinforced the concept that mammary tumorigenesis requires multiple genetic alterations. Cardiff (46) has argued per-suasively that tumors arising in mice with genetic alterations similar to those found in human breast cancers exhibit a similar histology. Thus, although the histological pattern of traditional mammary adenocarcinoma type B induced by MMTV is infrequently observed in human tumors, mouse and human tumors with a defect in ErbB2 show a similar histological pattern. Further, some of the models exhibit premalignant pathology and metastatic capabilities similar to human breast cancers (46). Finally, and perhaps, most importantly, the models provide the opportunity to examine functional changes in normal mammary development due to single genes that subsequently affect tumorigenesis. For instance, both TGFα and wnt-1 transgenic mammary glands are hyperplastic in a nonpregnant hormonal environment (22, 47). In contrast, TGFβ and p53$^{172Arg-His}$ transgenic glands are blocked in development (48).

Despite these advantages, the transgenic mouse has several limitations. First, classical transgenic mice reflect germ line alterations that do not accurately recapitulate somatic muta-tions. Second, expression levels of the transgene are often many-fold higher than expression of the wild type or naturally occurring mutant gene. Third, the promoters that target gene expression to the mammary gland provide for constitutive expression and are driven primar-ily by hormones. Thus, in order to obtain expression with either the whey acidic protein or β-lactoglobulin promoter, one needs a pregnancy-type hormonal stimulation. Although the MMTV promoter is expressed in the virgin animal, expression is markedly enhanced by pregnancy-type hormones. Thus, regulated expression is limited with these promoters. Finally, the promoters are not entirely mammary specific, or they are leaky. Thus, the MMTV-myc mice develop salivary gland and T-cell lymphomas that can interfere with studies on mammary tumorigenesis. To avoid complications, it is advantageous to have on–off switch-ing of expression localized to the mammary gland and capable of regulation at any time of

development. The Cre-*lox* system provides this potential for both gene activation and deletion (49); see Chapter 24 by Wagner *et al.* in this volume).

Gene-deletion mice (i.e., knockout) are a special case of transgenic mice in which the
gene is engineered to be nonfunctional in embryonic stem cell lines. This powerful approach
provides the opportunity to examine the effects of the absence of a specific gene. The impact
on mammary tumorigenesis can be stunning, as provided in the cyclin D1 knockout mouse
where the effect of cyclin D1 gene deletion was manifest only on the failure of the gland to
differentiate in pregnancy (50), but had no effect on growth of the gland in virgin mice. Similarly, the estrogen receptor knockout (ERKO) (51) and progesterone receptor knockout (52)
are very interesting models to use for examining specific gene function in mammary tumorigenesis. Although many of the knockouts relevant to mammary gland function are embryonic lethals, as is the case for *Brca* genes (5), it is possible to rescue the mammary epithelium
from some embryonic lethals (see Chapter 26 by Robinson *et al.* in this volume). However,
the need for conditional gene-deletion models is paramount and a primary objective for future
studies.

SUMMARY

The mouse models for mammary cancer have provided the basis for the establishment
of fundamental concepts in understanding the multistage nature of cancer development. Thus,
the concepts of genetics–hormone–virus interactions in tumorigenesis, Fould's concept of
tumor progression, gene activation, and the role of preneoplasia are all derived from the traditional models. These models have provided assays for pathogenesis, carcinogen identification, dietary modulation, and chemoprevention of mammary cancer. Further understanding
of the molecular basis of mammary cancer as well as the mechanistic basis of chemoprevention will be attained by the use of the mouse models that more closely mimic human breast
cancers. Thus, models now exist that overexpress *neu*, c-*myc*, and cyclin D1 genes and
$p53^{172\text{Arg-His}}$, each representative of a subset of human breast cancers. As new genes are identified in human breast cancer, it will be important to develop appropriate transgenic or gene-
deletion mice. It is worthwhile to emphasize that human breast cancer is not a single set of
genetic alterations, but many subsets of multiple genetic alterations. In the future, there should
be many murine models of mammary cancer, each reflecting a subset of the human disease.
One urgently needed technology is the ability to generate gene deletion or activation singly
and in combination so that such models can be utilized in studies on pathogenesis, gene function, genetic instability, and chemoprevention.

REFERENCES

 1. B. L. Slagle and J. S. Butel (1987). Exogenous and endogenous mouse mammary tumor viruses: replication
    and cell transformation. In D. Medina, W. Kidwell, G. Heppner, and E. Anderson (eds.), *Cellular and
    Molecular Biology of Mammary Cancer*, Plenum Press, New York, pp. 275–306.
 2. D. Medina (1982). Mammary tumors in mice. In H. L. Foster, J. D. Small, and J. G. Fox (eds.), *The Mouse
    in Biomedical Research*, Vol. IV, Academic Press, pp. 373–396.
 3. R. D. Cardiff (1996). The biology of mammary transgenes: Five rules. *J. Mam. Gland Biol. Neoplasia*
    1:61–74.
 4. L. A. Donehower, M. Harvey, B. Slagle, M. McArthur, C. Montgomery, J. S. Butel, and A. Bradley (1992).
    p53-Deficient mice are developmentally normal but susceptible to tumors. *Nature* **356**:215–221.

5. R. Hakem, J. L. de la Pompa, and T. W. Mak (1998). Developmental studies of B*rca1* and *Brca2* knock-out mice. *J. Mam. Gland Biol. Neoplasia* **3**:431–445.

6. R. Nusse and H. E. Varmus (1982). Many tumors induced by the mouse mammary tumor virus contain a provirus integrated in the same region of the host genome. *Cell* **31**:99–109.

7. C. Dickson and G. Peters (1983). Mouse mammary tumor virus. *Curr. Top. Microbiol. Immunol.* **106**:1–34.

8. A. Marchetti, F. Buttitta, S. Miyazaki, D. Gallahan, G. H. Smith, and R. Callahan (1995). *Int-6*, a highly conserved, widely expressed gene, is mutated by mouse mammary tumor virus in mammary preneoplasia. *J. Virol.* **69**:1932–1938.

9. C. A. MacArthur, D. B. Shankar, and G. M. Shackleford (1995). *Fgf-8*, activated by proviral insertion, cooperates with the *Wnt-1* transgene in murine mammary tumorigenesis. *J. Virol.* **69**:2501–2507.

10. D. Medina, and H. W. Lane (1983). Stage specificity of selenium-mediated inhibition of mouse mammary tumorigenesis. *Biol. Trace Element Res.* **5**:297–306.

11. E. L. Huguet, J. A. McMahon, A. P. McMahon, R. Bicknell, and A. L. Harris (1994). Differential expression of human *Wnt* genes 2, 3, 4, and 7B in human breast cell lines and normal and disease states of human breast tissue. *Cancer Res.* **54**:2615–2621.

12. R. V. Iozzo, I. Eichstetter, and K. G. Danielson (1995). Aberrant expression of the growth factor *Wnt-5A* in human malignancy. *Cancer Res.* **55**:3495–3499.

13. S. D. Hursting, T. J. Slaga, S. M. Fischer, J. DiGiovanni, and J. M. Phang (1999). Mechanism-based cancer prevention approaches: targets, examples, and the use of transgenic mice. *J. Natl. Cancer Inst.* **91**:215–225.

14. M. M. Fluck and S. Z. Haslam (1996). Mammary tumors induced by polyomavirus. *Breast Cancer Res. Treat.* **39**:45–56.

15. M. A. Webster, J. N. Hutchinson, M. J. Rauh, S. K. Muthuswamy, M. Anton, C. G. Tortorice, R. D. Cardiff, F. L. Graham, J. A. Hassell, and W. J. Muller (1998). Requirement for both Shc and phosphatidylinositol 3′ kinase signaling pathways in polyomavirus middle T–mediated mammary tumorigenesis. *Mol. Cell Biol.* **18**:2344–2359.

16. A. G. Liebelt and R. A. Liebelt (1967). Chemical factors in mammary tumorigenesis. In *Carcinogenesis: A Broad Critique*, Annual Symp. Fundamental Cancer Res., William and Wilkins, Baltimore, Maryland, pp. 315–345.

17. D. Medina, J. S. Butel, S. H. Socher, and F. L. Miller (1980). Mammary tumorigenesis in 7,12-dimethylbenzanthracene-treated C57BL × DBA/2f F1 mice. *Cancer Res.* **40**:368–373.

18. M. Taketo, A. C. Schroeder, L. E. Mobraaten, K. B. Gunning, G. Hanten, R. R. Fox, T. H. Roderick, C. L. Stewart, F. Lilly, C. T. Hansen *et al.* (1991). FVB/N: an inbred mouse strain preferable for transgenic analyses. *Proc. Natl. Acad. Sci. U.S.A.* **88**:2065–2069.

19. M. F. Fisher, C. J. Conti, M. Locniskar, M. A. Belury, R. E. Maldve, M. L. Lee, J. Leyton, T. J. Slaga, and D. H. Bechtel (1992). The effect of dietary fat on the rapid development of mammary tumors induced by 7,12-dimethylbenz[*a*]anthracene in Sencar mice. *Cancer Res.* **52**:662–666.

20. W.-G. Qing, C. J. Conti, M. LaBate, D. Johnston, T. J. Slaga, and M. C. MacLeod (1997). Induction of mammary cancer and lymphoma by multiple, low oral doses of 7,12-dimethylbenz[a]anthracene in SENCAR mice. *Carcinogenesis* **18**:553–559.

21. D. Medina and F. S. Kittrell (1987). Enhancement of tumorigenicity with morphological progression in a BALB/c preneoplastic outgrowth line. *J. Natl. Cancer Inst.* **79**:569–576.

22. R. J. Coffey, Jr., K. S. Meise, Y. Matsui, B. L. Hogan, P. J. Dempsey, and S. A. Halter (1994). Acceleration of mammary neoplasia in transforming growth factor alpha transgenic mice by 7,12-dimethylbenzanthracene. *Cancer Res.* **54**:1678–1683.

23. B. Li, K. L. Murphy, R. Laucirica, F. Kittrell, D. Medina, and J. M. Rosen (1998). A transgenic mouse model for mammary carcinogenesis. *Oncogene* **16**:997–1007.

24. D. Medina (1974). Mammary tumorigenesis in chemical carcinogen-treated mice. II: Dependence on hormone stimulation for tumorigenesis. *J. Natl. Cancer Inst.* **53**:223–226.

25. J. W. Jull (1954). The effects of estrogens and progesterone on the chemical induction of mammary cancer in mice of the IF strain. *J. Path. Bact.* **68**:547–559.

26. S. M. Swanson, R. C. Guzman, T. Tsukamoto, T. T. Huang, C. D. Dougherty, and S. Nandi (1996). *N*-Ethyl-*N*-nitrosourea induces mammary cancers in the pituitary-isografted mouse which are histologically and genotypically distinct from those induced by *N*-methyl-*N*-nitrosourea. *Cancer Lett.* **102**:159–165.

27. R. W. Wiseman, C. Cochran, W. Dietrich, E. S. Lander, and P. Söderkuist (1994). Allelotyping of butadiene-induced lung and mammary adenocarcinomas of B6C3F1 mice: frequent losses of heterozygosity in regions homologous to human tumor-suppressor genes. *Proc. Natl. Acad. Sci. U.S.A.* **91**:3759–3763.

28. M. Chatterjee and M. R. Banerjee (1982). *N*-Nitrosodiethylamine-induced nodule-like alveolar lesion and its prevention by a retinoid in BALB/c mouse mammary glands in the whole organ in culture. *Carcinogenesis* **3**:801–804.

29. Q. J. Tonelli, R. P. Custer, and S. Sorof (1979). Transformation of cultured mouse mammary glands by aromatic amines and amides and their derivatives. *Cancer Res.* **39**:1784–1792.

30. C. S. Watson, D. Medina, and J. H. Clark (1979). Characterization and estrogen stimulation of cytoplasmic progesterone receptor in the ovarian-dependent MXT-3590 mammary tumor line. *Cancer Res.* **39**:4098–4104.

31. K. Szepeshazi, A. V. Schally, A. Nagy, G. Halmos, and K. Groot (1997). Targeted cytotoxic luteinizing hormone releasing hormone (LH-RH) analogs inhibit growth of estrogen independent MXT mouse mammary cancers *in vivo* by decreasing cell proliferation and inducing apoptosis. *Anticancer Drugs* **8**:974–987.

32. F. Darro, P. Cahen, A. Vianna, C. Decaestecker, J. M. Nogaret, B. Leblond, C. Chaboteaux, C. Ramos, M. Petein, V. Budel, A. Schoofs, B. Pourrias, and R. Kiss (1998). Growth inhibition of human *in vitro* and mouse *in vitro* and *in vivo* mammary tumor models by retinoids in comparison with tamoxifen and the RU-486 anti-progestogen. *Breast Cancer Res. Treat.* **51**:39–55.

33. E. Stickeler, F. Kittrell, D. Medina, and S. M. Berget (1999). Stage-specific changes in alternative splicing of CD44 and SR splicing factors in mammary tumorigenesis. *Oncogene* **18**:3574–3582.

34. D. J. Jerry, J. S. Butel, L. A. Donehower, E. J. Paulson, C. Cochran, R. W. Wiseman, and D. Medina (1994). p53 mutations occur infrequently in 7,12-dimethylbenzanthracene-induced mammary tumors in BALB/c and hemizygous p53 mice. *Mol. Carcinogenesis* **9**:175–183.

35. Y.-R. Lou, Y.-P. Lu, J.-G. Xie, P. Yen, D. Lane, and M.-T. Huang (1996). Detection of p53 and Rb proteins in DMBA-induced breast tumors of Sencar mice. *Proc. Am. Assoc. Cancer Res.* Abstract #691.

36. D. J. Jerry, M. A. Ozbun, F. S. Kittrell, D. P. Lane, D. Medina, and J. S. Butel (1993). Mutations in p53 are frequent in the preneoplastic stage of mouse mammary tumor development. *Cancer Res.* **53**:3374–3381.

37. C. M. Aldaz, Q. Y. Liao, A. Paladugu, S. Rehm, and H. Wang (1996). Allelotypic and cytogenetic characterization of chemically induced mouse mammary tumors: high frequency of chromosome 4 loss of heterozygosity at advanced stages or progression. *Mol. Carcinogenensis* **17**:126–133.

38. H. W. Lane, J. S. Butel, C. Howard, F. Shepherd, R. Halligan, and D. Medina (1985). The role of high levels of dietary fat in 7,12-dimethylbenzanthracene-induced mouse mammary tumorigenesis: Lack of an effect on lipid peroxidation. *Carcinogenesis* **6**:403–407.

39. M. T. Huang, Y. R. Lou, J. G. Xie, W. Ma, Y. P. Lu, P. Yen, B. T. Zhu, H. Newmark, and C. T. Ho (1998). Effect of dietary curcumin and dibenzoylmethane on formation of 7,12-dimethylbenz[*a*]anthracene-induced mammary tumors and lymphomas/leukemias in Sencar mice. *Carcinogenesis* **19**(9):1697–1700.

40. C. W. Welsch (1987). Dietary retinoids and the chemoprevention of mammary gland tumorigenesis. In D. Medina, W. Kidwell, G. Heppner, and E. Anderson (eds.), *Cellular and Molecular Biology of Mammary Cancer*, Plenum Press, New York, pp. 495–508.

41. R. L. Ullrich, N. D. Bowles, L. C. Satterfield, and C. M. Davis (1996). Strain-dependent susceptibility to radiation-induced mammary cancer is a result of differences in epithelial cell sensitivity to transformation. *Radiat. Res.* **146**:353–355.

42. B. Ponnaiya, M. N. Cornforth, and R. L. Ullrich (1997). Radiation-induced chromosomal instability in BALB/c and C57BL/6 mice: the difference is as clear as black and white. *Radiat. Res.* **147**:121–125.

43. S. P. Ethier and R. L. Ullrich (1982). Detection of ductal dysplasia in mammary outgrowths derived from carcinogen-treated virgin female BALB/c mice. *Cancer Res.* **42**:1753–1760.

44. D. Medina, L. C. Stephens, P. J. Bonilla, C. A. Hollmann, D. Schwahn, C. Kuperwasser, D. J. Jerry, J. S. Butel, and R. E. Meyn (1998). Radiation-induced tumorigenesis in preneoplastic mouse mammary glands *in vivo*; significance of p53 status and apoptosis. *Mol. Carcinogenesis* **22**:199–207.

45. P. K. Pattengale, T. Stewart, A. Leder, E. Sinn, W. Muller, I. Tepler, E. Schmidt, and P. Leder (1989). Animal models of human disease: pathology and molecular biology of spontaneous neoplasms occurring in transgenic mice carrying and expressing activated cellular oncogenes. *Am. J. Pathol.* **135**:39–61.

46. R. D. Cardiff and S. R. Wellings (1999). The comparative pathology of human and mouse mammary glands. *J. Mam. Gland Biol. Neoplasia* **4**:105–122.

47. A. S. Tsukamoto, R. Grosschedl, R. C. Guzman, T. Parslow, and H. E. Varmus (1988). Expression of the *int-1* gene in transgenic mice is associated with mammary gland hyperplasia and adenocarcinomas in male and female mice. *Cell* **55**:619–625.

48. B. Li, F. S. Kittrell, D. Medina, and J. M. Rosen (1995). Delay of dimethylbenz(α)anthracene-induced mammary tumorigenesis in transgenic mice by apoptosis induced by an unusual mutant p53 protein. *Mol. Carcinogenesis* **14**:75–83.

49. K.-U. Wagner, R. J. Wall, L. St.-Onge, P. Gruss, L. Garrett, A. Wynshaw-Boris, M. Li, P. A. Furth, and L. Hennighausen (1997). Cre mediated gene deletion in the mammary gland. *Nucleic Acids. Res.* **25:**4323–4330.

50. P. Sicinski, J. L. Donaher, S. B. Parker, T. Li, A. Fazeli, H. Gardner, S. Z. Haslam, R. T. Bronson, S. J. Elledge, and R. A. Weinberg (1995). Cyclin D1 provides a link between development and oncogenesis in the retina and breast. *Cell* **82:**621–630.

51. K. S. Korach (1994). Insights from the study of animals lacking functional estrogen receptor. *Science* **266:**1524–1527.

52. J. P. Lydon, F. J. DeMayo, C. R. Funk, S. K. Mani, A. R. Hughes, C. A. Montgomery, Jr., G. Shyamala, O. M. Conneely, and B. W. O'Malley (1995). Mice lacking progesterone receptor exhibit pleiotropic reproductive abnormalities. *Genes Devel.* **9:**2266–2278.

Chapter 2

Methods for the Induction of Mammary Carcinogenesis in the Rat Using either 7,12-Dimethylbenz[α]anthracene or 1-Methyl-1-Nitrosourea

Henry J. Thompson

Abstract. Numerous animal model systems for investigating breast cancer exist, and new experimental approaches using transgenic and knockout strategies are resulting in the development of models with specific pathogenetic characteristics. Nonetheless, chemically induced mammary carcinogenesis has been investigated for over 50 years, and the results of experiments using this approach continue to provide important insights about the genesis, prevention, and treatment of breast cancer. This chapter provides a detailed account of the methods utilized to implement the two most widely studied chemically initiated models of mammary carcinogenesis in the rat. They are induced by treatment of female rats with either 7,12-dimethylbenz[α]anthracene or 1-methyl-1-nitrosourea.

Abbreviations. Institutional Biohazard Committee (IBC); Institutional Animal Care and Use Committee (IACUC); 7,12-dimethylbenz[α]anthracene (DMBA); 1-methyl-1-nitrosourea (MNU).

INTRODUCTION

The 7,12-dimethylbenz[α]anthracene (DMBA)- and the 1-methyl-1-nitrosourea (MNU)-induced rat mammary carcinogenesis models are currently in widespread use in the study of human breast cancer (1, 2). A brief historical account of the development of these models can be found in Ref. 3. DMBA is a proximate carcinogen that requires metabolic activation by the mixed function oxidase system to become carcinogenic. MNU is a direct-acting carcinogen that spontaneously decomposes to an alkylating agent at physiologic pH. This difference allows investigators to study various aspects of the initiation and promotion phases of mammary carcinogenesis using these models.

Generically, referral to either a DMBA- or MNU-induced rat mammary carcinogenesis model includes a surprisingly large array of approaches to route of carcinogen administration, dose and frequency of carcinogen administration, and age at which carcinogen is

Henry J. Thompson **Center for Nutrition in the Prevention of Disease, AMC Cancer Research Center, Lakewood, Colorado 80214.**

Methods in Mammary Gland Biology and Breast Cancer Research, edited by Ip and Asch. Kluwer Academic/Plenum Publishers, New York, 2000.

administered. Most of these approaches are discussed in Ref. 3. In this chapter consideration of these models is limited to those in which a single dose of carcinogen is administered. Relative to DMBA, we will discuss the i.g. (intragastric) route of carcinogen administration, because this approach is the most widely used and is technically achieved with the greatest ease. However, procedures have been published in which DMBA is injected i.v. (3). For the MNU model we will discuss the i.p. method of administration because, technically, this approach is the most efficient and has been reported to reduce the interanimal variability in carcinogenic response (4). However, reference will also be made to the i.v. and s.c. methods of carcinogen delivery since all three approaches are used and all involve the same method of preparing MNU for administration (5). The intent of this chapter is to provide a detailed guide to the methods used to implement the most widely studied chemically induced rat models of mammary carcinogenesis.

MATERIALS AND INSTRUMENTATION: DMBA MODEL

Chemicals

- DMBA, purity >97% (Sigma D3254) (chemical properties reviewed in Ref. 6)
- Reagent-grade sesame oil (Sigma S3547)

Materials

- Graduated cylinder, 100 ml (Fisher Scientific 08-550E)
- Polypropylene beaker, 120 ml (Fisher Scientific 02-591E)
- Watch glass (Fisher Scientific 02-610-5C)
- Hot plate with magnetic stirrer (Fisher Scientific 11-496-8)
- Stir bar, Teflon coated (Fisher Scientific 14-511-94)
- Stir bar retriever (Fisher Scientific 14-511-86)
- Glass syringe, 1 ml with 0.1 ml graduation, luer lock (Kimble Kontes H81301)
- Beveled tubing adapter (Popper and Sons 6251)
- Nelaton catheters (cat. no. 402100, size Ch. 8, Rusch, Kernen, Germany) or a premature infant feeding tube, size 5 French (local hospital supply company)
- A stable wide-mouthed glass container from which carcinogen can be removed for intubation (Fisher Scientific 03-320-7A)
- Biohazard waste disposal bags (Lab Safety 8B-11481)

Instrumentation

- Glove box equipped with an analytical balance and approved for weighing carcinogen
- Chemical fume hood or biological safety cabinet approved by IBC for preparation of carcinogen
- Chemical fume hood or biological safety cabinet approved by IBC and IACUC for administration of carcinogen to animals
- UV light, handheld (Fisher, 11-984-20, wavelength 254–365 nm)

MATERIALS AND INSTRUMENTATION: MNU MODEL

Chemicals

- MNU (Ash Stevens, ASI-701) (chemical properties reviewed in Ref. 7)
- Sodium chloride (Sigma S9888)
- Acetic acid (Fisher Scientific A38-212)

Materials

- Glass injection vial (Fisher-Wheaton 223745)
- Septum for injection vial (Fisher-Wheaton 224100-202)
- Aluminum seals (Fisher-Wheaton 224183-01)
- Crimper (Fisher-Wheaton 224303)
- Tuberculin syringe, 1 ml volume with 0.1 ml gradations (Becton Dickinson 309602)
- Needle, 26 gauge, 3/8 inch, intradermal bevel (Becton Dickinson 305110)
- Biohazard waste disposal bags (Lab Safety 8B-11481)

Instrumentation

- Glove box equipped with an analytical balance and approved for weighing carcinogen
- Chemical fume hood or biological safety cabinet approved by IBC for preparation and chemical inactivation of carcinogen
- Chemical fume hood or biological safety cabinet approved by IBC and IACUC for administration of carcinogen to animals

Notes. MNU should be obtained from a source that properly handles the compound during storage and shipping. MNU is sensitive to humidity and light, and storage at temperatures below −10°C is recommended. Thus MNU should be shipped by the vendor on dry ice. Ash Stevens, Detroit, MI, or the chemical repository at the National Cancer Institute are reliable sources of MNU.

METHODS FOR DMBA

Reagent Preparation

1. Before beginning preparation of carcinogen, examine the work area with a hand-held UV light to ensure that the surfaces are free of detectable contaminants.
2. Cover with disposable paper (Benchkote) the work surfaces in the glove box on which the bottle containing DMBA will be opened during the weighing process. This will facilitate the cleanup procedure.
3. Weigh DMBA in a glove box designated for this purpose.
   a. DMBA is a very lightweight powder that can be easily dispersed during the weighing process and contaminate work surfaces.
   b. To minimize the handling of DMBA in its powder form, weigh it directly into a container that can be covered (e.g., beaker with watch glass cover) and in which it will be dissolved in oil.

    c.   To make 100 ml of carcinogen solution, if a dose of 20 mg DMBA per rat is to be delivered, weigh 2 g of DMBA into a beaker.

4. Measure 100 ml of sesame oil using a graduated cylinder.
5. Slowly add the sesame oil to the DMBA so as to minimize dispersal of DMBA into the air. Ensure complete transfer of the oil into the beaker. (This procedure can be performed in the glove box.)
6. Transfer beaker to a hood approved for carcinogen preparation.
7. Protect the beaker from light and place on a hot plate equipped with a magnetic stirrer. (We prefer to wrap the beaker containing the DMBA and oil with aluminum foil so as to be able to easily monitor the dissolution of the DMBA in the oil.)
8. Carefully add a magnetic stir bar to the beaker.
9. Heat gently with stirring. Gentle heating facilitates dissolution; however, avoid high temperatures since they can change the chemical structure of the DMBA.
10. Once the DMBA appears to be in solution, continue stirring for at least 1 h to ensure DMBA is completely dissolved.
11. Transfer DMBA solution to an appropriate vessel (one that will not easily tip over) for delivery of the carcinogen to the animals.
12. Examine all work areas with handheld UV light source to detect contamination of work surfaces with DMBA. Use cotton gauze (or similar absorbent material) wetted with alcohol to remove DMBA from work surfaces. Thereafter, wash work surfaces with appropriate detergent.
13. Put all waste materials into biohazard bag and label. In general, all materials used in the preparation of the DMBA can be placed in a biohazard bag for subsequent incineration. An alternative to incineration is chemical inactivation of waste reagents.

Detailed Procedures for DMBA Administration

1. In facilities with a room specifically designed for carcinogen administration, animals are transported from their holding room to the carcinogen administration room. If such a room does not exist, it is critical to develop a procedure meeting the approval of both the IBC and the IACUC.
2. DMBA is administered to animals by gavage using a Nelathon catheter (this is a urinary catheter with a solid round end and the orifice on the side, size 8 French).
3. Cut the catheter (filling end), which is approximately 16 inches long, to an appropriate length, depending on the size of the animal. Given that animals are of the same age, one length of catheter is generally sufficient. Length can be determined by estimating the distance between the animal's mouth and its stomach (usually 4–5 inches).
4. Attach the cut catheter to a 1-ml glass syringe with a beveled tubing adapter.
5. Fill the syringe to the appropriate volume, being sure to exclude bubbles of air.
6. Pick up an animal by using a conventional grasp with the index and middle fingers placed around the neck and over the front legs. The thumb and index finger of the hand holding the animal are used to open the animal's mouth, and the catheter is inserted in the mouth and passed to the stomach. If the catheter is cut to the appropriate size, its entire length can be inserted into the animal. This increases the ease with which the carcinogen is delivered.
    a.   An experienced animal technician can perform carcinogen administration without using any type of restraining device.

      b.   Speed of the procedure can be increased if one technician is responsible for filling syringes and a second technician focuses on the intubation process.

7. The carcinogen is instilled into the stomach and then the catheter is removed. The entire procedure takes less than 15 s per animal.

8. Carcinogen is administered in a volume of 1 ml unless it is given per unit of body weight. The concentration of the carcinogen in the sesame oil needs to be calculated based on dose to be delivered and whether carcinogen is delivered in equal amounts to all animals or per unit body weight.

9. Solvent-treated control animals receive only the sesame oil in which the DMBA is dissolved.

10. Following carcinogen administration, animals are returned to the holding room. The hood in which carcinogen was administered should be decontaminated as discussed previously.

11. In general, it is recommended that access to the animal holding room in which treated animals are maintained be limited for 14 days following carcinogen administration because carcinogen metabolites can be detected in animal tissues or in urine and feces during this period. During this time all animal bedding is collected for incineration.

12. In some laboratories disposable animal caging is used so that at the end of the 14-day period, it can be incinerated.

13. Procedures for handling carcinogen-treated animals and the caging in which they are housed are generally specified by an institution's IBC and IACUC.

Notes

1. Although not widespread among all laboratories, some investigators have fasted animals for 12 h prior to gastric intubation of DMBA in order to improve uptake of carcinogen.

2. As an alternative to the urinary catheter, a premature infant feeding tube, size 5 French, can be used to instill carcinogen.

3. Although a disposable syringe is permissable, accuracy and ease of administration are improved if a glass syringe is used.

4. The use of a rubber tube (e.g., Nelathon catheter) rather than an intubation needle was recommended in the original work of Huggins (1). This approach minimizes the likelihood of injuring an animal's esophagus.

DOSES OF CARCINOGEN. DMBA dose is selected based on the incidence and multiplicity of mammary tumors desired. The range of doses of carcinogen administered to animals is, in general, between 5 and 20 mg per rat. If an investigator chooses to administer carcinogen per kilogram of body weight, then the average weight of the population of animals to be administered carcinogen can be assessed and the dose of carcinogen can be set accordingly. For example, in our hands a group of 30 female Sprague Dawley rats, of specified date of birth, obtained at 21 days of age and fed purified diet, will weigh, on average, 160 g at 50 days of age. Thus, a 20-mg dose of DMBA adjusted to body weight results in delivery of 125 mg DMBA/kg body weight. Depending on the strain of animal selected for carcinogen administration, the carcinogen dose can be chosen so that a control group of animals will have a desired carcinogenic response. Sprague Dawley and Wistar–Furth rats have the greatest susceptibility to chemically induced mammary carcinogenesis, F344 rats have intermediate sensitivity, and Copenhagen rats are resistant (8). Within 6 months of carcinogen administration, in highly susceptible rat strains, doses between 15 and 20 mg DMBA per rat should give a carcinogenic response in excess of 90% of treated animals, 10 mg should give a carcinogenic response in 50–70% of treated animals, and 5 mg should give a carcinogenic response in approximately 20–30% of treated animals. Note that the same methods can be used in the preparation of DMBA for administration to mice, except that the dose of DMBA delivered will differ.

METHODS FOR MNU

Reagent Preparation

1. Cover with disposable paper (Benchkote), the work surfaces in the glove box on which the bottle containing MNU will be opened during the weighing process. This will facilitate the cleanup procedure.
2. Remove MNU from the freezer for weighing, place in a covered ice bucket, and transfer to a glove box approved for weighing carcinogen.
3. Weigh MNU directly into a glass injection vial, stopper vial with septum, wrap vial in aluminum foil, and place vial on ice.
4. Immediately prior to administration, remove the vial from the ice bucket and add the appropriate volume of 0.9% (w/v) NaCl, pH < 5.0 to the injection vial. (The sodium chloride solution is acidified, prior to its addition to the MNU, by the dropwise addition of acetic acid to the solution with stirring; pH is checked with pH-sensitive paper.)
5. Reseal the vial with the septum and secure septum in place with an aluminum closure and crimper.
6. Dissolve the MNU in the saline solution by warming the vial under hot tap water with vigorous shaking.

Notes
1. As indicated, MNU is sensitive to light and humidity. Storage below −10°C is recommended. We store MNU at −80°C.
2. In general, we prepare carcinogen in a 25-ml injection vial to which is added 280 mg of MNU and 20 ml of solvent. Thus, the concentration of MNU is 14 mg/ml. This represents the maximum solubility of MNU in aqueous solution.
3. The MNU, protected from light, at acidic pH is reasonably stable; nonetheless, we generally prepare it immediately prior to injection and use it within an hour of preparation.

Detailed Procedures for MNU Administration

1. Weigh and record animal weights on the day of carcinogen administration.
2. In facilities with a room specifically designed for carcinogen administration, transport animals from their holding room to the carcinogen administration room. If such a room does not exist, it is critical to develop a procedure meeting the approval of both the IBC and the IACUC.
3. Administer MNU to animals i.p., using a 26 gauge, 3/8-inch needle. Carcinogen is administered per kilogram of body weight.
4. An experienced animal technician can perform carcinogen administration without using any type of restraining device.

5. Pick up the animal by using a conventional grasp with the index and middle fingers placed around the neck and over the front legs. The injection is made at the midline of the animal adjacent to the fifth pair of mammary glands. The entire procedure takes less than 15 s per animal.

6. Following carcinogen administration, animals are returned to the holding room, and the hood in which the carcinogen was administered is decontaminated.

7. Because MNU has a short half-life *in vivo* and no metabolites are known to be eliminated from the animal, no special precautions need to be taken. Nonetheless, specific additional measures may be required by either an institution's IBH or IACUC. Procedures for handling carcinogen-treated animals are generally specified by an institution's IACUC.

DOSES OF CARCINOGEN.   The dose of MNU to be injected is selected based on the incidence and multiplicity of mammary tumors desired. The range of doses is, in general, between 10 and 50 mg MNU/kg body weight. Depending on the strain of animal selected for carcinogen administration, the carcinogen dose can be chosen so that a control group of animals will have a desired carcinogenic response. Sprague Dawley and Wistar rats have the greatest susceptibility to chemically induced mammary carcinogenesis, F344 rats have intermediate sensitivity, and Copenhagen rats are resistant (8). Within 6 months of carcinogen treatment, in highly susceptible rat strains, injection with doses of MNU between 35 and 50 mg/kg body weight should give a carcinogenic response in excess of 90% of treated animals, 25 mg/kg should give a carcinogenic response in approximately 50–70% of treated animals, and 12.5 mg/kg should give a carcinogenic response in approximately 25–30% of treated animals. Note that the same methods can be used in the preparation of MNU for administration to mice, except that the dose of MNU delivered will differ.

ROUTE OF MNU ADMINISTRATION.   As noted, published procedures document that mammary carcinogenesis can be induced by a single injection of MNU delivered intravenously, subcutaneously, or intraperitoneally (4, 5). We recommend the i.p. route because of its simplicity and because we have observed a reduction in interanimal variation in tumor response with this approach. We attribute the reduction in variability to improved accuracy in carcinogen administration. Some laboratories inject MNU into the jugular vein; this approach requires anesthetization of the animal and the involvement of several technicians if large numbers of animals are to be injected on a given day. Administration via the tail vein requires greater skill and animal manipulation than i.p. administration. The s.c. route of administration was developed by our laboratory and is comparable to the i.p. method in terms of ease of administration (5). Nonetheless, discussions with some investigators using this approach have indicated a few problems with carcinogen delivery and leakage of carcinogen from the site of injection. While such problems are easily remedied, the i.p. route of administration is least problematic and most easily adapted by investigators with limited experience in working with laboratory animals.

GENERAL ISSUES AND COMMENTS

Animal-Related Preparations

Some protocols in which DMBA is given involve dosing each animal with the same amount of carcinogen, irrespective of body weight, as reported by Huggins (1), whereas others provide an amount of DMBA per kilogram of body weight. MNU is administered per kilogram of body weight. Accordingly, it may be necessary to weigh animals prior to carcinogen administration. A top-loading balance with 1-g accuracy is sufficient for this purpose. In addition, use of a computer-generated spreadsheet that provides the volume of carcinogen to be administered to an animal based on carcinogen dose, concentration of the working solution of carcinogen, and the animal's body weight can be prepared in advance of carcinogen administration, thereby reducing the time to administer the carcinogen while improving the accuracy of the procedure. In general, multiple animals are housed per cage. Therefore, in the carcinogen administration room, it is of value to have an additional empty cage for holding animals that have been injected with carcinogen so that no confusion arises as to which animals in a given cage have been injected.

Carcinogen and Carcass Disposal

A number of approaches exist to carcinogen inactivation and to disposal of biohazardous waste resulting from carcinogen preparation and administration. Most aspects of these activities are regulated by IBC and IACUC. In general, what is required is an approved hood for inactivating carcinogen should a chemical inactivation method be used or access to a biohazard waste disposal service approved for incinerating materials at temperatures in excess of 982°C. Either chemical inactivation or incineration can be used to dispose of DMBA or MNU. References 9 and 10 deal with disposal of these carcinogens.

Personal Protective Equipment

Standards have been set for the use of personal protective equipment that complements the physical environment in which carcinogen is used. Important issues include protection against any type of exposure, including ingestion or inhalation of carcinogen due to work surface contamination, aerosol formation during carcinogen preparation and administration, and protection against contact of carcinogen with body surfaces. Facilities should be provided for showering following work with carcinogens. Use of disposable personal apparel is generally recommended. Institutional procedures should be followed. For specific current information contact www.nih.gov (use the NIH search engine and research on chemical safety) and www.osha-slc.gov/OshStd (OSHA fact sheet 95-33, "Occupational Exposure to Hazardous Chemicals in Laboratories"). OSHA Standard 29 CFR should also be consulted.

Palpation, Recording Tumor Occurrence, and Time Course

Mammary carcinogenesis models can be applied in many ways. The question the model is being used to address will in part dictate how animals are monitored following carcinogen treatment. However, the occurrence of mammary tumors is generally detected by the palpation of the mammary gland chains of an animal for masses. An experienced technician can detect a mass the size of a pinhead. Such masses begin to emerge as early as 21–28 days following a high dose of DMBA or MNU. Tumor appearance is delayed at lower doses of carcinogen. We generally begin palpating animals two times per week at least 1 week before tumor emergence is anticipated. This allows animals to become accustomed to the type of handling that palpation entails. No type of physical restraining device is used for palpation.

In his original publication Huggins noted that when rats were given a 20-mg dose of DMBA, essentially all animals would have one or more palpable mammary tumors within 60 days (1). A similar result is obtained with the 50-mg/kg dose of MNU (6). Depending on the purpose for which the model is intended, it has been customary to observe the carcinogenic response for 6 months following carcinogen treatment. In general, this is done by palpating rats twice per week for mammary tumor detection and recording in a palpation logbook the location and date of initial detection of a palpable mass. Continued presence of a palpated tumor is confirmed on each palpation; if a tumor regresses to a point where it is no longer detected, this also is recorded. In general, when an experiment is concluded, euthanized rats are skinned and the skin is examined under translucent light. Using the palpation log as a guide, all detected masses, as well as those not detected by palpation, are excised and a piece of each lesion is processed for histopathological classification.

Tumor Measurement

Some protocols require estimation of tumor growth rate. The tumor is measured with a vernier caliper (Bel-Art H13415-0000). In general, this is most easily achieved without the use of anesthesia and with only brief restraint of the animal, which is limited to holding the animal so that tumor measurements can be obtained. Two researchers are required. One holds the animal while the other inspects the tumor and uses a vernier caliper to measure the tumor's two largest perpendicular axes. These measurements are used to compute tumor volume, using the formula for an ellipsoid ($V = \frac{4}{3}\pi a^2 b$). Considerable day-to-day variation occurs in the measurement of an animal's tumor. This variation can be reduced if the same individuals hold and measure the same tumors each day.

Age of Animals

DMBA.   In considering data published in Ref. 1 and the extensive literature review in Ref. 3, age is important in determining the sensitivity of the mammary gland to carcinogenic insult with a polycyclic aromatic hydrocarbon such as DMBA. Optimal sensitivity has been reported to range between 50 and 65 days of age. Treatment prior to this age has been shown to give a lower carcinoma yield and a greater percentage of benign mammary tumors. The mammary gland becomes increasingly refractory to carcinogenic insult after 65 days of age (3). In an effort to standardize the effects of age in a given protocol and for work conducted over periods of years, our approach has been to obtain rats of specified date of birth and to treat animals with carcinogen at 50 days of age. This approach was used by Huggins in the original report of the DMBA model (1). The disadvantage to this approach is that it can increase the cost of animal purchasing, and it requires that the vendor be given a longer lead time when an animal order is placed. The alternative approach is to obtain animals that have a range of birth dates, usually ±2 days. Thus, some laboratories inject rats between 50 and 55 days of age.

MNU.   For many years the same approach to age of carcinogen treatment that had been used with DMBA was used with MNU, i.e., limiting carcinogen treatment to the window of optimal sensitivity as defined by Huggins (1). The mammary gland becomes increasingly refractory to MNU beyond 65 days of age. However, in several papers our laboratory has shown that the mammary glands of young animals are very sensitive to carcinogenic initiation using MNU (11, 12). We have recently reported that injection of 21-day-old female Sprague Dawley rats with MNU offers the opportunity to study premalignant as well as malignant stages of mammary carcinogenesis over a very short timeframe, i.e., 35 days (12). Animals of specified date of birth should be used if carcinogen is injected at 21 days of age.

Rat Strain and Source

Consideration also should be given to the source of the animals used for either model system. It is desirable to maintain the same genetic profile over time, especially if experiments completed during different time frames are to be compared. Differences in responsiveness of animals to carcinogen have periodically been attributed to different vendors of the same rat strain, and even when animals are obtained from different colonies operated by the same vendor. This is not particularly surprising since strain differences among rats are well documented to influence responsiveness to carcinogen administration (8).

Animal Housing

For most studies, animals are housed three per cage in solid-bottomed polycarbonate cages. Because light intensity in an animal room can vary from shelf level to shelf level, and some evidence suggests that light intensity may influence carcinogenic response in the mammary gland, we house cages of animals in a particular experimental group so that all potential levels of light exposure are equally represented in each experimental group in a study.

Randomization

Although compelling rationale can be developed for many different approaches to randomizing animals into various experimental groups, our usual approach has been to randomize following carcinogen administration. Our primary stratification variable is body weight. If multiple bottles of carcinogen are used because of the size of the study, a secondary stratification factor is the bottle from which an animal is injected.

Other Factors

Over the last 20 years, the author has had many investigators inquire about procedures discussed in this chapter because they have had difficulty in inducing mammary tumors when injecting MNU or DMBA. The majority of inquiries have been with the MNU model. In general, problems have been identified in the proper handling of carcinogen prior to injection, use of the proper technique in administering carcinogen, obtaining animals of the appropriate age, controlling the level of noise in the environment in which animals were housed, and the introduction of unnecessary disturbances of animals in the animal facility.

It is hoped that by following the guidelines outlined here that investigators using chemically initiated models of mammary carcinogenesis in the rat will be highly successful in inducing tumor occurrence.

REFERENCES

1. C. B. Huggins, L. C. Grand, and F. P. Brillantes (1961). Mammary cancer induced by a single feeding of polynuclear hydrocarbons and its suppression. *Nature (London)* **189**:204–207.
2. P. M. Gullino, H. M. Pettigrew, and F. H. Grantham (1975). *N*-Nitrosomethylurea as mammary gland carcinogen in rats. *J. Natl. Cancer Inst.* **54**:401–414.
3. C. W. Welsch (1985). Host factors affecting the growth of carcinogen-induced rat mammary carcinomas: a review and tribute to Charles Brenton Huggins. *Cancer Res.* **45**:3415–3443.

4. H. J. Thompson and H. Adlakha (1991). Dose-responsive induction of mammary gland carcinomas by the intraperitoneal injection of 1-methyl-1-nitrosourea. *Cancer Res.* **51**:3411–3415.

5. H. J. Thompsonand and L. D. Meeker (1983). Induction of mammary gland carcinomas by the subcutaneous injection of 1-methyl-1-nitrosourea. *Cancer Res.* **43**:1628–1629.

6. International Agency for Research on Cancer (1985). *Dibenzanthracene.* IARC Monograph on the Evaluation of Carcinogenic Risk of Chemicals to Man, Vol. 3, pp. 178–196.

7. International Agency for Research on Cancer (1985). *Nitrosoureas.* IARC Monograph on the Evaluation of Carcinogenic Risk of Chemicals to Man, Vol. 1, pp. 125–134.

8. M. N. Gould and R. Zhang (1991). Genetic regulation of mammary carcinogenesis in the rat by susceptibility and suppressor genes. *Environ. Health Perspectives* **93**:161–167.

9. International Agency for Research on Cancer (1985). Laboratory decontamination and destruction of carcinogens in laboratory wastes: some *N*-nitrosamides. *IARC Sci. Publ.* **55**:1–65.

10. International Agency for Research on Cancer (1983). Laboratory decontamination and destruction of carcinogens in laboratory wastes: some polycyclic heterocyclic hydrocarbons. *IARC Sci. Publ.* **49**:1–81.

11. H. J. Thompson, H. Adlakha, and M. Singh (1992). Effect of carcinogen dose and age at administration on induction of mammary carcinogenesis by 1-methyl-1-nitrosourea. *Carcinogenesis* **13**:1535–1539.

12. H. J. Thompson, J. N. McGinley, K. Rothhammer, and M. Singh (1995). Rapid induction of mammary intraductal proliferations, ductal carcinoma *in situ* and carcinomas by the injection of sexually immature female rats with 1-methyl-1-nitrosourea. *Carcinogenesis* **16**:2407–2411.

Chapter 3

A Comparison of the Salient Features of Mouse, Rat, and Human Mammary Tumorigenesis

Daniel Medina and Henry J. Thompson

Abstract. This chapter briefly discusses the salient features of models of breast carcinogenesis. It is intended not to be an extensive encyclopedia of all models in the literature but to emphasize key features of the main models. The information presented here is very much the authors' interpretations of selected data in the literature, which, hopefully, will stimulate spirited discussion and new ideas.

Abbreviations.   loss of heterozygosity (LDH); ductal carcinoma *in situ* (DCIS).

INTRODUCTION

Chapters 1 and 2 have discussed the induction of mammary tumors in rodents by various etiological agents. Because the rodent models provide fundamental information on cellular and molecular pathways altered in neoplastic development, it is essential to ask how accurately these models mimic the human disease. This chapter discusses the salient features of animal models of breast carcinogenesis. As such, the discussion is a continuation of the information presented in the foregoing chapters, and, where appropriate, reference will be made to those chapters (1, 2). In this discussion, it is important to remember that human breast cancer is heterogeneous at the morphological, genetic, and molecular levels. Since premalignant and invasive breast lesions are divided into several types and compounded with known multiple molecular lesions, one must view human breast cancer as a subset of diseases. Given this perspective, it is unreasonable to expect any given animal model to faithfully mimic the spectrum of human breast cancers. At best, animal models mimic major subsets and major morphological pathways.

Daniel Medina   Department of Molecular and Cell Biology, Baylor College of Medicine, Houston, Texas 77030.   Henry J. Thompson   Center for Nutrition in the Prevention of Disease, AMC Cancer Research Center, Lakewood, Colorado 80214.

Methods in Mammary Gland Biology and Breast Cancer Research, edited by Ip and Asch. Kluwer Academic/Plenum Publishers, New York, 2000.

COMPARATIVE BIOLOGY AND PATHOGENESIS

The first five properties are given in Table 3-1 and refer to the comparative pathogenesis and biology of mammary cancer in the three species. Several points are of interest. First, it is clear that, with the exception of ionizing radiation (2), we do not know the etiological agent for the vast majority of human breast cancers. Currently, there is little direct and compelling evidence for a role of viruses or specific chemical carcinogens in the initiation of the human disease. However, the overall biology of the disease is remarkably similar among these species. The target cells for carcinogenic initiation are the luminal epithelial cells (or their progenitor cells) of the mammary gland. Upon initiation, these cells attain the potential to progress and appear as ductal hyperplasias, ductal carcinoma *in situ* (DCIS), and invasive breast cancer through the processes of clonal selection and clonal expansion. (See Ref. 3 for a discussion of the cellular origin of DCIS.) This progression is observed in chemical-carcinogen-treated rats and mice, hormone-treated mice, and irradiated mice. The virus-infected mammary gland shows transformation of the differentiated alveolar cell, probably a rare event in human disease. The ease of inducing alveolar hyperplasias in comparison to ductal hyperplasias in the mouse and the focus on understanding the mechanisms of oncogenic transformation have led to the preponderance of information on the biology of the former set of lesions in mouse mammary tumorigenesis. However, the recent extensive description of ductal hyperplasia and ductal carcinoma *in situ* in the rat, as reviewed in Ref. 1, provides a readily accessible model to study the cellular and molecular biology of these lesions.

The precursor relationship of hyperplasias to tumors has been proven by transplantation studies with the lesions in the mouse and rat and is inferred in the case of the human. Genetic characterization of DCIS and invasive breast cancer show a lineage relationship; however, the neoplastic potentials of the atypical ductal hyperplasias (ADH) lesions have not been directly demonstrated by transplantation analysis (3).

Hormone dependence of the mammary tumors in the three species varies widely. As discussed in Chapter 1, mice exhibit a low but measurable frequency of hormone-dependent tumors, rats exhibit a high frequency of about 70–80%, and humans exhibit around 50–60%. The explanation for the low frequency in the mouse is not clear and cannot be explained solely on the basis of known etiological agents. Although hypotheses have been presented to explain the differences in frequency of hormone dependence (4), such hypotheses have not been rigorously tested.

Perhaps one of the biggest misconceptions about rodent tumors has been the belief that metastasis is rare. This misconception is widely held, although there is extensive data that mouse mammary tumors readily metastasize to lung and liver (Chapter 1 this volume). The frequency of metastases varies with the tumor model but ranges from 29% in spontaneous

Table 3-1. Comparison of Mouse, Rat, and Human Mammary Tumorigenesis

Property	Mouse	Rat	Human
Carcinogen	MMTV, chem. carc., radiation	Chem. carc., radiation	Radiation
Precursor	AH, DH, DCIS[a]	DH, DCIS	DH, DCIS
Relationship	Proven	Proven	Inferred
Hormone dependence	Rare	Frequent	60%
Metastasis	Yes (lung)	Yes (lung)	Yes (brain, bone, lung)

[a]AH = alveolar hyperplasia; DH = ductal hyperplasia; DCIS = ductal carcinoma *in situ*.

BALB/c tumors to 63% in BALB/c/C3H tumors (1) (Chapter 1). Old data indicate some rat mammary tumors metastasize to lymph node, lung, and liver (6). This result has recently been confirmed by data demonstrating that rat mammary tumors metastasize to lung in a specific model (Thompson, unpublished results). The only outstanding question is whether metastases to bone occur in the rodent models.

In summary, the biology and pathogenesis of the diseases in mouse and rat show remarkable similarity to that in human, and one can choose among different models to examine the cellular and molecular bases for the particular property of interest.

GENETIC AND MOLECULAR COMPARISONS

Cytogenetic and chromosomal analyses of rodent mammary tumors indicate that the vast majority are diploid with an occasional loss of heterozygosity (LOH) (1, 8), whereas premalignant lesions and human breast cancers exhibit LOH at multiple loci. Common LOH in both classes of lesions strongly suggests a precursor–product relationship (7). More recent results in rodents suggest that given appropriate molecular changes or sufficient time for tumor progression, mouse mammary tumors will exhibit the diverse LOH and extensive aneuploidy common in human breast tumors. Studies with rat mammary tumors have been limited to just a few chemical carcinogens. It is likely that with the use of different etiological agents or selection of subsets of very aggressive tumors, aneuploidy and LOH will be detected as common events.

Table 3-2 lists the commonly examined genes in the three model systems. One can approach this issue in two ways. If one asks the question, "Are the same genes involved in human breast cancer as in mouse and chemically induced rat models?", the answer is, as one might predict, yes and no. Tumor suppressor genes are a good example. For instance, *p53* is mutated frequently in human cancers, but infrequently in rat mammary tumors and occasionally in mouse mammary tumors (Chapter 1 this volume). Tumor suppressor genes *Rb*, *Brca1*, and *Brca2* are altered in significant subsets of human breast cancers but, so far, have not been shown to be altered in rat or mouse breast cancers. On the other hand, the expression of the putative tumor suppressor gene gelsolin is down-regulated in all models of rodent breast cancer as well as human breast cancer (8). The cellular targets for gelsolin then merit further research to determine the exact role of this gene product in neoplastic initiation and progression.

Table 3-2. Comparison of Mouse, Rat, and Human Mammary Tumorigenesis

Property	Mouse	Rat	Human
wnt activation	MMTV (*wnt-1*) (*wnt-10b*)	UN[a]	*wnt-2, 5a, 7b*
fgf	MMTV (*fgf-3, 4, 8*)	UN	UN
ras activation	Chem. carc.	Chem. carc.	Infrequent
p53 mutation	Yes (variable)	No (chem. carc.)	Yes (frequent)
Brca mutation	No	No	Yes (germ line)
Gelsolin	Decreased	Decreased	Decreased
Growth factors/growth factor receptor[b]	EGF family	TGFα, ErbB2	EGF family, ErbB2
Cell cycle[a]	Cyclin B, D1, E	Cyclin D1	Cyclin D1, E, Rb
LOH/aneuploidy	Yes (in specific models)	Rare	Yes

[a]UN = unknown.
[b]The expression for these genes is generally increased at the mRNA or protein level.

Depending on carcinogen dose, *ras* mutation occurs in a relatively high frequency in chemical-carcinogen-induced mouse and rat tumors but infrequently in human. Conversely, *c-myc* expression is altered in a significant subset of human breast cancers but not noticeably in mouse tumors. The MMTV-activated genes *fgf3*, *fgf4*, and *fgf8* and *wnt-1* represent two families of genes important in mouse mammary tumorigenesis (9), but their respective roles in chemically induced mouse and rat tumors and in human breast cancer is uncertain, with the exception of the small percentage of human cancers exhibiting *wnt* gene activation (10). The EGF family of growth factors and their receptors exhibit major increases in gene expression in human breast cancer for EGFR, ErbB2, amphiregulin, and cripto, and in rat mammary cancers for TGFα and ErbB2 (11), but the altered expression of these genes in mouse models is still basically unclear.

The altered regulation of cell cycle genes is common in all models, human and rodent, particularly for cyclin D1. The mechanisms underlying the altered expression may be different, since the gene amplification observed in human tumors has not been detected in rodent tumors. In summary, outside of gelsolin and cyclin D1, few genes commonly are altered among the three models. This lack of commonality is not surprising given the heterogeneous nature of the human disease in comparison to the rather homogeneous nature of tumors induced in genetically similar animals by limited exposure to a single carcinogenic agent.

If one asks the question, "Can defects in genes involved in human breast carcinogenesis induce mammary cancer in rats and mice?", then the answer is yes. There is no doubt that the first round of transgenic mice demonstrated that the alteration of gene expression of *c-myc*, *p53*, *c-neu*, and cyclin D1 resulted in mammary hyperplasia and tumorigenesis. As new methods are developed that allow one to create models that replicate the multiple genetic defects detected in the human disease, it is likely that nearly all the genes implicated in human breast cancer can be modeled in the mouse and in the rat.

CONCLUSION

Where then lies the value of current models? Current models, whether they be conventional carcinogen-induced rat and mouse models or specific transgenic models, serve an important role in studies on mechanisms of chemopreventive agents, in assays for putative oncogenic agents, in studies on pathogenesis due to specific treatment regimens or the interaction of two "suspect" genes, in mechanisms of aneuploidy and of tumor progression, and in numerous other types of traditional studies in carcinogenesis. The radiation models of both mouse and rat are tremendously understudied especially in view of the fact that radiation is the only well-documented human carcinogen (2, 12).

Where lies future model development? The future lies in the development of models that emulate the combination of gene dysregulations that apply to major subsets of breast cancers. The establishment of these models will require the ability to develop conditional nulls and inducible mutants in specific groups of somatic cells, in this case luminal mammary epithelial cells. With this capability, one can dissect the timing and significance of chromosomal and genetic changes occurring in neoplastic development and progression and define the downstream molecular-pathways altered by the genetic changes. With such understanding, one can develop mechanistic-based and gene-pathway-specific chemopreventive and therapeutic approaches that selectively target the major subsets of human disease. Such models require the development of new technology, information on additional gene alterations in human disease, and the commitment to examine these models by using specific criteria.

Such specific criteria would include, minimally, the induction of ductal hyperplasias with progression to DCIS and invasive breast cancer, early onset of genetic instability, the presence of hormone-dependent and hormone-independent tumors, and metastasis to distal sites. Alterations of different gene combinations should mimic different subsets of human disease.

Do we need animal models at all if we know the key genetic alterations in humans? The answer is still yes for several reasons. There will be a critical research niche that only animal models can fill. First, they are necessary to screen new therapeutic or prevention modalities. The use of cell lines *in vitro* is often artificial and does not provide the appropriate environment for the complex cell–cell and cell–substrate interactions that dictate functional properties of *in situ* mammary epithelial cells. Animal models are needed so that the complex systemic effects of such agents on drug metabolism, host defense, and the endocrine system can be factored into a compound evaluation. Second, animal models provide the opportunity to examine cause and effect relationships in an *in situ* environment fully impacted by all other systemic factors. Third, to date, the technical difficulties associated with the analysis of small early lesions and the difficulty of studying human preneoplasia *in vivo* have precluded efforts to characterize the functional consequences of early genetic or chromosomal changes in human breast cancer. Such studies can be accomplished with animal models. Fourth, a common genetic background in animals removes a great source of uncontrolled variability naturally present in the outbred human population and provides the opportunity to manipulate genes and determine the effects of such alterations on the course of the disease. In the final analysis, appropriate animal models are economical, save time, and are necessary to circumvent the ethical issues that prohibit the investigation of many questions in human subjects. The focus of continuing investigations should be on the appropriate use of existing systems and on the intensive development of new animal models that are built upon the experience of the past and the promise of the emerging technology.

REFERENCES

1. D. Medina (2000). Mouse models for mammary cancer. Chapter 1, this volume.
2. H. J. Thompson (2000). Methods for the induction of mammary carcinognesis in the rat using either 7,12-dimethylbenzanthracene or 1-methyl-1-nitrosourea. Chapter 2, this volume.
3. M. Tokunaga, C. E. Land, S. Tokuoka, I. Nishimori, M. Soda, and S. Akiba (1994). Incidence of female breast cancer among atomic bomb survivors, 1950–1985. *Radiation Res.* **138**:209–223.
4. R. D. Cardiff and S. R. Wellings (1999). The comparative pathology of human and mouse mammary glands. *J. Mam. Gland Biol. Neoplasia* **4**:105–122.
5. S. Nandi, R. C. Guzman, and J. Yang (1995). Hormones and mammary carcinogenesis in mice, rats and humans: a unifying hypothesis. *Proc. Natl. Acad. Sci. USA* **92**:3650–3657.
6. W. Kim (1970). Metastasizing mammary carcinomas in rats: induction and study of their immunogenicity. *Science* **167**:72–74.
7. J. D. Haag, G. M. Brasic, L. A. Shepel, M. A. Newton, C. J. Grubbs, R. A. Lubet, G. J. Kelloff, and M. N. Gould (1999). A comparative analysis of allelic imbalance events in chemically induced rat mammary, colon and bladder tumors. *Mol. Carcinogenesis* **24**:47–56.
8. P. O'Connell, V. Pekkel, S. A. W. Fuqua, C. K. Osborne, and D. C. Allred (1998). Analysis of loss of heterozygosity in 399 premalignant breast lesions at 15 genetic loci. *J. Natl. Cancer Inst.* **90**:697–703.
9. Y. Dong, H. L. Asch, D. Medina, C. Ip, M. M. Ip, R. Guzman, and B. B. Asch (1999). Concurrent deregulation of gelsolin and cyclin D1 in the majority of human and rodent breast cancers. *Int. J. Cancer* **81**:930–938.
10. C. A. MacArthur, D. B. Shankar, and G. M. Shackleford (1995). *Fgf-8*, activated by proviral insertion, cooperates with the *wnt-1* transgene in murine mammary tumorigenesis. *J. Virol.* **69**:2501–2507.

11. E. L. Huguet, J. A. McMahon, A. P. McMahon, R. Bicknell, and A. L. Harris (1994). Differential expression of human *Wnt* genes 2, 3, 4 and 7B in human breast cell lines and normal and disease states of human breast tissue. *Cancer Res.* **54:**2615–2621.

12. R. B. Dickson and M. E. Lippman (1995). Growth factors in breast cancer. *Endocrine Rev.* 16:559–589.

13. P. E. Goss and S. Sierra (1998). Current perspectives on radiation-induced breast cancer. *J. Clin. Oncol.* **16:**338–347.

Chapter 4

Xenograft Models of Human Breast Cancer Lines and of the MCF10AT Model of Human Premalignant, Proliferative Breast Disease

Fred R. Miller and Gloria H. Heppner

Abstract. Immune deficient mice may be used to study the development, growth, and metastasis of human breast cancer. Progression of the MCF10 premalignant human breast epithelial cell lines occurs in xenografts, providing a model to study early events in human breast disease. Tumorigenicity of breast cancer cell lines may be enhanced either by suspending cells in Matrigel prior to injection into the subcutis or by injecting the cells into a mammary fat pad. Metastasis is enhanced by implanting breast cancer xenografts into mammary fat pads.

Abbreviations. atypical hyperplasia (AH); ductal carcinoma *in situ* (DCIS); severe combined immune deficiency (SCID); x-linked immune deficiency (xid).

INTRODUCTION

Xenograft Systems

Several immune deficient mouse strains are available that accept grafted tissue from other species (xenografts), including human cancer cell lines. Each immune deficient strain has different immunological characteristics (Table 4-1). The nude mouse, for example, although deficient in T cells, has quite high NK activity. Nude–beige mice are available with both T-cell and NK deficiencies, but the NK deficiency is not as severe as in beige mice. SCID (severe combined immune deficiency) mice have T- and B-cell deficiencies but retain NK activity. Triple deficient mice are available with the nude, beige, and xid (x-linked immune deficiency, a B-cell defect) mutations. Although human xenografts have been successfully established in all of these mutant strains, significant differences in tumorigenic doses, incidence, latency, and metastasis have been observed for several cancer lines among the strains. Human tumors have been reported to grow better in SCID mice than in nude mice, requiring two log fewer cells to produce tumors in some cases (1). A *lacZ*-transduced variant of MDA-MB-435 was reported to metastasize in 96% of SCID mice and in only 26% of nude mice (2). Thus, SCID

Fred R. Miller and Gloria H. Heppner   Karmanos Cancer Institute, and School of Medicine, Wayne State University, Detroit, Michigan 48201.

Methods in Mammary Gland Biology and Breast Cancer Research, edited by Ip and Asch. Kluwer Academic/Plenum Publishers, New York, 2000.

Table 4-1. Immune Characteristics of Mice Commonly Used for Xenografting Human Cells

Immune deficient mouse	T-cell deficiency	B-cell deficiency	NK-cell deficiency
Nude	×		
Nude–beige	×		×
Triple deficient (nude–beige–xid)	×	×	×
SCID	×	×	
SCID–beige	×	×	×

mice may be most optimal for human cancer xenograft studies. Additional immune suppression by whole-body irradiation (1), treatment with anti-AsGM1 or anti-interleukin-2 receptor beta chain antibodies (3), or treatment with etoposide (4) further enhances tumorigenicity and metastasis in SCID mice.

Breast Cancer Xenograft Models

It is difficult to establish cell lines from human breast cancer, and many established lines are very poorly tumorigenic in immune deficient mice. However, cell lines have been established that form tumors when xenografted (5), and tumorigenic potential can be improved by suspending cells in Matrigel prior to injection (6). Most human breast carcinoma lines are estrogen independent, but exceptions include MCF-7, T47D, and ZR75–1, which respond to estrogen supplementation of the host mice. Indeed, MCF-7 requires estrogen supplementation for tumor growth (7). Most human breast cancer cell lines that are able to form tumors in immune deficient mice do not metastasize spontaneously from primaries growing in subcutaneous sites, nor do they form experimental metastases (lung colonies) following intravenous injection. Notable exceptions include the lines MDA-MB-435 and MDA-MB-231 (8). However, metastatic efficiency can often be improved by implantation of tumor cells into the natural site of origin (orthotopic site). Thus, human breast cancer cells metastasize more readily when implanted into mammary fat pads than when injected subcutaneously (8). Because neoplastic mammary cells are not inhibited by normal mammary epithelium, fat pads do not need to be cleared (see the sequel).

The MCF10AT Xenograft Model

We have derived a series of human breast epithelial cell lines that form premalignant lesions when xenografted into immune deficient mice. The parental line, MCF10A, was derived by spontaneous immortalization of breast epithelial cells from a patient with fibrocystic disease (9). It does not form persistent xenografts. MCF10A cells were transfected with a mutant C-Ha-*ras* to produce the MCF10AneoT cell line (10), which does produce xenografts. The MCF10AT model is a family of lines produced by culturing cells from xenografts of MCF10AneoT and from xenografts of later transplant generations (11, 12).

The initial histology of MCF10AT xenografts is benign. Simple ducts and cysts with simple epithelium coexist with ducts displaying tufting or papillary infolding. Simple ducts become proliferative within the xenografts, displaying varying degrees of epithelial hyperplasia, including atypical hyperplasia (AH) and ductal carcinoma *in situ* (DCIS). In advanced lesions, benign areas, both simple and hyperplastic, coexist with DCIS and invasive carcinoma. The early cancers grow slowly, mimicking human breast cancer development. However, by prolonging the natural history of the MCF10AT tumors via serial trocar implantation of advanced lesions, researchers have derived rapidly growing MCF10CA tumor lines with metastatic potential (13, Santner *et al.*, manuscript submitted).

The MCF10AT model presents a histological spectrum of outgrowths—AH, DCIS, and invasive cancer—that is remarkably similar to that found in women, both in regard to morphology and to intraspecimen heterogeneity. AH and DCIS are indicative of an enhanced risk of developing invasive cancer in women, and MCF10AT xenografts develop invasive cancer as well, following a sporadic time course again similar to that in women, albeit in an abbreviated time frame (several months in mice versus years in women). Although the xenografts persist and progress in the absence of estrogen supplementation, MCF10AT cells express functional estrogen receptors, and estrogen exposure markedly enhances development of high-risk lesions and invasive carcinomas in MCF10AT xenografts. Thus, MCF10AT lesions are estrogen responsive but not estrogen dependent. In this chapter we review the methods that we use in our xenograft studies with the MCF10AT model.

MATERIALS

Culturing Breast Epithelial Cells

Note: It is very important to use the appropriate medium for any breast epithelial cell line being used. When obtaining a cell line from another laboratory or source, it is important to follow the recommended culture conditions. The MCF10 family of cell lines illustrates this very well (Table 4-2). The mortal MCF10 cells can only be maintained in medium with low calcium, the immortal MCF10A cells require hydrocortisone and epidermal growth factor, the MCF10AneoT cells do not require EGF but grow faster with it added, whereas the MCF10AT variants do not respond to EGF at all. The MCF10CA variants are maintained in monolayer culture with no added supplements (13, Santner *et al.*, manuscript submitted).

- Dulbecco's modified Eagle's medium (DMEM) (GIBCO, Grand Island, NY)
- Ham's nutrient mixture F-12 (GIBCO, Grand Island, NY)
- Cholera toxin (ICN Biomedicals, Cleveland, OH)

Table 4-2. Media Components for Monolayer Culture of MCF10 Cell Lines

Media component	MCF10MS	MCF10A	MCF10AneoT	MCF10AT variants (premalignant)	MCF10CA variants (malignant)
DMEM / Ham's F-12 (1:1)	×	×	×	×	×
5% serum (horse or calf)	×	×	×	×	×
*Streptomycin (100 µg/ml)	×	×	×	×	×
*Penicillin (100 units/ml)	×	×	×	×	×
*Fungizone (0.5 µg/ml)	×	×	×	×	×
Insulin (10 µg/ml)	×	×	×	×	
EGF (20 ng/ml)	×	×	×	*	
Cholera toxin (100 ng/ml)	×	×	×	×	
Hydrocortisone (0.5 µg/ml)	×	×	×	×	
Calcium (0.04 mM)	×				
Calcium (1.05 mM)		×	×	×	×

*Optional additives.

- Epidermal growth factor (EGF) (Collaborative Research, Bedford, MA)
- Hydrocortisone (Sigma, St. Louis, MO)
- Insulin (Sigma, St. Louis, MO)

Enzymes for Disaggregation of Tissue

- Digestion mixture to recover organoids from MCF10AT lesions: 125 U/ml collagenase (Sigma Chemical Co., St. Louis, MO) in 70% Hanks' minimal essential medium (GIBCO, Grand Island, NY) and 30% Earle's minimal essential medium (GIBCO, Grand Island, NY) supplemented with 7.5% serum (horse or calf) and 10 μg/ml insulin.
- Enzyme mixture to obtain single-cell suspensions from organoids: 12.5 mg/ml protease type IX (Sigma Chemical Co., St. Louis, MO) in serum-free 70% Hanks' minimal essential medium and 30% Earles minimal essential medium.

Surgical Materials

- Stainless steel wound clips: Clay Adams 9-mm Autoclips, applicators, and removers are distributed by Becton Dickinson (Sparks, MD).
- Cavitron thermocautery manufactured by Burton Division, Cavitron Corp. (Van Nuys, CA). Matrigel basement membrane matrix is obtained from Becton Dickinson Labware (Franklin Lakes, NJ).
- Estradiol slow-release pellets and 10-gauge stainless steel trocar are obtained from Innovative Research of America (Sarasota, FL).

METHODS

Pathological Assessment of Stage of MCF10AT Xenografts

Although MCF10AT xenografts closely resemble human high-risk breast lesions, differences in stroma and overall structure exist. For example, there is no lobular organization of the MCF10AT ductular elements and, although the MCF10AT cells are stem cells capable of differentiating into a myoepithelial layer as well as a luminal epithelial layer (14), the myoepithelial layer is neither distinct nor always discernible. Table 4-3 describes the criteria we have used to classify the xenograft lesions and is broadly based on criteria outlined by Page and Anderson (15).

The stromal elements in the xenografts are of mouse origin. If orthotopic injections are used, one must be careful not to confuse mouse mammary gland epithelium with the xenografted epithelium. We have used fluorescent *in situ* hybridization with human centromeric probes to confirm the human origin of specific cells in xenografts (14).

Transplantation of Breast Cancer and MCF10AT Cells

Any of the immune deficient strains of mice may be used to establish premalignant MCF10AT xenograft lesions. We have used nude, nude–beige, SCID, and SCID–beige mice. Although the use of female mice seems natural, and is recommended, male mice also support the development and progression of the MCF10AT lesions. We have always used mice aged 4–12 weeks to initiate lesions, but older mice may also suffice.

Table 4-3. Criteria for Grading of Proliferative Breast Lesions

Grade 0	Simple epithelium	Small ducts with single layer of luminal epithelium, no nuclear enlargement, no nucleoli or mitoses
Grade 1	Mild hyperplasia	Small ducts, 2 or more layers of epithelial cells,[a] no significant bridging, variable nuclear contours
Grade 2	Moderate hyperplasia	Mildly distended ducts, 4 or more layers of epithelial cells,[a] irregular papillary proliferation, bridging by nonuniform cells, irregularly shaped lumens, no solidly filled spaces, indistinct cell boundaries, variable nuclear contours, bland chromatin, small nucleoli
Grade 3	Atypical hyperplasia	Grossly distended ducts, regular micropapillary configuration, marked cellular proliferation often forming regularity (roundness) of spaces, some loss of polarity, luminal mass, some cells become monotonous, tendency to clear cytoplasm with distinct borders, enlarged, nonround hyperchromatic nuclei, small nucleoli, occasional mitoses
Grade 4	Carcinoma *in situ*	Distended ducts filled with uniform cells, rigid intraluminal bridges forming round spaces, occasional central necrosis, distinct cell boundaries, uniform round, hyperchromatic, enlarged nuclei, prominent nucleoli, frequent mitoses
Grade 5	Invasive carcinoma	Glandular, squamous, or undifferentiated

[a]Due to the inconspicuous nature of the myoepithelial cells in many of the specimens, they were not considered as a layer.

IMPLANTATION OF TISSUE PIECES. The most reliable means of generating tumors in immune deficient mice is to transplant pieces of tumor. The disadvantages are that individual pieces are likely to consist of multiple components and the different pieces may be very different from each other due to heterogeneity. For this procedure a 10-gauge trocar can be used. However, we prefer to anesthetize mice (we use 80 mg/kg ketamine and 7 mg/kg zylazine, i.p.), make a 2–3 mm incision in the skin, and place the piece of tissue under the skin with sterile forceps. The incision is closed with a stainless steel surgical clip that is removed after 10–14 days.

INJECTION IN MATRIGEL. We recommend that cells be suspended in Matrigel before injecting into the subcutis because the tumorigenic potential of human cells in immune deficient mice is markedly increased by Matrigel (6). The cells should be pelleted by centrifugation, and the volume of the pellet should be noted. All media should be poured off and cells resuspended by snapping the tube with a finger. A volume of undiluted Matrigel equal to the volume of the cell pellet is added and gently pipetted to mix cells with Matrigel. Care must be taken to avoid bubbles while pipetting, because a minimum surface of the pipette is to be used to avoid loss of cells. For MCF10AT cells the final mixture yields approximately 10^7 cells per 0.15 ml. We use a 21-gauge needle for injecting mice. It is difficult to force the cell and Matrigel slurry through smaller-gauge needles. We insert the needle to its full length and twist the needle as it is removed following injection, to minimize loss of cells through the needle track.

ORTHOTOPIC INJECTION. Mice are anesthetized, the skin is incised (1 cm), and the skin flap is laid back to expose a No. 4 mammary gland. Cells (10^3 to 10^5) are injected in a volume of 0.02 ml into the mammary gland with a 27-gauge needle. The injected material should be clearly visible as a bubble within the fat pad. It is also possible to place a piece of tissue into an exposed mammary fat pad by making a small incision in the fat and inserting the transplanted tissue. The skin is aligned and stapled with stainless steel surgical clips. The clips are removed 2 weeks later.

Assessment of Metastasis by Breast Cancer Xenografts

Metastasis is a series of events or obstacles that tumor cells must be able to overcome before metastatic nodules can develop. Spontaneous metastasis refers to the ability to break free of a primary tumor, enter a transport system (intravasation)—either the blood-stream or lymphatic vessel—survive the trauma encountered during transport, arrest, extravasate, and grow at the metastatic site. The lung is by far the most common site for metastasis of xenografted human breast cancer, but additional sites may be involved as well.

Experimental metastasis, in which cells are injected directly into the bloodstream, leads only to the latter stages of the process. Cells that are unable to form experimental metastases after intravenous injection invariably fail to metastasize spontaneously. However, a number of cell lines that are not able to metastasize spontaneously can colonize the lungs following intravenous injection.

SPONTANEOUS METASTASIS. Tumor cells are injected either into fat pads or into Matrigel in the subcutis as described earlier. Because metastases are established subsequent to growth of primary tumors, primary tumors are often large before metastases can be detected. In some cases mice die before metastases can be detected. Therefore, the primary must be removed and mice maintained for an extended period to allow growth of any metastases that may have been present at the time of surgery. After tumors reach a diameter of 12–18 mm (this depends on the cell model being used), mice are anesthetized, tumors are swabbed with disinfectant, and the tumors and overlying skin are surgically removed with sterile (autoclaved) instru-ments. Bleeding is controlled with an electrocautery. The skin is aligned and stapled with sterile clips. The mice are placed on sterile gauze pads in cages on heating pads until recov-ery (2–3 h). Surgical clips are removed 2 weeks later. Animals are observed for signs of dis-tress associated with metastatic disease, including weight loss, scruffy coat, labored breathing, hunching, and overall loss of activity. When symptoms appear, mice are sacrificed and organs assessed for the presence of metastases.

EXPERIMENTAL LUNG COLONIZATION (EXPERIMENTAL METASTASIS). Groups of immune deficient mice are warmed by placing the cage (with minimal bedding) on a heating pad for approximately 30 min. This results in dilation of the tail vein to facilitate injection. We prefer this method to heat lamps or hot swabs because discomfort to the animal is minimal and there is no chance of injuring it. Each mouse is then placed inside a clean cage with the tail pulled externally between two lid wires for injection. We prefer this method over plastic restrainers because the animals appear to be less stressed by this means of restraint. Once injected, the animal is simply released and drops to the bottom of the cage. Up to 5×10^6 cells in a total volume of 0.2 ml of isotonic medium or saline can be injected with a 25-gauge needle.

In general, it takes 3–10 weeks for lung colonies to form, assuming the cell line is able to colonize lungs. Mice are monitored for signs of distress associated with lung metastasis, sacrificed, and lungs assessed for the presence of metastases.

Estrogen Supplementation

Normal mice have endogenous estradiol levels (varying between 10 and 60 pg/ml during the estrous cycle) (16) comparable to the follicular phase of premenopausal women (about 50–100 pg/ml) (17). Estrogen-depleted animals can be used to simulate postmenopausal conditions. Estrogen pellet supplementation does not mimic the cyclic spikes of serum estrogen levels but can provide serum levels of estradiol equivalent to those of premenopausal women. Silastic tubing or silastic elastomer can be used to make slow-release estradiol pellets (16). Placing different amounts of estradiol in the pellets allows different serum levels of estradiol to be achieved. Slow-release estradiol pellets are available commercially (Innovative Research of America, Sarasota, FL). The manufacturer provides 0.72-mg pellets to achieve 300–400 pg/ml estradiol levels, which are comparable to levels in women in mid-cycle, and 1.7-mg pellets to achieve 700–900 pg/ml, equivalent to the highest peak seen in premenopausal women that occurs the day before the luteinizing hormone peak (17). The 0.72-mg pellets are commonly used to support MCF-7 growth in nude mice (18). The 1.7-mg pellet accelerates progression of MCF10AT cells (19).

Mice are oophorohysterectomized and have estradiol or placebo slow-release pellets implanted in the subcutis. Pellets may be placed at the time of surgery; cells may be xenografted at that time or a week later. Ovariectomy is sufficient for short-term experiments of up to 2 months, but elevated estrogen levels cause severe uterine hypertrophy and mice do not do well for more extended experiments. Thus, we recommend oophorohysterectomy. Development and progression of MCF10AT proliferative lesions are accelerated by elevated estrogen levels in that the numbers and stages of lesions seen after 70 days in mice implanted with estrogen pellets are comparable to those after 210 days in mice not supplemented with estrogen (19).

To implant pellets in anesthetized mice, one makes an incision through the skin between the shoulder blades with sterile (autoclaved) scissors. The pellet (approximately 2 mm in diameter) is placed under the skin with sterile forceps and the skin is closed with sterile stainless steel wound clips. Mice are placed in cages on paper towels until recovery. Wound clips are removed 10 days later. If it is necessary to maintain elevated estrogen levels for extended periods, pellets should be replaced every 75 days.

Establishment of Cultured Cells from MCF10AT Xenografts

All cell cultures derived from xenografts must be characterized to ensure their origin. We have used DNA fingerprinting as well as karyotyping to confirm the MCF10 lineage of our variants (11, 12). Collagenase is used to disrupt lesions into small organoid aggregates of cells. Lesions are enzymatically dissociated with collagenase (125 U/ml of collagenase in 70% Hanks' minimal essential medium, 20% Earle's minimal essential medium, and 7.5% equine serum supplemented with 10 mg/ml insulin, 100 IU/ml penicillin, 100 mg/ml streptomycin, and 0.5 mg/ml amphotericin B). Small lesions weighing less than 200 mg are placed in 10 ml of digestion medium in capped T25 flasks on a rocking platform at 37°C. As organoids are released, they are removed and plated onto plastic and the digestion medium is replenished in the digestion flask. This process is repeated until the tissue is essentially dispersed, which requires 6–72 h. We have no difficulty in establishing premalignant cultures from hyperplastic xenografts even though less than 20 mg of tissue is typically used as starting material.

We have also cloned cells directly from the xenograft lesions. Organoids were obtained as already described and were further dissociated by treating for 15–20 min with 12.5 mg/ml protease type IX and then pipetted to break up clumps. By making single-cell suspensions of xenografts and plating at various dilutions into dishes containing plastic cover slips, we successfully obtained clones from carcinomas that have karyotypes different from the typical MCF10AT stem cell. Cover slips with single slow-growing clones are isolated simply by removing the cover slip and placing in a new well.

Chemoprevention Studies

The premalignant MCF10AT cells provide a unique model to test the ability of putative chemopreventive agents to inhibit progression of high-risk human breast lesions. Because the MCF10AT model is accelerated in estradiol supplemented mice, one can test chemopreventive agents in both estrogen-depleted animals, to simulate postmenopausal conditions, and in estrogen-supplemented animals. Differential activity of chemopreventive agents in estrogen-depleted versus estrogen-supplemented conditions might suggest preferential use in postmenopausal or premenopausal women.

Although the incidence of AH, DCIS, and invasive carcinoma increases with time, reasonable numbers of each can be detected by 200 days after xenografting in mice that have not been implanted with estradiol pellets (Figure 4-1). Figure 4-1 shows there is an incidence of 20% invasive carcinoma at day 200 versus 26% final incidence, 36% DCIS plus invasive carcinoma at day 200, and 48% AH plus carcinoma *in situ* plus invasive carcinoma at day 200 versus 56% final incidence.

In estrogen-supplemented (serum levels 900 pg/ml) mice at day 70 the incidence of invasive cancer is 15%, the incidence of DCIS plus invasive carcinoma is 53%, and the incidence of AH plus carcinoma *in situ* plus invasive carcinoma is 90% (Figure 4-2).

The number of implants needed for chemoprevention studies depends on the size of the effect one is willing to accept, determined by statistical power calculations, and whether one is interested in a reduction in incidence of invasive cancer or a reduction in the incidence of the high-risk lesions (note: up to four lesions/mouse are feasible; we routinely use two).

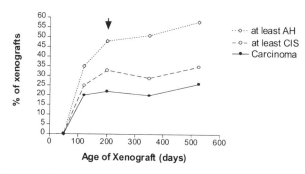

Figure 4-1. Cumulative incidence of lesion pathology in MCF10AT3B xenografts without estrogen. At day 50, all xenografts consisted of benign ducts with no atypical features. At each time point depicted, all lesions to date were included in the calculation, not just the lesions taken at that time point. By 200 days, 52% of lesions had no areas graded as AH, DCIS, or invasive cancer. Of the remaining 48% of lesions, 20% had progressed to invasive carcinoma, 16% to DCIS, and 12% to AH.

Figure 4-2. The cumulative incidence of lesion pathology in MCF10AT1 xenografts at day 70 in estradiol-supplemented mice. Only 1/13 (8%) of lesions had no areas graded as AH, DCIS, or invasive cancer. Of the remaining lesions, 2 (15%) contained areas of invasive cancer, 5 (38%) contained DCIS, and 5 (38%) contained AH. Each bar indicates the percent of lesions with at least the indicated grade. Thus, 91% of lesions had progressed to AH or worse.

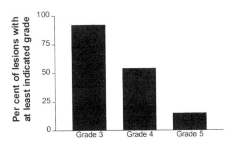

For example, consider two alternatives for the proportion of lesions for each level of the ordinal response variable (benign, AH, DCIS, and invasive carcinoma): (1) 50% decrease in the proportion of lesions observed to be AH, DCIS, and invasive, each compared to the absence of any change, and (2) a 50% decrease in only the proportion of lesions observed to be invasive (with no change in the other two) compared to the absence of any change. The probabilities for the null hypothesis for the chi-square goodness-of-fit test comparing the ordinal response variable for a treatment group compared to the control group (which has a chi-squared distribution with 3 degrees of freedom) is as follows. (1) From data illustrated in Figure 4-1, estrogen-depleted mice are assumed to be 0.52, 0.12, 0.16, 0.20 for benign, AH, DCIS, and invasive carcinoma, respectively. The calculation allows for all six possible comparisons between the control group and the three treatment groups by selecting a significance level of <0.01 by using Bonferroni's technique. Under these conditions, 176 lesions have a power of at least 90% for both alternative hypotheses. (2) From data presented in Figure 4-2, estrogen-supplemented mice are assumed to be 0.08, 0.38, 0.38, and 0.15 for benign, AH, DCIS, and invasive carcinoma, respectively. The calculation allows for all six possible comparison between the control group and the three treatment groups by selecting a significance level of <0.01 by using Bonferroni's technique. Under these conditions, 64 lesions have a power of at least 90% for both alternative hypotheses.

Thus, it would be possible to detect inhibition of progression to each level of disease allowing discrimination between agents that prevent development of high-risk lesions from those that only prevent late-stage progression to carcinoma.

Carcinogen Testing

Potential carcinogens are tested with cell cultures or animals. Treatment of human breast epithelial cells with benzo[a]pyrene *in vitro* was found to extend the life span of the cells in culture and occasionally resulted in emergence of an immortalized line (20). No cell line was tumorigenic in nude mice. Treatment of the immortalized human breast epithelial cell line MCF10F with a number of carcinogens (including DMBA and NMU) *in vitro* resulted in transformation as assessed by anchorage-independent growth. None of the transformed populations or clones was tumorigenic in immune deficient mice. Eventually, after cloning and subcloning of a culture treated with benz[a]pyrene, a subclone was reported to form tumors in immune deficient mice (21). This single tumorigenic clone arose 498 days after treatment with carcinogen. Clearly, the in vitro assay provides insufficient means of assessing carcinogen activity. The high-risk, but premalignant, MCF10AT xenograft model could be a valuable tool for carcinogenesis studies. The final incidence of invasive carcinoma in untreated MCF10AT xenografts is ~25%. If a threefold increase in carcinoma incidence is accepted as a positive response to carcinogen (from 25% incidence to more than 75%), power analysis, using an α of 0.05 and 90% power, indicates that 20 lesions are necessary.

COMMENTS

Other Xenograft Models of Premalignant Breast Disease

A number of publications describe implantation of pieces of normal breast, hyperplastic breast, or carcinoma *in situ* into immune deficient mice (16, 22–28). Sheffied and Welsch (23) were able to establish small ductular organoids of normal human breast epithelium in nude mice by injecting enzymatically dissociated breast cells into cleared fat pads. A total of 68% of fat pads injected with 2×10^5 cells grew small organoids that persisted up to 180 days. The largest number of organoids observed in a single fat pad was 23, and total xenograft volumes approximated $1 mm^3$ per fat pad. Although expansive growth was never observed and no evidence of progression to proliferative stages occurred, in these experiments, a modest but statistically significant response to estrogen and progesterone was demonstrated.

Pieces of normal human breast were also found to respond to estradiol, but not progesterone, as determined by increased thymidine labeling in nude mice (16). Estradiol serum levels at concentrations comparable to human levels during the follicular phase induced progesterone receptor expression but were not mitogenic for the xenografts, whereas treatment with estradiol to achieve luteal phase concentrations induced progesterone receptor expression and proliferation in the xenografts (25).

Jensen and Wellings (22) transplanted pieces of breast tissue into nude mice for up to 27 weeks. Survival of epithelial xenografts was somewhat higher if transplanted into cleared mammary fat pads (80%) than if transplanted subcutaneously (70%). Samples were obtained from cancerous breast and contralateral noncancerous breasts, and supravital staining was used to determine whether each sample appeared normal or atypical. None of the xenografts increased in size or were able to fill cleared fat pads, as do mouse hyperplastic alveolar nodules. However, intraductal proliferation did occur with some loss of organization, an event the authors termed "dedifferentiation." There was no difference in the incidence of dedifferentiation between normal lobules from the cancer-associated breast (5/33) and normal lobules from the contralateral breast (9/66) when samples were taken from patients under 50 years of age. Very few samples were tested from contralateral breasts of patients over age 50, but it appeared that samples from cancer-associated and contralateral breasts dedifferentiated at a higher frequency than samples from younger patients (15/28 from cancer associated and 2/3 from contralateral). Atypical samples dedifferentiated at similar frequencies to normal lobules in both age groups. However, in these experiments progression to structures resembling AH, DCIS, or invasive cancer was not reported.

A recent report demonstrated that samples from breast carcinoma *in situ* survive in xenografts better than do samples of invasive carcinoma (24). No increase in size or progression in stage of the lesions during the 56 days of engraftment was noted. This study also demonstrated a proliferative response to estradiol by estrogen-receptor-positive DCIS (3 cases) but not by estrogen-receptor-negative DCIS (10 cases). Measurement of proliferation by staining with antihuman Ki-67 antibody demonstrated an increase from an initial 2%

positive cells to 15% at 14 days after xenografting, a time when host serum estrogen levels were highest, resembling the human premenopausal midcycle level. Although not specifically addressed by the authors, the DCIS samples were presumably taken from postmenopausal women because in control mice with follicular phase levels of estradiol, Ki-67 staining increased to 4% in the estrogen-receptor-positive xenografts.

The MCF10AT model consists of a panel of cell lines that are amenable to genetic manipulation. The unique feature of MCF10AT is the establishment of hyperplastic lesions and carcinomas *in situ* that sporadically progress to invasive carcinomas of different histologic types. The progression is accelerated by estrogen supplementation that provides peak premenopausal human estradiol serum levels. The model provides a means to test specific mechanisms in progression to invasive cancer and metastasis by introducing functional genes into cells at the appropriate stage of progression or by knocking out gene function. The model may also prove valuable for detecting agents that promote breast cancer and for screening chemopreventive agents.

Orthotopic Tissue Interactions

Tissue interactions in the normal mammary gland are important for homeostasis. In the case of murine mammary cells, both normal and preneoplastic mammary epithelia are stroma dependent; that is, they only grow in mammary fat pads and not at ectopic sites. The growth of normal and preneoplastic cells is inhibited by normal mammary epithelium. Thus, to obtain growth of normal or preneoplastic mouse mammary epithelia, the cells must be transplanted into mammary glands free of glandular elements, i.e., "cleared" fat pads (ones from which mammary epithelium was surgically removed by the age of 3 weeks to prevent development of epithelial structure; see Chapter 6 by L. J. T. Young, this volume). Mouse mammary tumors are obviously not mammary stroma dependent because tumors grow after subcutaneous implantation and at metastatic sites. However, we found that tumor formation in the fat pad requires approximately ten-fold fewer cells than at subcutaneous sites (29), and thus even tumor cells are "stromal responsive." Furthermore, mouse mammary tumor cells are stimulated rather than inhibited by normal mammary epithelium as evidenced by their enhanced growth in intact fat pads versus growth in cleared fat pads (29, 30). The preferential metastasis from the orthotopic site that we originally described for mouse mammary tumors (31) has been described for human breast carcinoma cells implanted into mammary fat pads of nude mice (8). For these reasons, we recommend that the orthotopic site be utilized for human cancer xenografts when possible.

Unfortunately, MCF10AT cells do not consistently form persistent epithelial lesions when injected into cleared or intact mammary fat pads, in contrast to the formation of lesions when injected subcutaneously in Matrigel. A possible explanation is that 10^7 cells can be injected subcutaneously in Matrigel compared to $<10^6$ in fat pads because of the limited volume (0.02 ml) that can be injected into a fat pad without leakage. Furthermore, due to the small needle gauge required for fat pad injections, Matrigel cannot be used.

Derivation of Malignant Variants of MCF10

We readily establish cells in culture from MCF10AT lesions of all histologic stages. Interestingly, the cells established from MCF10AT xenografts containing invasive carcinoma are premalignant; when injected into nude–beige mice, simple ducts form that progress to hyperplastic lesions and sporadically form cancers. The karyotypes as well as the premalignant phenotypes are the same irrespective of the histology of the lesion from which the cultured cells are derived. Thus, it appears that the premalignant stem cell remains in the xenograft even after progression to carcinoma and that this stem cell has a growth advantage *in vitro*.

We reasoned that in order to isolate cancer cells from the stem cell we must serially transplant pieces of tumor from one mouse to the next with no intervening *in vitro* selection. In this manner we hoped to eliminate the premalignant stem cell by continuing *in vivo* selection pressure for the cancer cells. To lengthen the selection time for malignant variants, we serially transplanted pieces of lesions that had progressed to invasive carcinoma into immune deficient mice, avoiding an in vitro selective step. After three consecutive in vivo passes, malignant variants of MCF10 (MCF10CA lines) were derived successfully (13).

Future Directions

The MCF10 series of cell lines provides unique tools for determining molecular pathways of progression in breast cancer. Genetic alterations may be determined by comparing variants at different stages of progression by differential display, genetic array analysis, or protein expression analysis. Because different stages of progression are available, genetic manipulation for direct testing of gene function is possible. Thus, if an oncogene is found to be overexpressed in the MCF10CA variants, it can be determined whether overexpression of that oncogene in MCF10AT variants result in a malignant phenotype.

Because MCF10AT xenografts spontaneously progress to invasive cancer 25% of the time, treatment of xenografted animals can be used to test for suspected human breast carcinogens. Do xenografts in carcinogen-treated mice progress at a higher incidence than xenografts in control groups? Alternatively, treatment of xenografted animals can be used to determine the ability of chemopreventive agents to inhibit progression of the xenografts.

ACKNOWLEDGMENTS. Work of authors supported in part by USPHS grants CA61230 (FRM) and CA28366 (FRM) and a grant from the Elsa U. Pardee Foundation (GHH).

REFERENCES

1. A. Taghian, W. Budach, A. Zietman, J. Freeman, D. Gioioso, W. Ruka, and H. D. Suit (1993). Quantitative comparison between the transplantability of human and murine tumors into the subcutaneous tissue of NCr/Sed-nu/nu nude and severe combined immunodeficient mice. *Cancer Res.* **53**:5012–5017.
2. X. Xie, N. Brunner, G. Jensen, J. Albrectsen, B. Gotthardsen, and J. Rygaard (1992). Comparative studies between nude and scid mice on the growth and metastatic behavior of xenografted human tumors. *Clin. Exp. Metastasis* **10**:201–210.
3. S. Yano, Y. Nishioka, K. Izumi, T. Tsuruo, T. Tanaka, M. Miyasaka, and S. Sone (1996). Novel metastasis model of human lung cancer in SCID mice depleted of NK cells. *Int. J. Cancer* **67**:211–217.
4. S. Visonneau, A. Cesano, M. H. Torosian, E. J. Miller, and D. Santoli (1998). Growth characteristics and metastatic properties of human breast cancer xenografts in immunodeficient mice. *Am. J. Pathol.* **152**:1299–1311.
5. R. Clarke (1996). Human breast cancer cell line xenografts as models of breast cancer. The immunobiologies of recipient mice and the characteristics of several tumorigenic cell lines. *Breast Cancer Res. Treat.* **39**:69–86.

6. R. Fridman, M. C. Kibbey, L. S. Royce, M. Zain, T. M. Sweeney, D. L. Jicha, J. R. Yannelli, G. R. Martin, and H. K. Kleinman (1991). Enhanced tumor growth of both primary and established human and murine tumor cells in athymic mice after coinjection with Matrigel. *J. Natl. Cancer Inst.* **83:**769–774.

7. C. K. Osborne, K. Hobbs, and G. M. Clark (1985). Effect of estrogens and antiestrogens on growth of human breast cancer cells in athymic nude mice. *Cancer Res.* **45:**584–590.

8. J. E. Price, A. Polyzos, R. D. Zhang, and L. M. Daniels (1990). Tumorigenicity and metastasis of human breast carcinoma cell lines in nude mice. *Cancer Res.* **50:**717–721.

9. H. D. Soule, T. M. Maloney, S. R. Wolman, W. D. J. Peterson, R. Brenz, C. M. McGrath, J. Russo, R. J. Pauley, R. F. Jones, and S. C. Brooks (1990). Isolation and characterization of a spontaneously immortalized human breast epithelial cell line, MCF-10. *Cancer Res.* **50:**6075–6086.

10. F. Basolo, J. Elliott, L. Tait, X. Q. Chen, T. Maloney, I. H. Russo, R. Pauley, S. Momiki, J. Caamano, A. J. P. Klein-Szanto, M. Koszalka, and J. Russo (1991). Transformation of human breast epithelial cells by c-Ha-ras oncogene. *Mol. Carcinogen.* **4:**25–35.

11. F. R. Miller, H. D. Soule, L. Tait, R. J. Pauley, S. R. Wolman, P. J. Dawson, and G. H. Heppner (1993). Xenograft model of human proliferative breast disease. *J. Natl. Cancer Inst.* **85:**1725–1732.

12. P. J. Dawson, S. R. Wolman, L. Tait, G. H. Heppner, and F. R. Miller (1996). MCF10AT: a model for the evolution of cancer from proliferative breast disease. *Am. J. Pathol.* **148:**313–319.

13. S. J. Santner, F. Miller, P. Dawson, L. Tait, H. Soule, J. Eliason, and G. Heppner (1998). MCF-10CA1 cell lines: New highly tumorigenic deribvatives of the MCF-10AT system. *Proc. Am. Assoc. Cancer. Res.* **39:**202–203.

14. L. Tait, P. J. Dawson, S. R. Wolman, and F. R. Miller (1996). Multipotent human breast stem cell line MCF10AT. *Int. J. Oncol.* **9:**263–267.

15. D. L. Page and T. J. Anderson (1987). *Diagnostic Histopathology of the Breast*, Churchill Livingstone, Edinburgh.

16. I. J. Laidlaw, R. B. Clarke, A. Howell, A. W. Owen, C. S. Potten, and E. Anderson (1995). The proliferation of normal human breast tissue implanted into athymic nude mice is stimulated by estrogen but not progesterone. *Endocrinology* **136:**164–171.

17. K. Fotherby (1984). Endocrinology of the menstrual cycle and pregnancy. In H. L. J. Makin (ed.), *Biochemistry of Steroid Hormones*, Blackwell Scientific Publications, Oxford, pp. 409–440.

18. Y. Liu, D. El-Ashry, D. Chen, I. Y. F. Ding, and F. G. Kern (1995). MCF-7 breast cancer cells overexpressing transfected c-erbB-2 have an in vitro growth advantage in estrogen-depleted conditions with reduced estrogen-dependence and tamoxifen-sensitivity *in vivo*. *Breast Cancer Res. Treat.* **34:**97–117.

19. P. V. M. Shekhar, P. Nangia-Makker, S. R. Wolman, L. Tait, G. H. Heppner, and D. W. Visscher (1998). Direct action of estrogen on sequence of progression of human preneoplastic breast disease. *Am. J. Pathol.* **152:**1129–1132.

20. M. R. Stampfer and J. C. Bartley (1985). Induction of transformation and continuous cell lines from normal human mammary epithelial cells after exposure to benzo[a]pyrene. *Proc. Natl. Acad. Sci. U.S.A.* **82:**2394–2398.

21. G. Calaf and J. Russo (1993). Transformation of human breast epithelial cells by chemical carcinogens. *Carcinogenesis* **14:**483–492.

22. H. M. Jensen and S. R. Wellings (1976). Preneoplastic lesions of the human mammary gland transplanted into the nude athymic mouse. *Cancer Res.* **36:**2605–2610.

23. L. G. Sheffield and C. W. Welsch (1988). Transplantation of human breast epithelia to mammary-gland-free fat-pads of athymic nude mice: influence of mammotrophic hormones on growth of breast epithelia. *Int. J. Cancer* **41:**713–719.

24. P. A. Holland, W. F. Knox, C. S. Potten, A. Howell, E. Anderson, A. D. Baildam, and N. J. Bundred (1997). Assessment of hormone dependence of comedo ductal carcinoma *in situ* of the breast. *J. Natl. Cancer Inst.* **89:**1059–1065.

25. R. B. Clarke, A. Howell, and E. Anderson (1997). Estrogen sensitivity of normal human breast tissue *in vivo* and implanted into athymic nude mice: analysis of the relationship between estrogen-induced proliferation and progesterone receptor expression. *Breast Cancer Res. Treat.* **45:**121–133.

26. R. B. Clarke, A. Howell, and E. Anderson (1997). Type I insulin-like growth factor receptor gene expression in normal human breast tissue treated with oestrogen and progesterone. *Br. J. Cancer* **75:**251–257.

27. N. K. Popnikolov, J. Yang, R. C. Guzman, and S. Nandi (1995). Reconstituted human normal breast in nude mice using collagen gel or Matrigel. *Cell. Biol. Int.* **19:**539–546.

28. S. N. Zaidi, I. Laidlaw, A. Howell, C. S. Potten, D. P. Cooper, and P. J. O'Connor (1992). Normal human breast xenografts activate *N*-nitrosodimethylamine: identification of potential target cells for an environmental nitrosamine. *Br. J. Cancer* **66:**79–83.

29. F. R. Miller, D. Medina, and G. H. Heppner (1981). Preferential growth of mammary tumors in intact mammary fatpads. *Cancer Res.* **41:**3863–3867.

30. F. R. Miller and D. McInerney (1988). Epithelial component of host–tumor interactions in the orthotopic site preference of a mouse mammary tumor. *Cancer Res.* **48:**3698–3701.

31. F. R. Miller (1981). Comparison of metastasis of mammary tumors growing in the mammary fatpad versus the subcutis. *Invasion Metastasis* **1:**220–226.

Chapter 5

Implantation and Characterization of Human Breast Carcinomas in SCID Mice

Yan Xu, Stephen B. Edge, Thelma C. Hurd, Elizabeth A. Repasky, and Harry K. Slocum

Abstract. To establish a better animal model for the study of human breast carcinomas, we investigated the growth and metastatic potential of surgical specimens of human breast carcinomas in SCID mice, using the large abdominal (gonadal) fat pad as an implantation site. Previously, we have shown that 12 (25%) out of 48 xenografts grew and reached a size of 1–2 cm within 2–6 months; these tumors were then sequentially passaged in SCID mice. In addition, we observed that the majority (8 out of 12) of these transplantable tumors became metastatic (e.g., to liver and lung) in the second or third passage. In this chapter we describe the protocol, in detail, for growing human breast carcinomas in the gonadal fat pad (GFP) of SCID mice from receiving and processing of surgical specimens to tumor implantation, passage, and archiving. We have also carefully examined and characterized these human tumor xenografts by histological analysis. Further, we identified the presence of human lymphocytes and human immunoglobulin in SCID mice bearing human breast carcinomas. The merits, potential applications, and pitfalls of this model are discussed.

Abbreviations. dimethyl sulfoxide (DMSO); Epstein–Barr virus (EBV); estrogen receptor (ER); fetal bovine serum (FBS); gonadal fat pad (GFP); hematoxylin and eosin (H&E); institutional review board (IRB); *in situ* hybridization (ISH); phosphate-buffered saline (PBS); severe combined immunodeficient (SCID); tissue procurement facility (TPF).

INTRODUCTION

Most studies on human breast cancer using animal models rely on a few established human breast cancer cell lines due to a relatively low success rate for establishing human breast carcinomas either as stable cell lines *in vitro* or as xenografts in immunodeficient mice (1, 2). Because these cell lines were derived from the highly malignant cells found in pleural effusions, it is likely that they represent only the most aggressive subpopulations of breast cancer cells. Therefore, the data derived from these cellular and molecular studies on human breast cancer may be representative of only the latest stages of disease progression. To overcome the limitations of using these breast tumor cell lines, researchers have investigated the

Yan Xu and Elizabeth A. Repasky   Department of Immunology, Roswell Park Cancer Institute, Buffalo, New York 14263.   Stephen B. Edge and Thelma C. Hurd   Department of Surgical Oncology, Roswell Park Cancer Institute, Buffalo, New York 14263.   Harry K. Slocum   Tissue Procurement Facility, Department of Pathology, Roswell Park Cancer Institute, Buffalo, New York 14263.

Methods in Mammary Gland Biology and Breast Cancer Research, edited by Ip and Asch. Kluwer Academic/Plenum Publishers, New York, 2000.

growth of patients' breast carcinomas as xenografts in a variety of animal model systems, including the anterior chamber of the eye of guinea pigs, lethally irradiated or thymectomized mice, and nude or severe combined immunodeficient (SCID) mice (3–8). However, these approaches have yielded a disappointingly low percentage of breast tumor outgrowths compared to the growths obtained with other major cancers of epithelial origin. In a comprehensive study that evaluated the growth potential of 433 surgical specimens of human breast carcinomas in nude mice, Giovanella and colleagues reported only a 6.1% success rate (5). Recently, more successful growth and metastasis of human breast carcinomas have been achieved with approaches including orthotopic transplantation, Matrigel, or pretreatment of SCID mice with etoposide to inhibit innate immunity (9–13). For example, various studies have described the successful growth of a human breast carcinoma implanted orthotopically into the mammary fat pad (9, 10). However, in each of these studies, a tumor from only one patient was tested. When breast tumor biopsies were co-injected with Matrigel, a significant increase in tumor engraftment and metastasis to distant sites was observed (11). Visonneau *et al.* reported that they could improve the success of tumor engraftment (8 out of 16 breast carcinomas) to 50% when SCID mice were pretreated with etoposide and observed for tumor growth over a prolonged period (18 months) (13).

Several years ago, we started to evaluate various protocols of serial transplantation to increase the yield of human breast tumor growth and metastatic spread in SCID mice. After many unsuccessful attempts, we developed a technique whereby a small piece of breast tumor (2–3 mm in diameter) from a fresh surgical specimen was embedded into the large abdominal (gonadal) fat pad of a SCID mouse (14). Of 48 surgical specimens studied, 12 (25%) grew rapidly enough to allow repeated passage; i.e., the tumors reached a diameter of 1–2 cm within 2–6 months. After these tumors were passaged two or three times in SCID mice, 8 out of these 12 rapidly growing tumors metastasized to the SCID mouse liver, lung, diaphragm, and abdominal wall. Histological analysis of the remaining 36 tumors revealed that 25 (53% of the 48 studied) had microscopic growth of tumor cell clusters within the GFP. However, these tumors failed to reach passageable size (>7 mm in diameter) within 6 months to 1 year. The remaining 11 patients' tumors (23% of the total 48) showed no evidence of tumor cell growth even at a microscopic level. The techniques we have developed for implanting breast tumors from patients in the GFP of SCID mice, thereby creating a better animal model for breast cancer research, are described in this chapter.

MATERIALS AND INSTRUMENTATION

Female CB17-SCID/SCID mice (8 weeks old or older) are obtained from Taconic Laboratories (Germantown, PA) and housed in microfilter cages (Lab Products, Maywood, NJ). All cages, water, and food (Teklad Mills, Wienfield, NJ) are autoclaved before use. The cages are maintained in an air-conditioned and light-controlled (12 h/day) room. All animal handling and operations are done in a laminar flow hood under sterile conditions. Ear tags for individual mouse identification are purchased from National Band and Tag (Newport, KY).

The general surgical materials and instruments, including scissors (4 inches), forceps (4 inches), and surgical needle holders, are purchased from VWR Scientific Products or Fisher Scientific. Surgical sutures (6-O Dexon) are obtained from Davis & Geck, Division of American Cyanamid Company (Wayne, NJ). Estrogen pellets (1.0–1.7 mg 17-β-estradiol, 60-day or 90-day release) are obtained from Innovative Research of America (Toledo, OH). Avertin (12.5 mg/ml) is used for anesthetizing mice. The Avertin solution is prepared by mixing 2.5 g of 2,2,2-tribromoethanol in 5 ml of *tert*-amyl alcohol (both of the materials are obtained from Aldrich Chemical Company, Inc., Milwaukee, WI). Double-distilled water is added to bring the solution volume up to 200 ml. The solution is then mixed with a magnetic stir bar for 2 h at room temperature and filtered through a 0.2-μm filter to sterilize. It is then kept in the dark at 4°C. The Avertin solution should be good for 3 months if stored appropriately.

For histological analysis, an automatic tissue processor (Autotechnicon Mono, Technicon Corporation, NY) is used to process tumor tissues. The tissues are then embedded in paraffin and sections are made on a standard microtome (American Optical Company, Instrument Division, NY). Hematoxylin and eosin are obtained from Richard–Allan Scientific (Kalamazoo, MI). Formaldehyde is purchased from Fisher Scientific (Springfield, NJ). H&E staining of tumor tissue sections can also be done by commercial services, e.g., the histological staining lab in the department of pathology at Roswell Park Cancer Institute. The *in situ* hybridization (ISH) detection system kit for detecting human DNA (Alu sequence) is purchased from BioGenex (San Ramon, CA). The kit contains all the reagents and a detailed procedure for the assay.

METHODS

Receiving and Processing Surgical Specimens

In order to achieve successful growth of patients' breast tumors in SCID mice, the critical role of the tissue procurement facility (TPF) and of the interdisciplinary collaboration in the management of surgical specimens must be appreciated. At Roswell Park, we have a TPF designed to assist investigators in obtaining human tissue for their research. This facility also provides assistance in the planning stages of the project and facilitates the involvement of appropriate surgical and pathology personnel. It also provides assistance in preparing the project for review by the Institutional Review Board (IRB) and Biosafety Office.

The pathologist involved in the case releases excess tissues for research and indicates that the sample is not needed for diagnosis or determination of extent of disease. To avoid potential mishandling of samples and confusion that could endanger clinical treatment, the TPF obtains documentation of this release.

Tissue procurement is also responsible for protecting patient anonymity, and to this end patient identifiers are removed and the tissue is renumbered before delivery to laboratory investigators (research protocols). This cross-registration is kept by the TPF, and if clinical information related to the specimen is needed, it is also provided with patient anonymity. Informed consent from the patient to provide anonymized discarded tissue for research is obtained at our institute when the patient is admitted to the hospital or when consenting for a surgical procedure.

The surgery and pathology staff are important collaborators in the tissue procurement process. The surgeon must ensure that the surgical specimen is handled in a sterile fashion and that it is sent to pathology immediately, even in cases where immediate clinical examination of the specimen is not necessary. We find that the best specimens are obtained when the surgeon interacts with the pathologist to select viable tumor tissue. With IRB approval and informed consent of the patient, blood samples can be obtained in the operating room to accompany the specimen for the tissue procurement program. Ongoing interaction with the clinical staff is critical to ensure continued identification of appropriate cases for tissue procurement and fair and appropriate triaging of cancer specimens to all investigators with IRB-approved research programs. Further, with IRB approval, the clinical staff can subsequently review the medical records to provide pathologic and cancer staging and outcome data to the researchers while maintaining patient confidentiality.

Review of surgical schedules and communication with surgical personnel enable the TPF to anticipate the release of tissue for research, so the pathology staff and the research personnel can anticipate the receipt of tissue. Provision of sterile containers for specimen transport, monitoring of the transport process to avoid delays, and provision of sterile equipment for cutting specimens to go to research labs are important functions of the TPF. Whenever possible, a piece of tumor tissue (0.2–0.6 g) is fixed in formalin, embedded in paraffin, and kept in the TPF as a reference for H&E stained slides.

When tumor specimens are delivered to our research lab by the staff of the facility, we sign their delivery book and then record the receipt of materials into our own tumor logbook. This log includes (1) the TPF number, which protects patient confidentiality, (2) the date of receipt, (3) the tumor type and weight, (4) the types of other tissues received from the same patient (i.e., lymph node or blood), (5) the number of mice implanted, and (6) whether or not a portion of tumor is stored in a −70°C freezer for future studies. Depending on its size, a breast tumor specimen is usually divided into three parts. One portion of tumor is further cut into three small pieces (2–3 mm in diameter) and implanted into the GFP of three female SCID mice as described later. The second part is snap-frozen for cellular and molecular analyses, and the third piece is processed for isolation of tumor cells and tumor-infiltrating lymphocytes. A blood sample from the same patient can also be used for isolation of lymphocytes to establish potentially tumor-specific cytotoxic lymphocyte lines.

Implantation of Patient Surgical Specimens into the GFP of SCID Mice

For tumor implantation, a fresh tumor specimen is placed in a cell culture dish containing RPMI 1640 cell culture medium with 10% FBS and cut into 2–3 mm pieces with a pair of scissors under aseptic conditions. The detailed tumor implantation procedure is illustrated in the series of photographs in Figure 5-1. A SCID mouse is anesthetized via intraperitoneal injection of 0.4–0.5 ml Avertin (12.5 mg/ml) or as per IACUC requirements. A 5-mm horizontal incision is made in the skin of the right lower abdomen through which the peritoneum can be visualized. A horizontal cut is made in the peritoneum and a GFP is gently exteriorized. One piece of tumor (2–3 mm) is placed on the GFP and then enclosed within it by wrapping the GFP around the tumor and fixing it in place with 6-O surgical suture. The tumor and GFP are gently replaced into the abdominal cavity. The peritoneum is carefully closed with a surgical suture, and the skin is closed with a surgical staple or suture. An estrogen pellet is implanted, subcutaneously, between the scapulae if the estrogen receptor (ER) status of the tumor is positive or unknown. A number tag is punched into the right ear of each mouse. After surgery, the mice are allowed to recover under mild heat from an infrared lamp or on a bench warmer (Thermolyne, IA) before being returned to their cages. The surgical staple is removed 7 days postoperation. A new estrogen pellet should be implanted if no tumor growth is observed after 60 or 90 days postimplantation, thereby allowing time for very slow growing tumors to become established.

Passage and Collection of Tumor Tissues Grown in SCID Mice

Tumor growth is assessed and recorded weekly by palpation of the implantation site. When a tumor reaches 1.5–2.0 cm in diameter, the mouse is sacrificed and the tumor is dissected from the GFP. Macroscopic and microscopic tumors grown in the GFP of SCID mice are shown in Figure 5-2. Figure 5-2A shows the symmetrical GFPs of a 2-month-old SCID mouse. Figure 5-2B shows a tumor grown in the GFP 8 weeks after the implantation of a

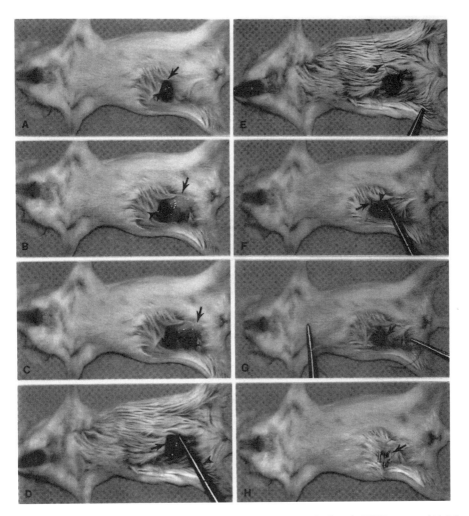

Figure 5-1. Implantation of a patient breast carcinoma in the GFP of a female SCID mouse. (A) A horizontal incision approximately 5 mm long is made in the skin of the lower part of the abdomen. An arrow indicates the cut edge of the skin; the arrowhead identifies the underlying peritoneum. (B) A horizontal cut is made in the peritoneum (arrowhead), exposing the white GFP, which is externalized and spread flat (arrow). (C) A surgical suture (not visible in this frame) is drawn from the underside of the fat pad (arrow) through its central region and through a 2–3 mm piece of fresh tumor (arrowhead) to hold the tumor in place. (D) A surgical needle holder (arrowhead) is used to draw the suture through the tumor (arrow). (E) The free edges of the fat pad are wrapped around the piece of tumor (arrow) and pulled over the end of the suture needle. Knotting the suture (arrowhead) ensures that the tumor piece remains wrapped in the fat pad. The wrapped tumor is then carefully replaced in the abdomen through the incision in the peritoneum. (F) The free edges of the peritoneum (arrowhead) are picked up on the suture needle (arrow). (G) The incision in the peritoneum may then be sutured (arrow). (H) Finally, a surgical staple is used to close the skin incision (arrow).

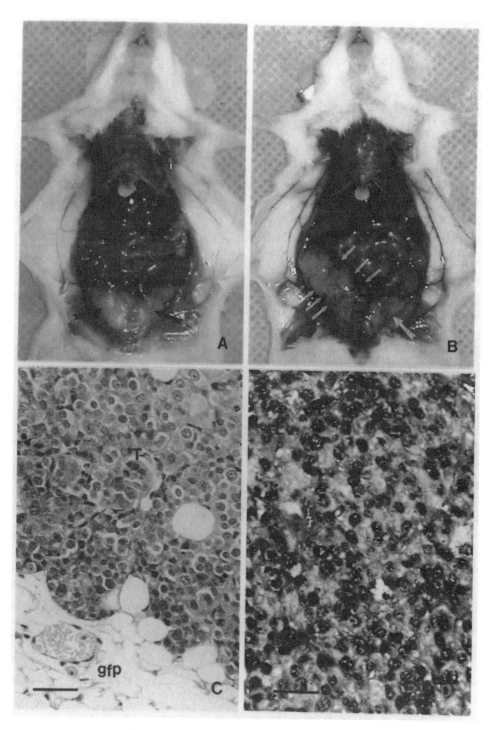

Figure 5-2. Gross and microscopic human breast tumors grown in the GFP of SCID mice. (A) Normal GFP of a 2-month-old SCID mouse showing its symmetrical positioning in the abdomen (arrows). (B) Small arrows indicate a tumor seen 8 weeks after the implantation of a surgical specimen (No. 10365). (C) Histology of the tumor shows a poorly differentiated tumor with a dense sheet growth pattern surrounded by adipocytes. (gfp = gonadal fat pad; T = tumor. Bar = 40 μm. (D) Identification of human Alu sequence in breast xenograft. Note that the human Alu sequence is detected in tumor cell nuclei by *in situ* hybridization (blue staining). Bar = 40 μm. (For a color representation of this, see figure facing page 56.)

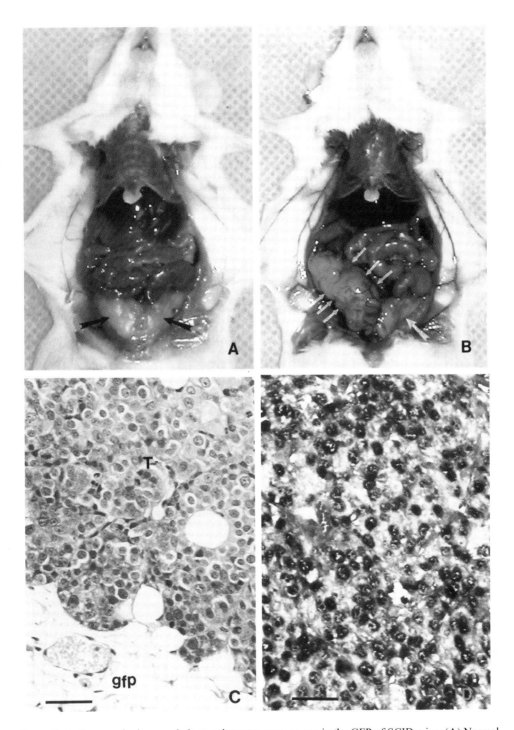

Figure 5-2. Gross and microscopic human breast tumors grown in the GFP of SCID mice. (A) Normal GFP of a 2-month-old SCID mouse showing its symmetrical positioning in the abdomen (arrows). (B) Small arrows indicate a tumor seen 8 weeks after the implantation of a surgical specimen (No. 10365). (C) Histology of the tumor shows a poorly differentiated tumor with a dense sheet growth pattern surrounded by adipocytes. (gfp = gonadal fat pad; T = tumor. Bar = 40 μm. (D) Identification of human Alu sequence in breast xenograft. Note that the human Alu sequence is detected in tumor cell nuclei by *in situ* hybridization (blue staining). Bar = 40 μm.

surgical specimen. Figure 5-2C reveals the histology of the tumor shown in Figure 5-2B. When a tumor-bearing mouse is sacrificed, the thoracic and peritoneal cavities are carefully examined to identify gross metastatic masses. Any gross metastases are saved for histological examination. Pieces of tumor removed from the host mouse are (1) passaged into other SCID mice (normally three mice), (2) stored in liquid nitrogen for reimplantation in the future (see the sequel), (3) fixed in 10% buffered formalin for histology, and (4) snap-frozen for cellular and molecular biological analyses. Generally, after a tumor has been passaged three times, we freeze 2–3 mm pieces of the tumor in RPMI 1640 medium with 10% DMSO and 40% FBS in a -70°C freezer overnight and then move the samples into a liquid nitrogen tank for long-term storage. The cryopreserved tissues can be reimplanted into SCID mice later as needed. When tumor xenografts remain in SCID mice for 6 months to 1 year without reaching 7 mm in diameter, the mice are sacrificed and the xenografts are excised with the surrounding GFP for histological analysis.

Assessment of Tumors by Histology and *in situ* Hybridization

For histopathological analysis, the excised tumors are fixed for at least 24 h in 10% buffered formalin, followed by an 18 h dehydration in an automatic dehydration processor (Autotechnicon Mono), and embedding in paraffin blocks. Paraffin tissue sections 5 μm thick are cut with a microtome, deparaffinized, rehydrated, and stained with hematoxylin and eosin. Light microscopic examination is routinely performed in the lab. The paraffin blocks and the histological slides are saved for future studies, such as *in situ* hybridization and immunohistochemical staining.

To confirm that tumors grown in SCID mice are human in origin, *in situ* hybridization (ISH) can be carried out on paraffin-embedded tissue sections, using an ISH detection system kit that detects a human genomic DNA (Alu) sequence. The detailed procedure is provided in the kit. Briefly, paraffin-embedded tissue sections (5 μm) are deparaffinized and rehydrated. The sections are treated with freshly diluted 1× proteinase K for 15 min at 37°C, followed by a 5-min wash in 1× PBS. Forty microliters of fluoresceinated Alu oligonucleotide are placed onto each tissue section. The sections are covered, heated in an oven for 10 min at 95°C, and then incubated at 37°C overnight. The slides are then washed in 2× sodium citrate buffer with sodium chloride (SSC). Next, the sections are sequentially incubated for 20 min each at room temperature with (1) mouse antifluorescein antibody, (2) biotinylated F(ab)2 fragments of goat antimouse immunoglobulins, and then (3) alkaline phosphatase-labeled streptavidin. Three 5-min washes with 1× PBS follow each of these incubations. Finally, the tissue sections are reacted with alkaline phosphatase substrate BCIP/NBT for 10 min for color development and counterstained with eosin. Positive Alu staining is indicated by blue staining in the nuclei of the tumor cells (Figure 5-2D).

DISCUSSION OF CRITICAL ISSUES AND EXPERIMENTAL APPLICATIONS

The quality of a tumor specimen is crucial for successful tumor growth in SCID mice, since tumor cells are distributed heterogeneously in patients' tumors. We have observed variation in success rate over the years. Several factors have been associated with this observed variation; the quality of tumor tissue being implanted is the most important factor. The varying quality of surgical specimens directly affects the success of tumor engraftment. Pieces from a solid tumor mass have more viable tumor cells than those pieces from the tumor margin, which have fewer tumor cells. The surgeons, pathologists, and TPF staff play critical roles in selecting tumor tissue with high engraftment potential.

The GFP location and the use of intact tumor tissues are two very important factors in support of human breast tumor growth. Breast carcinomas are derived from the epithelial cells of mammary glands that are normally surrounded by adipocytes (fat cells). The mouse GFP is highly vascularized and consists largely of white fat cells mixed with regions of brown fat and exhibits a histology similar to that of the human mammary fat pad, except that it is completely lacking in mammary epithelium. Unlike the small mammary fat pads, the GFP of the mouse is large enough to wrap around an intact piece of tumor, a factor we believe to be important for greater engraftment success. The GFP seems to provide a particularly favorable microenvironment that stimulates and maintains breast tumor cell growth. Rapid development of new blood vessels within the GFP may be one of the important factors involved in support of tumor cell growth.

Another crucial factor, which may stimulate breast tumor cell growth in the GFP, is estrogen synthesis by adipocytes, providing tumor cells with a high local concentration of estrogen (15–17). The fact that the growth of human colon carcinomas in the GFP of SCID mice does not result in better engraftment compared with other implantation sites, i.e., subcutaneous sites, supports the preceding hypothesis (our unpublished data). Implantation of an intact tumor piece, rather than cell suspensions, is essential for breast tumor cell growth in the mammary fat pad and the GFP of mice. This observation suggests that the extracellular matrix of the initially engrafted tumor is needed for human tumor cells to integrate more efficiently into the host murine environment (18). This notion is supported by the well-known fact that tumor growth is about 10 times faster when a tumor is implanted as a solid piece derived from an established cell line in comparison to injection of a cell suspension of the same cell line.

SCID mice, mouse gender, age, and estrogen supplementation affect tumor engraftment and growth rate. Utilization of the SCID mouse may offer the advantage of fewer graft rejections due to its deficiency of B and T lymphocytes compared to the more frequently utilized nude mouse, which is deficient only in T cells. The better engraftment of human tumors in SCID mice, rather than in nude mice, has been reported by many investigators (19). Female mice are essential for breast tumor growth in SCID mice (13–14). The age of mice (older than 8 weeks) is an important factor for support of breast tumor growth in the GFP, possibly because older female mice have larger GFPs, which makes it easier to wrap the tumor piece, and because fat cells of larger GFPs supply more endogenous estrogen locally to stimulate breast tumor growth (15–17). In addition, we have observed an estrogen-dependent growth of ER-positive tumors and an estrogen-independent tumor growth of ER-negative tumors (data not shown). However, we have also observed that ER-negative tumors grow faster with estrogen supplementation (data not shown).

A longer latency period for initial tumor growth is required. Generally speaking, a longer latency for the growth of human breast xenografts compared with other human solid tumors has been observed, although the latency period varies among tumor specimens and SCID mice. We observed an average latency of 3.5 months with an observation time of 6–12 months. This is in agreement with other investigators who have also demonstrated long latency periods in nude mouse models (5, 13). A recent study by Visonneau *et al.* observed better tumor engraftment when an extended observation time of 1–1.5 years was used. The large variation in latency periods may reflect the heterogeneity of tumor cell distribution in patients' tumors as well as the initial alterations in stromal cells, extracellular matrix, and the tumor angiogenic switch required for tumor cell growth in a new environment.

The tumors grown within the GFP of SCID mice maintain the histological features of the original human tumors, and disease progression is evidenced with sequential passages. In the last 6 years, we have archived most of the tumors implanted in SCID mice in paraffin blocks. Histopathological analysis of these tumors was performed. We found that the histopathological features, growth patterns, and heterogeneity of the original human breast carcinomas were maintained in this tumor model. Figure 5-3 shows the histology of human breast carcinoma xenografts in the GFP of SCID mice, and demonstrates histopathological features and growth patterns similar to those of the original human breast carcinomas (note that histology of the original surgical specimens is not shown in this figure). Figure 5-3A shows the histology of a tumor in the second passage derived from surgical specimen No. 9019. This is a well-differentiated adenocarcinoma characterized by ductlike structures forming tubules and glands. Figure 5-3B shows the histology of breast tumor No. 7764 in its first passage in a SCID mouse, displaying an intermediate histological growth pattern characterized by sheets of cells as well as some area consisting of glandular cells. Figure 5-3C shows the growth pattern of tumor No. 9720 in its third passage; this tumor is poorly differentiated. The cells in this tumor grow as sheets without evidence of tubule or gland formation. Figure 5-3D shows the histology of tumor No. 7722 in its third passage, displaying large tubular structures with central necrosis. Figure 5-3E shows a liver metastasis from the third tumor passage of surgical specimen No. 7722. The tumor has morphology similar to that of the tumor in the GFP shown in Figure 5-3D. Figure 5-3F shows the lung metastasis from tumor No. 7722 (third passage) also displaying morphology similar to the tumor shown in Figure 5-3D. With sequential passages, we have observed that some tumor xenografts become less differentiated and exhibit features that are more frequently associated with tumor progression, such as darker nuclear staining and greater numbers of mitotic figures. These observations suggest that disease progresses during sequential passaging in SCID mice. We have also observed that most of the passaged tumors metastasize to distant sites (Figure 5-3E, 5-3F) after being sequentially passaged in SCID mice, thus providing further evidence of tumor progression in this model.

The presence of immunocompetent human lymphocytes in tumor xenografts suggests that this model system has the potential to be used for studying human antitumor immune responses. During the course of the characterization of human breast tumor growth in SCID mice, we have carefully examined all of the tumor xenografts for the presence of human lymphocytes. In addition, we have collected the sera from most tumor-bearing mice every 2 weeks for the first 3 months after tumor implantation and then once again at time of sacrifice. All sera were analyzed for the presence of human immunoglobulin (Ig). The sera containing relatively high levels of human Ig were used for tumor antigen identification. We have frequently observed the presence of human lymphocytes and plasma cells in first-passage tumors (Figure 5-4A) and detectable levels (5–200 µg/ml) of human Igs in the sera of the tumor-bearing mice for at least 3 months (data not shown). These human Igs apparently come from tumor-infiltrating lymphocytes and plasma cells present in the surgical specimens, suggesting that tumor-infiltrating cells are co-engrafted into SCID mice along with the tumor. These data indicate that this animal model has the potential to be used for studying human immune responses against tumors. The long-term presence of plasma cells and resultant human Ig has been previously seen by our group in a SCID mouse–human lung tumor xenograft model (20). However, we did not see a correlation between the tumor growth rate and the level of human Ig found in the lung tumor-bearing SCID mice. Assuming that the lymphocytes present in the original surgical specimen might have been there because of some antitumor specificity, we believe that this model system may prove valuable for study of human antitumor immune

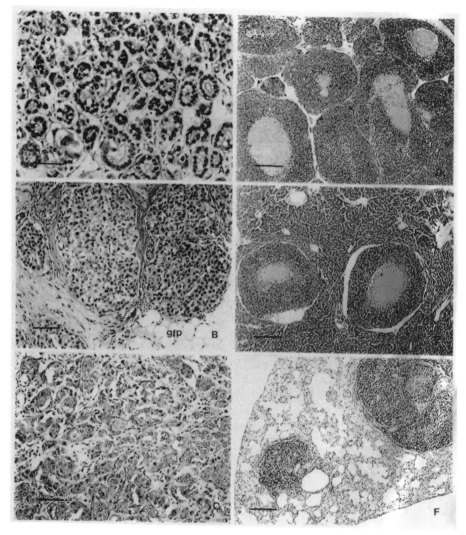

Figure 5-3. Histology of human breast carcinoma xenografts in the GFP of SCID mice. Several growth patterns of breast carcinoma xenografts grown in SCID mice are shown and display a close similarity to the growth patterns of original human breast carcinomas. (A) The histology of a second tumor passage derived from surgical specimen 9019. This is well-differentiated adenocarcinoma and characterized by ductlike structures forming tubules and glands. Bar = 80 μm. (B) The histology of breast tumor 7764 in its first passage in a SCID mouse, which displays an intermediate histological growth pattern characterized by sheets of cells as well as some glands. gfp = gonadal fat pad; T = tumor. Bar = 80 μm. (C) The histopathological growth pattern of tumor 9720 in its third passage. This tumor is poorly differentiated, and the cells in it grow as sheets without evidence of tubule or gland formation. Bar = 80 μm. (D) The histology of tumor 7722 in its third passage displays large tubular structures with central necrosis. Bar = 80 μm. (E) A liver metastasis from the third tumor passage of surgical specimen 7722. The tumor has similar morphology to the tumor in the GFP shown in Figure 5-3D. Bar = 80 μm. (F) A lung metastasis from tumor 7722 (third passage) also displays similar morphology to the tumor shown in Figure 5-3D. Bar = 200 μm.

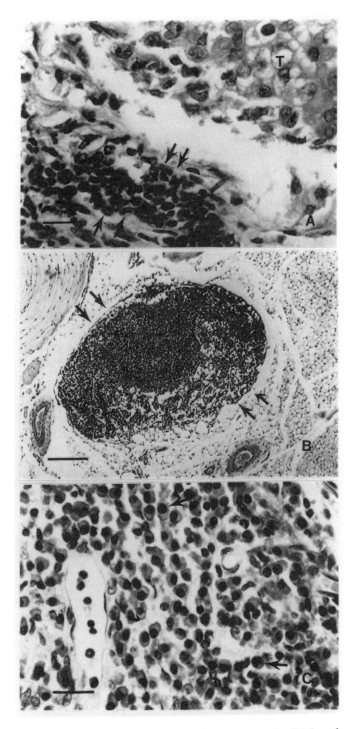

Figure 5-4. Presence of human immune cells in human breast xenografts. (A) Lymphocytes present in the first passage of human breast tumors in SCID mice. Arrows indicate lymphocytes (small, dark-blue-staining cells). T = tumor cells. Bar = 20 μm. (B) When tumor cells failed to grow in the GFP of SCID mice, a lymph-node-like structure has been often observed in the tumor implantation site. Components of this cellular aggregate include lymphocytes, neutrophils, and macrophages, and there are no tumor cells found in the structure. Arrows point to the lymph-node-like structure. Bar = 200 μm. (C) A high magnification of B showing typical plasma cells (arrows). Bar = 20 μm.

responses. Further, the study of the specificity of the antibodies derived from these cells may be a valuable tool for the identification of tumor-associated antigens. We have often seen lymph-node-like structures in xenografts in which tumor cells fail to grow (Figure 5-4B). These cellular aggregates consist of macrophages, neutrophils, and lymphocytes. In some cases, the structure is full of plasma-cell-like cells (Figure 5-4C). It seems that either the SCID mouse host innate immune system or the tumor-infiltrating lymphocytes from the patient destroyed the implanted tumor cells. This suggests the importance of the host innate immune system and antitumor activity of tumor-infiltrating lymphocytes in the growth of human tumor xenografts.

Human breast carcinoma xenografts grown in the GFP of SCID mice can be used for a variety of experimental studies on human breast cancer. Many cellular and molecular studies of human breast carcinomas have been hampered by the lack of a sufficient amount of tumor tissue. The successful growth and passage of human surgical specimens in the GFP of SCID mice allow us to produce a large amount of human breast tumor tissue that can be used for these studies. The SCID-mouse-propagated human tumor is more desirable than the currently available alternatives for performing a variety of human breast cancer studies, since tumor heterogeneity has been maintained. In addition, the relatively slow growth of human primary breast tumors in the GFP of SCID mice makes it an improved model for preclinical investigations, since one of the problems in using rodent tumor models is that tumors grow too fast to perform some evaluations. The evidence of human breast tumor progression in the GFP of SCID mice with passage suggests that this model also has potential to be used for prediction of patients' outcome and to be used for cellular and genetic studies of disease progression. The paraffin tumor blocks made from SCID-mouse-produced tumors can be used for a variety of immunohistochemical studies and hybridization analyses. The evidence that most of our fast-growing tumors developed distant metastases with passage in SCID mice suggests the potential of the model to be used to evaluate the metastatic potential of patients' breast carcinomas and to be used for establishment of *in vivo* metastatic models.

PITFALLS

As with all animal models, this model has some problems. One problem concerns estrogen supplementation. We observe occasional occurrence of urinary leakage or blockage in estrogen-treated tumor-bearing mice. Histopathological analysis reveals deposition of salts in the urinary bladder and uterine hyperplasia. The salt deposition in the urinary bladder and the compression from the hyperplastic uterus may contribute to the presentation of urination difficulties.

Another problem we occasionally encounter is the development of mouse stromal cell tumors or human lymphomas (presumably from EBV-positive, tumor-infiltrating lymphocytes) in sequentially passaged human tumors. The mechanism involved is unknown. Therefore, it is important to monitor every tumor grown in SCID mice by histopathological analysis of tumor H&E stained sections. Any tumors of questionable origin should be further analyzed by *in situ* hybridization staining for human DNA sequences to ascertain human origin or by immunohistochemical staining of human lymphoma markers to identify human lymphomas.

ACKNOWLEDGMENTS. We wish to thank Dr. Kàroly Tóth and Mrs. Nancy Reska of the Tissue Procurement Facility for their consistent help in obtaining tumor tissues. We wish to thank Ms. Michele Pritchard and Dr. Bonnie Hylander for their helpful discussion of the manuscript. We are also grateful to Ms. Ning-Ping Yang for her expert assistance in tissue preparation for histology and animal care. Many graduate students in Dr. Repasky's lab have extensively contributed to the establishment and maintenance of the SCID mouse colony. This work was supported by RPCI Core Grant (NCI Comprehensive Cancer Center Support Grant CA16056), the Department of Defense (No. 8570607), and NIH-CA71599.

REFERENCES

1. R. Clarke (1996). Animal models of breast cancer. In J. R. Harris, M. Morrow, M. E. Lippman, and S. Hellman (eds.), *Diseases of the Breast*, Lippincott–Raven, Philadelphia, pp. 221–235.
2. J. Taylor-Papadimitriou, F. Berdichevsky, B. D'Souza, and J. Burchell (1993). Human models of breast cancer. *Cancer Surveys* **16**:59–78.
3. B. C. Giovanella and J. Fogh (1985). The nude mouse in cancer research. *Adv. Cancer Res.* **44**:69–120.
4. S. Ethier (1996). Human breast cell lines as models of growth regulation and disease progression. *J. Mammary Gland Biol. Neopl.* **1**:111–121.
5. B. C. Giovanella, D. M. Vardeman, L. J. Williams *et al.* (1991). Heterotransplantation of human breast carcinomas in nude mice. Correlation between successful heterotransplants, poor prognosis and amplification of the HER-2/*neu* oncogene. *Inte. J. Cancer* **47**:66–71.
6. R. A. Phillips, M. A. S. Jewett, and B. L. Gallie (1989). Growth of human tumors in immune-deficient scid mice and nude mice. *Curr. Top. Microbiol. Immunol.* **152**:259–263.
7. A. Sabesteny, J. Taylor-Papadimitriou, R. Ceriani *et al.* (1979). Primary human breast carcinomas transplanted in the nude mouse. *J. Natl. Cancer Inst.* **63**:1331–1337.
8. B. Rae-Venter and L. M. Reid (1980). Growth of human breast carcinomas transplanted in nude mice and subsequent establishment in tissue culture. *Cancer Res.* **40**:95–100.
9. H. C. Outzen and R. P. Custer (1975). Growth of human normal and neoplastic mammary tissues in the cleared mammary fat pad of the nude mouse. *J. Natl. Cancer Inst.* **55**:1461–1466.
10. X. Fu, P. Le, and R. M. Hoffman (1993). A metastatic orthotopic-transplant nude-mouse model of human patient breast cancer. *Anticancer Res.* **13**:901–904.
11. R. R. Menta, J. M. Graves, G. D. Hart, A. Shilkaitis, and T. K. Das Gupta (1993). Growth and metastasis of human breast carcinoma with Matrigel in athymic mice. *Breast Cancer Res. Treat.* **25**:65–71.
12. A. Cesano, J. A. Hoxie, B. Lange, P. C. Nowell, J. Bishop, and D. Santoli (1992). The severe combined immunodeficient (SCID) mouse as a model for human myeloid leukemias. *Oncogene* **7**:827–836.
13. S. Visonneau, A. Cesano, M. H. Torosian, E. J. Miller, and D. Santoli (1998). Growth characteristics and metastatic properties of human breast cancer xenografts in immunodeficient mice. *Am. J. Pathol.* **152**:1299–1311.
14. T. Sakakibara, Y. Xu, H. L. Bumpers, F.-A. Chen, R. B. Bankert, M. A. Arredondo, S. B. Edge, and E. A. Repasky (1996). Growth and metastasis of surgical specimens of human breast carcinomas in SCID mice. *Cancer J. Sci. Am.* **2**:291–300.
15. E. Perel, M. E. Blackstein, and D. N. Killinger (1982). Aromatase in human breast carcinoma. *Cancer Res.* (*Suppl.*) **42**:3369–3372.
16. P. A. Beranek, E. J. Folkerd, M. W. Ghilchick, and V. H. T. James (1984). 17Beta-hydroxysteroid dehydrogenase and aromatase activity in breast fat from women with benign and malignant breast tumors. *Lin. Endocrinol.* **20**:205–212.
17. E. R. Simpson, J. C. Merrill, A. J. Hollub, S. Graham-Lorence, and C. R. Mendelson (1989). Regulation of estrogen biosynthesis by human adipose cells. *Endocrine Rev.* **10**:136–148.
18. J. Koh, T. Kubota, H. Sasano, M. Hashimoto, Y. Hosoda, and M. Kitajima (1998). Stimulation of human tumor xenograft growth by local estrogen biosynthesis in stromal cells. *Anticancer Res.* **18**(4A):2375–2380.
19. S. S. Williams, T. R. Alosco, B. A. Croy, and R. B. Bankert (1993). The study of human neoplastic disease in severe combined immunodeficient mice. *Lab. Anim. Sci.* **43**:139–146.
20. S. S. Williams, F. A. Chen, H. Kida, S. Yokata, K. Miya, M. Kato, M. P. Barcos, H. Q. Wang, T. Alsosco, T. Umemoto, B. A. Croy, E. A. Repasky, and R. B. Bankert (1996). Engraftment of human tumor-infiltrating lymphocytes and the production ofanti-tumor antibodies in SCID mice. *J. Immunol.* **156**(5):1908–1915.

Part II

Special Techniques for *In Vivo* Studies

The Cleared Mammary Fat Pad and the Transplantation of Mammary Gland Morphological Structures and Cells

Lawrence J. T. Young

Abstract. The mammary fat pad, when cleared of glandular tissues in female mice 3–4 weeks old, provides an ideal site for the transplantation of normal, hyperplastic, or malignant lesions of the mammary gland into syngeneic hosts. The cleared fat pad retains the microenvironment necessary for the normal morphological growth of transplanted mammary gland elements. The biological development of mammary gland structures can be evaluated and lesions can be tested for cancer risk. Serial transplantation into cleared fat pads can provide pools of the tissue of choice for biochemical, immunological, and molecular analysis, for tissue culture, and for the perpetuation of hyperplastic tissues for future use. With the advent of transgenic and knockout mice, the clearing technique has become a powerful biological system wherein the effect of genes and their interactions on mammary neoplasia can be determined. This chapter describes the clearing and transplantation technique for mammary tissues and cells.

INTRODUCTION

The morphological and biological development of normal mammary tissue and unique hyperplastic lesions found in the mouse mammary gland has been directly demonstrated by transplantation techniques into the "cleared" mammary fat pads. The availability of syngeneic strains of mice has made these transplantation studies possible. The transplantation technique of "clearing" the inguinal fat pads of the developing mammary parenchyma was described and pioneered by DeOme *et al.* (1). The concept of preventing the developing mammary gland from occupying the entire fat pad stemmed from an astute observation. It was noted that the mammary gland in a young C3H female mouse was readily outlined and seen due to the dark background of the agouti strain. Whole mounts of various ages of female mice indicated that the developing mammary parenchyma in the No. 4 pair of mammary glands did not extend beyond the lymph nodes in 3- to 4-week-old weanling mice weighing up to 14 g. Thus surgical removal of the developing glands in these mice resulted in the No. 4 fat pads remaining gland-free (cleared). The cleared fat pad provided the natural microenvironment

Lawrence J. T. Young   Center for Comparative Medicine, University of California-Davis, Davis, California 95616.

Methods in Mammary Gland Biology and Breast Cancer Research, edited by Ip and Asch. Kluwer Academic/Plenum Publishers, New York, 2000.

for mammary gland growth and proved to be an excellent transplantation site for the study of mammary tissue. Although all fat pads of the mouse can be cleared and utilized for transplantation, the No. 4 fat pad has been utilized exclusively because of its accessiblity. The thickness of the No. 4 fat pad also makes transplantation of mammary tissue easier because the transplant must be totally embedded in the fat in order for optimal growth to occur.

Transplantation of normal mammary gland tissues (2–6), dissociated mammary gland cells (7, 8), preneoplastic hyperplastic alveolar nodules (HAN) (9–11), and induced lesions after chemical carcinogens (12–14) have been reported. Whereas normal mammary gland tissue and hyperplastic outgrowths were confined to the mammary fat pad area (15), mammary tumors were capable of overgrowing both normal and hyperplastic tissue. Serial transplantation of normal mammary tissue demonstrated a finite life span, but the serial transplantation of HANs could be carried out indefinitely (2). Cells derived from primary mammary epithelial gland cultures have been transplanted (16, 17). Transplantation of hyperplastic alveolar nodules (HAN) into the cleared fat pads demonstrated that they were the lesions of high tumor risk (9–11). Human mammary gland lesions and human mammary cell lines have been transplanted into cleared nude mice fat pads (18, 19). The cleared fat pad is a powerful tool in the determination of the developmental and biological endpoint of different mammary gland structures.

MATERIALS

1. Dissecting microscope
2. Electric cautery, cautery pencil, and eye cautery tip or disposable cautery pencil (Artists Surgical Supply Co., 67 Lexington Ave, New York, NY 10010-1898; ELE 8-2 low-power transformer; ELE 8-4 cautery pencil handle; ELE 9-1 eye platinum tips with a 1inch shank)
3. Cork boards, $3 \times 4 \times \frac{1}{4}$ inch
4. Double-sided tape
5. Scissors, $4\frac{1}{2}$ to 5 inches, S/S
6. Dressing forceps, $4\frac{1}{2}$ inch (skin forceps, tissue forceps)
7. Forceps, angle, 4 to $4\frac{1}{2}$ inch
8. Forceps, jewelers, 45° angle, $4\frac{1}{2}$ inch for transplantion
9. Iris scissors, angle, $4\frac{1}{2}$ inch
10. Autoclips, Clay–Adams, 9 mm (wound clips)
11. Autoclip applicator
12. Autoclip remover
13. Cotton balls
14. Cotton swabs
15. 70% EtOH
16. Hamilton syringe, 100 µl
17. 0.6% Nembutal (sodium phenobarbital); Nembutal diluent: 50 ml 100% EtOH, 350 ml distilled water, 100 ml propylene glycol
18. 1-ml syringe
19. Syringe needles, 25 and 30 gauge
20. 3-week-old female mice
21. Appropriate donor(s)
22. Microscope lamps

23. Sterility of instruments, cotton swabs and balls, and autoclips not necessary; quickly dipping and wiping with 70% EtOH has proven to be sufficient against infection.

METHODS

1. Swab operating table surface with 70% EtOH.
2. Inject 3-week-old female mice IP with 0.6% Nembutal, 10 µl per gram body weight (60 mg/kg); mice will be anesthetized in 30 to 60 s and will remain so for 45 to 60 min.
3. Tape mice to corkboard, ventral side up.
4. Liberally wipe inguinal area of mice with 70% EtOH.
5. Locate No. 4 and No. 5 nipples.
6. Make a 1- to 1.5-cm midline incision beginning at a point between the No. 4 nipples; hold scissors so that blades are at a vertical and not at a horizontal plane or at an angle; cut toward the sternum, using care not to injure the abdominal musculature.
7. Make angled lateral incisions from the midline point between the No. 4 nipples and ending at a point between the No. 4 and No. 5 nipples so that the incision resembles an inverted Y (Figure 6-1a).
8. Use cotton swab and dressing forceps to loosen skin from body wall; pin one skin flap back to expose No. 4 and No. 5 fat pads (Figure 6-1b).
9. Using the dissecting microscope, locate and cauterize No. 4 nipple, blood vessel near junction by lymph node, and blood vessel at a point on the fat pad bridge between the No. 4 and No. 5 fat pads (Figure 6-1c). Location of the nipple can be done by tracing the primary duct back to the nipple, especially in albino strains of mice.
10. Use iris scissors to carefully excise and discard the triangular area defined by the cautery points. The developing mammary gland has not grown past the lymph node into the No. 4 mammary pad in 3- to 4-week-old female mice. Removal of the above triangular area will result in a "cleared" No. 4 mammary fat pad into which tissues can be transplanted without interference from the host's mammary epithelium.
11. Make sure incisions on the pad are precise and clean (Figure 6-1d).
12. Repeat gland-clearing operation on contralateral side.
13. Obtain donor animal or cells for implantation; size of tissue for transplantation should be 1–2 mm³; implantation of cells should be anywhere between 10^3 to 10^7 cells per 10 µl, depending on cells or cell line.
14. Use 45° jeweler's forceps for implanting tissue; use 100-µl Hamilton syringe for cells.
15. Prepare a pocket in the middle of the cleared fat pad (Figure 6-1e) for tissue implantation by holding points of jeweler's forceps together and carefully inserting the points into the fat pad such that they do not rupture the surrounding connective tissue layer on the underside; tension on the fat pad can be produced by holding fat pad near lymph node with another forceps, making it easier to insert jeweler's forceps.
16. Remove forcep points from cleared fat pad and insert tissue to be transplanted into the prepared pocket; remove forceps by releasing points; this allows the transplant tissue to slip into the pocket more snugly.

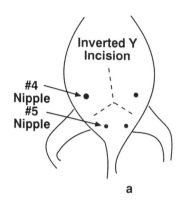

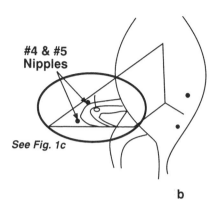

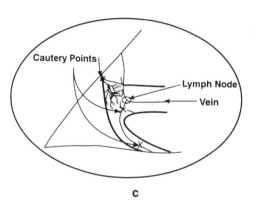

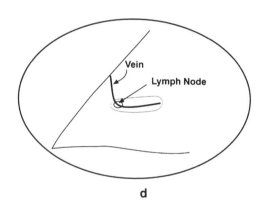

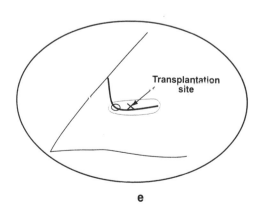

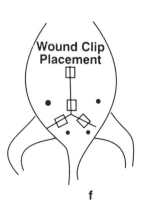

17. Cells are implanted in 10-µl volume with a 100-µl Hamilton syringe and 30-gauge needle into the middle of the cleared fat pad. No more than a 10-µl volume should be used to ensure that no leakage occurs after removal of the needle from the fat pad. The 10-µl volume can be visualized as a bolus after inoculation into the fat pad.

18. Repeat transplantation on contralateral side.

19. Suture skin flaps by using wound clips; generally only 4 wound clips are necessary (Figure 6-1f); care should be taken that the abdominal wall is not attached to skin; cut edges of skin should be aligned as closely to each other as possible. Place wound clips as close to the corners of the midline and lateral incisions as possible. The wound will heal within 2 to 4 days with no adverse effects.

20. Ear-tag mice and place in clean cage.

21. If mice are too deeply anesthetized (e.g., shallow breathing), place in clean cage and keep mice warm with a heat lamp. Be sure that heat lamp is not too close. Make sure that mice are shaded with a paper towel.

22. Give food and water after mice awaken.

23. Examination of the fat pads for growth can be done at any point after transplantation. Initial growth can be observed between 7 and 10 days posttransplantation. Most transplants will grow and fill the fat pads after 10 to 12 weeks.

Figure 6-1. a Schematic indicating the location of the inverted Y incision. Make a 1- to 1.5-cm midline incision beginning at a point between the no. 4 nipples toward the sternum followed by slightly angled lateral incisions from the midline point between the no. 4 nipples and ending at a point between the no. 4 and no. 5 nipples. Hold scissors so that blades are at a vertical, not a horizontal, plane in order to obtain clean, straight incisions so that wound clips can be easily placed and the wound heals properly. Use care not to puncture the abdominal musculature. **b** Use cotton swab and dressing forceps to loosen skin from body wall and position skin flap in order to expose the no. 4 and no. 5 fat pads. **c** Cauterize no. 4 nipple, blood vesssel near junction by lymph node, and blood vessel at a point on the fat pad bridge between the no. 4 and no. 5 fat pads (×). Use iris scissors to carefully excise and discard the triangular area defined by the cautery points. Developing mammary gland has not grown past the lymph node into the no. 4 mammary pads in 3- to 4-week-old female mice. Removal of the above triangular area will result in a cleared no. 4 mammary fat pad into which tissues can be transplanted without interference from the host's mammary gland. Transplant tissue of choice or cells approximately in the middle of the cleared fat pad. Position of the transplant is important in order to distinguish ingrowth (growth from host gland if not all of mammary parenchyma was successfully removed) from outgrowth. The resultant outgrowth from the transplanted tissue or cells will radiate out from the point of transplantation. Flow of ingrowth will be unidirectional from the lymph node. **d** The cleared fat pad. **e** Transplantation site. Prepare a pocket in the middle of the cleared fat pad for tissue implantation by holding points of jeweler's forceps together and carefully inserting the points into the fat pad such that they do not rupture the surrounding connective tissue layer on the underside; tension on the fat pad can be produced by holding fat pad near lymph node with another forceps, making it easier to insert jeweler's forceps. Remove forcep points from cleared fat pad, and insert tissue to be transplanted into the prepared pocket; remove forceps by releasing points; this allows the transplant tissue to slip into the pocket more snugly. Cells are implanted in 10-µl volume by using 100-µl Hamilton syringe and 30-gauge needle into the middle of the cleared fat pad. No more than a 10-µl volume should be used to ensure that no leakage occurs after removal of the needle from the fat pad. The 10-µl volume can be visualized as a bolus after inoculation into the fat pad. **f** Position of the wound clips after closing of the wound. Wound clips should be placed no more than 5 mm away from the corners of the flaps in order for proper skin closure to occur.

24.   Serial transplantation of hyperplastic outgrowths can be done by cutting a 1- to
      2-mm strip from the outer edge of the outgrowth and snipping 1- to 2-mm sec-
      tions from the strip to transplant. Serial transplantation of normal mammary tissue
      can be done by a 0.5- to 1.0-ml IP overnight inoculation of a 0.5% suspension of
      trypan blue in saline, especially for albino strains of mice. The trypan blue out-
      lines the ducts of the normal outgrowth.
25.   Prepare whole mounts of the transplanted pads by fixation in 10% formalin. Defat
      in acetone, stain with hematoxylin, and store in methyl salicylate. See Chapter 7
      by Rasmussen, Young, and Smith in this volume.

REFLECTIONS

The clearing and transplantation techniques described have been performed primarily
in mice because of the many inbred strains available and because of interest in the influence
of the mouse mammary tumor virus on mammary neoplasia. The cleared fat pad technique
provided a model that demonstrated the high risk factor in the preneoplastic HAN and
the concept of at least a two-step mammary tumorigenesis system. The ability to surgically
remove, transplant, and observe tumor progression of the HAN led to the conclusion that the
HAN was a morphological intermediate point, a preneoplastic lesion, in the tumorigenesis
process. The role of transplantation into the cleared fat pad for the study of the normal development and tumorigenesis of the mammary gland has been emphasized in several reviews
(20–22).

It is imperative that no residual host mammary gland tissue remain after the clearing process. Any remaining host glands will invade the cleared fat pad, become an ingrowth,
and prevent or alter the growth of the transplant. Ingrowth of the host mammary gland
makes it difficult to interpret the growth of the transplant and to select tissues for further
transplants.

Vascularization of mammary gland implants can be observed after 4 to 7 days. End bud
formation in normal mammary gland transplants can be recognized by day 7 and will fill the
cleared fat pad in 10 to 12 weeks. HAN transplants will fill the cleared fat pad in 8 to 12
weeks, and tumor transplants can be palpated in 7 to 10 days. HAN outgrowths can be serially transplanted even if tumors are present by carefully dissecting and transplanting only the
hyperplastic area. Tumor areas as small as 1 mm in diameter, which arise within the HAN
outgrowth, can be recognized because of their dense structures surrounded by thin connective tissue capsules.

Different morphological areas were observed within some hyperplastic outgrowths. If
these areas were transplanted selectively by serial passage, several hyperplastic outgrowth
lines could be developed from the primary hyperplastic outgrowth. Each line retained the
phenotype selected. Changes in the acquired mouse mammary tumor virus DNA were demonstrated in the individual lines (23).

Athymic mice provided a source of experimental mice for the analysis of lesions from
human mammary gland but with limited success because of the difficulties involved in tissue
growth (18, 19). Greater success was achieved with transplantation of human mammary
tumors into nude mice (24, 25).

Normal mammary gland and hyperplastic lesions in albino strains such as the BALB/c,
RIII, GR, etc., were difficult to visualize. It was found that most of the mammary tree in
albino strains was readily outlined by a 0.5- to 1.0-ml overnight inoculation of a 0.5% suspension of trypan blue in saline given intraperitoneally.

The clearing and transplantation technique was used in the development and analyses of the angiogenic property of nonmetastatic and metastatic mammary gland cell lines derived from wild type and a point mutation of Polyomavirus middle T transgenic mice (26). Future impetus should be focused on the mammary lesions found in transgenic mice and knockout mice (27–31). These tissues should give us important insights into the influence and the interactions of known genes on the normal development and neoplastic pathways of the mammary gland.

ACKNOWLEDGMENTS. I am grateful to Denise Waters of the Graphic Arts Department, Shriners Hospital for Children Northern California, who kindly produced the schematic drawings.

REFERENCES

1. K. B. DeOme, L. J. Faulkin, Jr., H. A. Bern, and P. B. Blair (1959). Development of mammary tumors from hyperplastic alveolar nodules transplanted into gland-free mammary fat pads of female C3H mice. *Cancer Res.* **19**:515–520.
2. C. W. Daniel, K. B. DeOme, L. J. T. Young, P. B. Blair, and L. J. Faulkin, Jr. (1968). The *in vivo* life span of normal and preneoplastic mouse mammary glands: a serial transplantation study. *PNAS* **61**:53–60.
3. L. J. T. Young, D. Medina, K. B. DeOme, and C. W. Daniel (1971). The influence of host and tissue age on life span and growth rate of serially transplanted mouse mammary gland. *Exp. Geront.* **6**:49–56.
4. C. W. Daniel and L. J. T. Young (1971). Influence of cell division on an aging process. Life span of mouse mammary epithelium during serial propagation *in vivo. Exp. Cell Res.* **65**:27–32.
5. K. Hoshino (1967). Transplantablity of mammary gland in brown fat pads of mice. *Nature* **213**:194–195.
6. K. Hoshino and W. U. Gardner (1967). Transplantablity and life span of mammary gland during serial transplantation in mice. *Nature* **213**:193–194.
7. K. B. DeOme, M. J. Miyamoto, R. C. Osborn, R. C. Guzman, and K. Lum (1978). Effect of parity on recovery of inapparent nodule-transformed mammary gland cells *in vivo. Cancer Res.* **38**:4050–4053.
8. K. B. DeOme, M. J. Miyamoto, R. C. Osborn, R. C. Guzman, and K. Lum (1978). Detection of inapparent nodule-transformed cells in the mammary gland tissues of virgin female BALB/cfC3H mice. *Cancer Res.* **38**:2103–2111.
9. K. B. DeOme. P. B. Blair, and L. J. Faulkin, Jr. (1961). Some characteristics of the preneoplastic hyperplastic alveolar nodules of C3H/CRGL mice. *Acta Union Int. Contre le Cancer* **17**:973–982.
10. K. B. DeOme and L. J. T. Young (1970). Hyperplastic lesions of the mouse and rat mammary glands. Proceedings, Tenth International Cancer Research Congress, Houston, TX; (1971) In R. E. Clark, R. W. Cumley, J. E. McCay, and M. M. Copeland (eds.), *Experimental Cancer Therapy* Yearbook Medical Publishers, Chicago, pp. 474–483.
11. D. Medina (1976). Preneoplastic lesions in murine mammary cancer. *Cancer Res.* **36**:2589–2595.
12. C. W. Daniel, B. D. Aidells, D. Medina, and L. J. Faulkin, Jr. (1975). Unlimited division potential of precancerous mouse mammary cells after spontaneous or carcinogen-induced transformation. *Proc. Fed. Am. Soc. Exp. Biol.* **34**:64–67.
13. L. J. Faulkin, Jr. (1966). Hyperplastic lesions of mouse mammary glands after treatment with 3-methylcholanthrene. *J. Natl. Cancer Inst.* **36**:289–297.
14. R. C. Guzman, R. C. Osborn, and K. B. DeOme (1981). Recovery of transformed nodule and ductal mammary cells from carcinogen-treated C57Bl mice. *Cancer Res.* **41**:1808–1811.
15. L. J. Faulkin, Jr., and K. B. DeOme (1960). Regulation of growth and spacing of gland elements in the mammary fat pad of the C3H mouse. *J. Natl. Cancer Inst.* **24**:953–969.
16. U. K. Ehmann, R. C. Guzman, R. C. Osborn, L. J. T. Young, R. D. Cardiff, and S. Nandi (1987). Cultured mouse mammary cells: Normal phenotype after implantation. *J. Natl. Cancer Inst.* **78**:751–757.
17. R. C. Guzman, R. C. Osborn, J. Yang, K. B. DeOme, and S. Nandi (1982). Transplantation of mouse mammary epithelial cells grown in primary collagen gel cultures. *Cancer Res.* **42**:2376–2383.
18. H. C. Outzen and R. P. Custer (1975). Growth of human normal and neoplastic mammary tissues in the cleared mammary fat pad of the nude mouse. *J. Natl. Cancer Inst.* **55**:1461–1466.
19. H. M. Jensen and S. R. Wellings (1976). Preneoplastic lesions of the human mammary gland transplanted into the nude athymic mouse. *Cancer Res.* **36**:2605–2610.

20. D. Medina (1996). The mammary gland: A unique organ for the study of development and tumorigenesis. *J. Mammary Gland Biol. Neoplasia* **1**:519.

21. R. D. Cardiff, S. R. Wellings, and L. J. Faulkin (1977). Biology of breast preneoplasia. *Cancer* **39**:2734–2746.

22. R. D. Cardiff, D. W. Morris, L. J. T. Young, and R. Strange (1986). MuMTV genotype, protoneo-plasia and tumor progression. In M. A. Rich, J. C. Hager, and J. Taylor-Papadimitriou (eds.), *Breast Cancer: Origins, Detection, and Treatment*, Martinus Nijhoff, Boston, pp. 156–166.

23. R. D. Cardiff, D. W. Morris, and L. J. T. Young (1983). Alterations of acquired mouse mammary tumor virus DNA during mammary tumorigenesis in BALB/cfC3H mice. *J. Natl. Cancer Inst.* **71**:1011–1019.

24. M. V. Pimm and T. M. Morris (1990). Growth rates of human tumours in nude mice. *Eur. J. Cancer* **26**:764–765.

25. H. Naundorf, I. Fichter, G. J. Saul, W. Haensch, and B. Buttner (1993). Establishment and characteristics of two new human mammary carcinoma lines serially transplantable in nude mice. *J. Cancer Res. Clin. Oncol.* **119**:652–656.

26. A. T. W. Cheung, L. J. T. Young, P. C. Y. Chen, C. Y. Chao, A. Ndoye, P. A. Barry, W. J. Muller, and R. D. Cardiff (1997). Microcirculation and metastasis in a new mouse mammary tumor model system. *Int. J. Oncol.* **11**:69–77.

27. G. H. Smith, R. Sharp, E. C. Kordon, C. Jhappan, and G. Merlino (1995). Transforming growth factor-alpha promotes mammary tumorigenesis through selective survival and growth of secretory epithelial cells. *Am. J. Pathol.* **147**:1061–1096.

28. N. Su, J. O. Ojeifo, A. MacPherson, and J. A. Zwiebel (1994). Breast cancer gene therapy: transgenic immunotherapy. *Breast Cancer Res. Treatment* **31**:349–356.

29. S. A. Eccles, G. Box, W. Court, J. Sandle, and C. J. Dean (1994). Preclinical models for the evaluation of targeted therapies of metastatic disease. *Cell Biophys.* **24–25**:279–291.

30. J. M. Bradbury, J. Arno, and P. A. Edwards (1993). Induction of epithelial abnormalities that resemble human breast lesions by the expression of the neu/erbB-2 oncogene in reconstituted mouse mammary gland. *Oncogene* **8**:1551–1558.

31. D. M. Ornitz, R. D. Cardiff, A. Kuo, and P. Leder (1992). Int-2, an autocrine and/or ultra-short-range effector in transgenic mammary tissue transplants. *J. Natl. Cancer Inst.* **84**:887–892.

Chapter 7

Preparing Mammary Gland Whole Mounts from Mice

Susan B. Rasmussen, Lawrence J. T. Young, and Gilbert H. Smith

Abstract. We present methods, fixation schedules, and stains for preparing whole mounts of murine mammary glands. We have included references to papers published 60 years ago as well as those in current journals. The use of this method has undergone a renaissance with the advent of transgenic and knock-in–knockout genetic mouse models relevant to the study of mammary growth, development, and neoplasia.

INTRODUCTION

A whole mount is a preparation for viewing the complete unsectioned organ to be studied. Whole mounts have been used to study developing tissues and organs in the embryo and to evaluate sub-gross changes in fully developed tissues excised from the mature organism. We will concentrate our focus upon the preparation of mammary gland whole mounts from the mouse.

One of the earliest reports of observations based on the mammary gland whole mount technique was by Gardner and Strong in 1935 (1). They examined mammary gland development in virgin mice of 10 different strains varying in their susceptibility to the development of spontaneous mammary neoplasms. Although they found no association between mammary cancer and structural development of the glands through postpubertal development (through ~70 days of age), they did confirm and extend earlier reports of the cyclic hypertrophy and regression of the mammary glands during the estrus cycle, a feature all too-often ignored in comparative studies of mammary structure and function. During estrus and postestrus the ducts were slightly distended, and in younger mice the terminal end buds were more numerous and distended, whereas during diestrous the opposite was true. In 1940, Taylor and Waltman compared hyperplasias of the mammary gland found in the human and in the mouse, listing detailed characteristics and whole mounts (2). Later, Huseby and Bittner used mammary gland whole mounts to demonstrate the presence of "precancerous nodules" and distinguished these from

Susan B. Rasmussen and Gilbert H. Smith   Laboratory of Tumor Immunology and Biology, National Cancer Institute, National Institutes of Health, Bethesda, Maryland 20892.   **Lawrence J.T. Young** Center for Comparative Medicine, University of California-Davis, Davis, California 95616.

Methods in Mammary Gland Biology and Breast Cancer Research, edited by Ip and Asch. Kluwer Academic/Plenum Publishers, New York, 2000.

"inflammatory nodules" in the glands of parous females of mouse strains exhibiting high susceptibility for mammary cancer development (3). Early analysis of the effect of diet and diethylstilbestrol on the histogenesis of the murine mammary gland as determined by whole mounts was published by Dalton in 1945 (4). DeOme *et al.* showed a correlation between the gross morphology of hyperplastic alveolar nodule transplants seen in whole mounts and the cellular detail seen with serial tissue sections (5). Widespread whole mount study of mouse mammary glands was inaugurated in the 1960s and 1970s. Some early publications on the morphology of mammary gland development adopted excessive descriptive language and copious measurements of phenomena to convey their evidence rather than images. A notable paper on the "biological and morphological characteristics of mammary tumors in GR mice" by R. Van Nie and Anna Dux contained no whole mount photographs or drawings with which to illustrate the morphological differences revealed so descriptively within the paper (6). In 1968, Daniel *et al.* published a seminal paper defining the *in vivo* life span of serially transplanted normal and preneoplastic mammary glands (7). This paper contained numerous whole mounts illustrating the percent fat pad filled and morphology associated with each transplantation. Several seminal articles contain detailed technique sections on whole mounting of murine mammary glands, including Rivera *et al.*, Banerjee *et al.*, Medina, and others (8–11). Whole mounts have been utilized to show the effect of transgenes or knockouts on mammary gland development and function (12, 13). Hence, mammary gland whole mounting is a technique integral to the illostiation of experimental results when evaluating growth, development, and malignant epithelium. In fact, it has maintained its status as the *methodologie de rigeur* for detailing the morphologic characteristics of mammary tissue. Some detailed protoeals for rapid whole mounting and for pelt preparation are given in the appendix.

MATERIALS AND METHODS

The reagents and materials listed here are only a guide as there are multiple ways to prepare excellent mammary whole mounts. The methods are listed in logical progression from mammary gland removal through all subsequent fixation, staining, clearing, and mounting steps. A very useful book on the basics of fixatives and stains is *Humason's Animal Tissue Techniques* (14). This book details the recipes for most fixatives and stains and lists the appropriate protocols for their use. The pros and cons for each protocol are also mentioned. Unless otherwise noted within the recipes, percentages are expressed as volume per volume measurements.

Materials

- Cork board (approximately 4.5 inch $\times$ 5.5 inch $\times \frac{1}{4}$ inch)
- 1-inch metal straight pins
- No. 2 lead pencil
- 3 $\times$ 5 index cards
- 10% formalin solution or other fixative
- Staining solution
- 70% ethanol in 500-ml wash bottle
- Clearing agent
- Mounting media
- Surgical instruments
  - Dissecting scissors, fine

       De Wecker's scissors (Roboz Instruments, Gaithersburg, MD)
       Rat-tooth forceps
       Scalpel with disposable blades
- Sterile cotton swabs
- Anesthesia (pentobarbital) or as required by the local Institute Animal Care and Use Committee
- 1-ml syringe and 23- or 25-gauge needle
- Binocular dissecting microscope
- Dissecting microscope lamp
- Microscope slides, frosted glass or plastic

Removal of Inguinal Mammary Glands for Whole Mount Analysis (see also Appendix)

Depending on experimental protocol, either anesthetize or euthanize the mouse as required by the local Institute Animal Care and Use Committee. The mouse is then placed in a recumbent position, ventral side up, on a cork board using a suitable method of restraint and is swabbed with 70% ethanol. Refer to Figure 7-1 for mammary gland location. A ventral midline inverted Y incision is made beginning midway between nipples 4 and 5 just above the genital area toward the thorax (about 2.5 cm) and laterally to each leg (about 1.5 cm) between the nipples (Figure 7-2). The skin flaps, with mammary glands attached, are carefully separated from the peritoneum with a blunt-edged instrument. The free edge of each skin flap is secured to the cork board, thereby exposing the adherent mammary glands. Mammary glands can then be carefully excised from the skin flap by using de Wecker

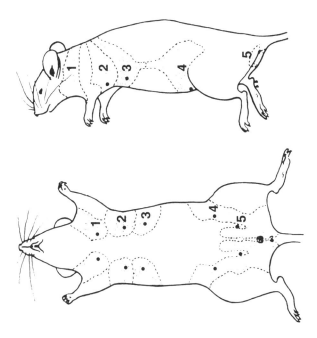

Figure 7-1. Diagram of murine mammary gland location, ventral and lateral aspect respectively. Large black dots represent the nipples, and the stippled areas the mammary glands. Numbers are marked on each mammary gland according to currently used terminology. Thoracic glands are 1–3 and inguinal glands are 4–5. [Reprinted with permission from McGraw Hill Companies (23)].

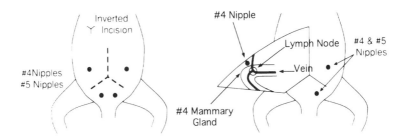

Figure 7-2. Inguinal mammary gland diagrams. Dotted line designates placement of the inverted Y incision. Expanded diagram shows placement of nipple, lymph node, and vein within the no. 4 inguinal mammary gland.

scissors. For survival surgery, incisions can be closed with wound clips or some other suitable method. For a more thorough removal of all mammary glands, refer to Method 3 in the appendix.

Slides

Glass slides are most commonly used for mounting single mammary glands. It is preferred that the slides have frosted edging for labeling purposes and, on occasion, specialized coating material. Plastic slides may also be used; however, this material is soluble in organic solvents and becomes more brittle with age. For most whole mounting of mouse mammary glands, plain glass slides are suitable.

Labeling

An accurate system of labeling is essential when starting and maintaining a whole mount collection. In principle, a specimen should be given an identifying number or name at the time it is prepared for fixation. A record book should be kept in which is written the source of the specimen, specimen number, date of sample collection, and any other data that may be relevant, such as fixing and staining solutions, etc. One can use either a lead pencil to denote sample name on the glass slide or a permanent marker. Paper labels resistant to organic solvents may also be employed. Alternatively, a diamond-tipped pencil may be used to etch the code on the slide.

Fixative

Fixation changes the appearance, texture, and reactivity of tissues. Fats are preserved by an aqueous fixative, whereas polysaccharides are preserved by fluids with high alcohol content. Neutral fats of adipose tissue are removed by fixation with alcohol or acetone. Fixation also acts upon tissue to preserve its original form and prevent decomposition and autolysis. Air-drying of the fat pad onto the slide for several seconds ensures adhesion of the tissue to the glass slide. To ensure proper preservation, the sample must be placed into fixative as soon as possible after removal from the animal, otherwise deterioration of the cells through tissue autolysis may start to occur (15). However, there may be some disadvantages associated with tissue fixation. For example, the use of alcohol-based fixatives sometimes leads to excessive sample dehydration and shrinkage. Nevertheless, after fixation, the tissue is generally more permeable to fluids than in its natural state, thereby allowing tissue staining to occur more readily.

Many fixatives are available for use; however, several fixatives are used predominantly the mammary gland literature (16). Formaldehyde solution, approximately 40% formaldehyde gas in water, called formalin, is treated as a 100% solution in making other formalin percent solutions (i.e., 10 ml formalin and 90 ml H_2O produce a 10% formalin solution) (17). Formalin fixative is the simplest of all recipes. It consists of 10% formaldehyde (36–38% stock solution) in a buffered aqueous solution, such as sodium phosphate [4 g NaH_2PO_4(monobasic), 6.5 g Na_2HPO_4(dibasic) in a solution of 100 ml formalin (37–40% stock solution) and 900 ml distilled water]. Formalin is buffered to counteract the formation of formic acid, to which formalin is oxidized over time.

A modification of this basic recipe, often referred to by its original maker Tellyesniczky, consists of 10% formaldehyde, 5% glacial acetic acid, and 85% ethanol (70% stock solution). However, this recipe is often used in varying ratios, such as 5–15% formaldehyde, 2–10% glacial acetic acid, and 30–80% ethanol (70% stock solution).

An often-used fixative is Carnoy's formula 1 and formula 2 (15, 18). Formula 1 consists of a v/v solution of 25% glacial acetic acid and 75% absolute ethanol. Formula 2 contains 10% glacial acetic acid, 30% chloroform, and 60% absolute ethanol. Carnoy's fixatives allow rapid fixation of tissues and preserve glycogen and improve nuclear staining. These fixatives also dehydrate and, in the case of mammary glands, remove lipids as well as fix the tissue. It is claimed that they may cause excessive tissue shrinkage, although we have not experienced this in our mammary gland samples.

Another fixative used to preserve fine structural detail is a solution of 2% (w/v) paraformaldehyde and 2.5% glutaraldehyde in 0.1 M sodium cacodylate, pH 7.3 (19). This fixative is suggested for use when preserving whole mounts for electron microscopy (see Method 2). Staining with trypan or methylene blue creates a more delicate appearance than seen in typical hematoxylin whole mount staining. This may be due to a tendency to overstain with hematoxylin. This modified protocol allows the use of the same whole mount for both macroscopic evaluation and electron microscopy on specific areas selected from the whole mount. This technique often eliminates wasteful sectioning through entire blocks of tissue searching for a particular feature.

Mammary glands can be fixed from 4 to 24 h, depending on the tissue thickness and temperature at which fixation takes place. After fixation, the general rule is to transfer the samples to a medium comparable to the solvent of the dye being used. For example, if the dye is in a water solution, the samples are hydrated through a series of decreasing alcoholic solutions to 50% alcohol, then finally they go into water. Conversely, if the dye is dissolved in a 50% alcoholic solution, the samples are only carried into 50% alcohol before going into the dye solution.

Stains

Staining solutions contain mordants, which are substances that provide a linkage or bonding between a tissue component and a dye. Mordants often are heavy metals such as iron or aluminum. These metals increase the tissues' affinity for the dye, allowing staining to occur more rapidly and thoroughly. Again, there are numerous staining solutions available for use. The most widely used stains for mammary gland tissue are hematoxylin, carmine alum, and trypan blue.

HEMATOXYLIN (16).   The different types of hematoxylin solution are determined chiefly by the chemical used as a mordant and the method used to oxidize hematoxylin to hematein. Ferric salts act as mordants and oxidizers; hence, no additional oxidation is needed when they are included in a formula. Hematoxylin produces a blue stain, in an alkaline medium, of most nuclei and connective tissue. Collagen and other intercellular substances stain yellow, pink, or brownish red. In an acidic medium, hematoxylin stains nuclei red. Hematoxylin solutions are available commercially from Sigma (St. Louis, MO) and Fisher (Pittsburgh, PA).

Iron Hematoxylin (20)
>   *Hematoxylin stock*: 10 g hematoxylin in 100 ml ethanol (190 proof) (let stand overnight before use).
>   *Working hematoxylin solution*: 1.6 g ferric chloride in 240 ml water
>   290 ml 1 N HCl
>   20 ml hematoxylin stock
>   1810 ml ethanol (190 proof)

Mayer's Hematoxylin (21, 22)
>   1 g hematoxylin crystals
>   0.2 g sodium iodate
>   50 g aluminum ammonium sulfate (ammonium alum)
>   1 g citric acid
>   50 g chloral hydrate
>   Distilled water to 1 liter

Dissolve the alum in water, without heat; add and dissolve the hematoxylin in this solution. Then add the sodium iodate, citric acid, and the chloral hydrate; shake until all components are in complete solution. The final color of the stain is a reddish violet. This solution can be stored at room temperature for several months. Color changes in the stock solution indicate its efficacy. When purple, the hematoxylin solution is most vigorous; as it oxidizes the solution turns brown and is no longer useful. Hematoxylin may be used successfully on whole mounts fixed in any of the fixatives described earlier in this Chapter. Of the several formulations for hematoxylin stain, we recommend Mayer's formulation for mammary gland whole mounts.

TRYPAN BLUE.   As its name implies, this stain causes the epidermal tissue to turn blue. This stain is mainly used *in vivo* to illuminate the position of mammary glands, particularly in virgin mice. Trypan blue is made as a 0.5% (w/v) solution in normal saline. Staining should be done overnight. Alternatively, 0.4% (w/v) trypan blue solution can be obtained commercially from companies that supply tissue culture reagents, for example Gibco BRL (Gaithersburg, MD).

CARMINE ALUM (16).   Carmine is a red compound derived from the dried pulverized bodies of the cochineal insect, *Coccus cacti*. It is available as cochineal, carmine, or carminic acid, which represent, from lowest to highest, the three degrees of purity of the coloring agent. Like hematoxylin, carmine staining solutions can be used with or without a mordant mixed with them. Carmine itself is practically insoluble in water, but it is soluble in acids or alkalis. Its activity as a stain is strongly affected by aluminum, iron, and other metal salts. These salts are usually added to the staining solution or used as a mordant on the tissue to be stained. Fixation in acid and alcohol is required for good staining.

Carmine Alum Stain. Weigh 1 g carmine and 2.5 g aluminum potassium sulfate and place into 450 ml distilled water. Boil mixture for 20 min. Adjust volume to 500 ml with distilled water. Cool solution and filter solution through Whatmann paper no. 1. A crystal of thymol may be added as a preservative. Refrigerate stain. This stain solution can be used for several months. Discard stain when color becomes weak. Carmine alum is a progressive stain that colors nuclei selectively. Staining intensity varies from batch to batch, so staining should be monitored closely. Destaining is possible using a 1% solution of 1 N HCl (Russell Hovey, personal communication).

CLEARING (15). Clearing refers to delipidation and subsequent increased transparency of tissue. This is often achieved by using toluene, xylene, or methyl salicylate. This rapid process creates a sharper delineation between structures in the mammary gland and clearer images for photographic purposes. Yet it does cause excessive shrinkage of delicate tissues, and clearing can only be done from absolute alcohol or 74 O.P. spirit if toluene or xylene is used. Methyl salicylate is also used as a storage medium for the whole mounts. The use of scintillation vials is excellent for this purpose. We have found that clearing in Fisher Hema-D, a citrus-peel-based, nontoxic clearing agent results in bleaching of the stain over longer periods of storage even after mounting with balsam and a coverslip.

Mounting Media

Many resinous materials can be used for permanently mounting the whole mammary gland to the slide and a cover slip. Traditionally, natural resins were employed, such as gum dammar and Canadian balsam. However, these resins have an inherent acidity, causing basic stains (such as hematoxylin) to fade rapidly. In addition, natural resins often yellow with age.

Currently, many synthetic resins, such as Permount and Clearmount, are available on the market that preserve tissues without the effects seen with traditional resins. A good mounting media should be a synthetic resin viscous enough to coat with 1 or 2 drops that dries quickly with a clear transparent finish. Ensure that the solvent of the mounting media is miscible with the clearing agent. Before mounting, mammary glands need to be thoroughly dehydrated unless they are to be mounted in water-soluble medium. Failure to remove all the water may cause staining to fade rapidly and mounting media or tissue to become cloudy. Cover slides are placed on top of mammary glands after the addition of mounting media and firmly pushed to ensure even distribution of adhesive. Warming the coverslip a bit before applying to the slide often minimizes the presence of bubbles. Lastly, baking slides for 20 min at 60°C quickly dries mounting media.

When the need arises for restaining slides, it becomes necessary to remove the coverslips, and this can be done in one of several ways (17). When using any one of these methods, remember that the older the slide, the longer it will take to remove the coverslip. The first method involves placing the slide in xylene until the coverslip detaches of its own accord. Leave slide in xylene until all of the mounting media is dissolved. Hydrate slide to water and stain as desired.

A second method uses heat to remove the coverslip. Heat the underside of the slide around the coverslip edges by passing over an open flame (Bunsen burner, cigarette lighter, etc.) about two times a second. Do not hold slide directly over the flame as the whole mount may be burned and the slide will crack if the flame is directed to any spot for any length of time. Coverslip may be eased off the slide with forceps when the first air bubble is noted beneath the coverslip. If the coverslip does not move easily, flame slide until it does. Do not force the coverslip because the whole mount may be damaged. Cool to room temperature. Place slide in xylene until all the mounting media is dissolved. Hydrate to water and stain as desired.

The last method employs the use of heat and xylene. Place slide in a coplin jar filled with xylene. Close coplin jar with lid and place at 60°C. Check slides every 30 min until coverslip is off. After mounting media is completely dissolved, hydrate to water and then stain as desired.

RESULTS AND DISCUSSION

The subcutaneous position of the mouse mammary glands allows their examination in either living animals or postmortem. For animals in which ongoing experiments are being done, one may excise a portion of the no. 4–5 glands for interim analysis by a small cutaneous incision and turning back the skin without seriously incapacitating the animal. At the conclusion of an experiment, the remaining mammary glands may be harvested for subsequent analysis. This versatility enables the researcher to examine mammary glands from the same experimental mouse, thereby limiting potential intraspecies variability. Due to the bilateral symmetry of the mouse mammary glands (Figure 7-1), controls can be placed in contralateral glands for transplantation or similar experiments. Whole mounts may be used to isolate and identify regions for subsequent histopathological, immunocytochemical, and ultrastructural evaluations.

Problems associated with whole mounting mammary glands include cloudiness, air pockets, and excessive hair. Opaque mammary gland whole mounts are caused by insufficient dehydration of the mammary gland. It is imperative to dehydrate the mammary gland fully before attempting clearing and application of mounting media. When opacity occurs, return whole mounts to xylene, dissolve all mounting medium, and then place into absolute ethanol (acetone may also be used), clear, and remount. Air pockets beneath the mammary glands are often created by the movement of the samples between staining media. Air pockets can be alleviated by firmly attaching mammary glands to the slide before applying mounting media. Lastly, the problem of excessive hair on mammary gland whole mounts is solved by using cotton-tipped applicators to carefully remove any hair before applying mounting media (N. Kenney, personal communication).

APPENDIX

Method 1: Simple Protocol for Rapid Whole Mounting of Mammary Gland

Spread mammary gland on glass slide, making sure to extend the margins of the gland to expose as much area as possible to the glass surface to ensure flatness. Fix glands in Carnoy's fixative (formula 2) for 2–4 h at room temperature. Wash in 70% ethanol for 15 min. Change gradually to distilled water: Wash in 50% ethanol for 15 min. Wash in 25% ethanol for 15 min. The glands are rinsed in tap water for 5 min and then stained in carmine alum overnight until stain has permeated the mammary gland (staining clearly apparent on both faces of the mammary gland). Wash in 70%, 95%, and absolute ethanol for 15 min each. Clear mammary glands in xylene for two changes of 30 min each (the last xylene clearing step can be done overnight). Mount with Permount (Fisher Scientific, Pittsburgh, PA) and coverslip. Representative whole mounts made using this technique are found in Figure 7-3.

Method 2 (19): Preparation of Whole Mounts for Subsequent Analysis Using Electron Microscopy

Fix mammary glands overnight at 4°C in freshly made 2% (w/v) paraformaldehyde–2.5% glutaraldehyde in 0.1 M sodium cacodylate, pH 7.3. Glands are then placed into a 0.2 M cacodylate–HCl, pH 7.5, for 24–72 h. The glands are then passed twice in acetone for 24 h each to defat mammary glands. Then the glands may be stained in either 0.5% (w/v) methylene blue in saline or 0.5% (w/v) trypan blue in saline overnight. Next they are serially passed through 50%, 70%, and 95% ethanol for 24 h each. Finally, the slides are placed twice into absolute ethanol for 2 h each. The glands can then be photographed in absolute ethanol. These glands can then be whole-mounted onto slides or processed for electron microscopy.

Method 3: Pelt Preparation for Mammary Gland Whole Mounts (10)

Euthanize mouse as required by the local Institute Animal Care and Use Committee. Pin mouse to cork board ventral side up by placing pins through base of tail and upper jaw. Thoroughly wet hair with 70% ethanol. Make a midline incision through skin, from external genitalia papillae at base of tail to top of the lower jaw, taking care not to penetrate the peritoneum. Make dorsoventral incisions on both sides of external genitalia papillae from the top to the base of the tail. Skin mouse by gently pulling the body wall away from the skin. This can be done by holding the skin with rat-tooth forceps or finger while peeling body with the other hand. The mammary fat pads will be exposed and remain with the skin. Skin mouse in quadrants, starting with the inguinal region (Figure 7-1). Pull skin flap as far from body as possible and pin to cork board; this maneuver will expose the no. 4 and no. 5 fat pads (Figures 7-1 and 7-2). Gently dissect no. 5 fat pad away from the leg muscles. Pull leg through skin and cut off paw if necessary. Place pins through skin and cork board so that skin is taut. Repeat maneuver on the opposite side. Free skin from thoracic region; pin skin to cork board to expose pads 1, 2, and 3. Pull limbs through the skin, cutting off the leg at paws if necessary. Pick up both hind limbs and sever spinal column at the tail base. Carefully pull carcass away from skin by lifting and peeling toward head. Snip the intrascapular brown fat away from the body to thoroughly free carcass from skin. Snip skin from the head by cutting behind ears, freeing the carcass from the skin. Place pins through edge of skin to keep skin taut. Discard carcass in plastic bag and dispose of appropriately. Immerse skin and cork board in excess Tellyesniczky or 10% formalin fixative skin side down. Use a weight to totally immerse cork board in fixative. Fix at least overnight. The next day, discard fixative and wash skin in running water until most of the fixative is removed. Use a No. 3 or 4 scalpel blade and lightly score the mammary fat pad side into quarters, making sure that the skin is not cut through; the right 1, 2, and 3 fat pads should be contained in one quarter and the corresponding left side should be in another; the right 4 and 5 fat pads should be in one of the quarters and the corresponding left side in another quarter (Figure 7-1). Using the handle of scalpel holder, gently scrape mammary fat pads from skin. Place the quarters into staining cassettes with the appropriate identification. Place cassettes in acetone to defat at least overnight; one or two changes of acetone may be required. Process and stain whole mounts manually as in Method 1. The staining process can be automated by using an Autotechnicon Duo (Technicon Instruments, Tarrytown, NY).

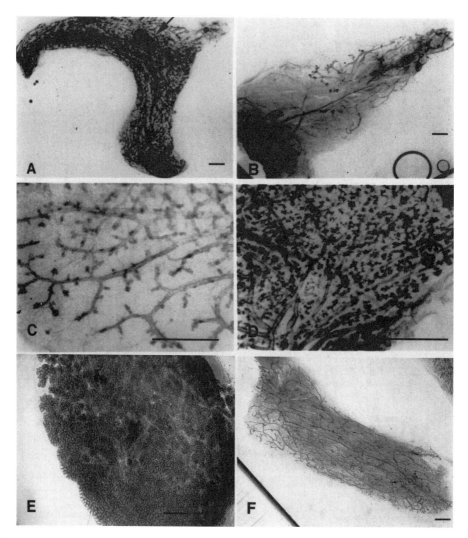

Figure 7-3. Representative mammary gland whole mounts. Fixation was done in Carnoy's fixative (5 h to overnight) and stained overnight with carmine alum. Bar represents 1 mm. (A) An inguinal mammary fat pad (4–5 mammary gland) taken from a normal 13-week-old virgin FVB strain female. The arrow points to the lymph node present within the no. 4 mammary gland portion of the whole mount. (B) An inguinal gland from a 25-week-old virgin *Int3* transgenic littermate. The major feature is the lack of normal ductal development as well as the absence of terminal growing end buds and a lymph node in the mature *Int3* virgin. (C) A normal outgrowth developed in an *Int3* mammary fat pad that had been surgically cleared of transgenic epithelium, indicating that normal growth and ductal branching are supported by the transgenic host. (D) Lobular development induced by treatment with a slow-release pellet (60-day exposure) containing 10 mg progesterone, 0.1 mg estradiol, and 1.0 mg hydrocortisone in a normal FVB virgin host. (E) Lobular development induced by full-term gestation in a normal FVB host. (F) Represents a senescing outgrowth (14 weeks after implantation) in a lactating normal host where a complete branched ductal network has developed; however, alveolar development is essentially absent. This observation suggests that ductal branching morphogenesis and secretory lobulogenesis age independently of one other in serially passaged normal outgrowths (Smith, unpublished observations).

REFERENCES

1. W. U. Gardner and L. C. Strong (1935). The normal development of the mammary glands of virgin female mice of ten strains varying in susceptibility to spontaneous neoplasms. *Am. J. Cancer* **25**:282–290.
2. H. C. Taylor and C. A. Waltman (1940). Hyperplasias of the mammary gland in the human being and in the mouse. Morphologic and etiologic contrasts. *Arch. Surgery* **40**:733–820.
3. R. A. Huseby and J. J. Bittner (1946). A comparative morphological study of the mammary glands with reference to the known factors influencing the development of mammary carcinoma in mice. *Cancer Res.* **6**:240–255.
4. A. J. Dalton (1945). *Histogenesis of the Mammary Gland of the Mouse*, The Science Press Printing Company, Lancaster, PA.
5. K. B. DeOme, L. J. Faulkin, H. A. Bern, and P. B. Blair (1959). Development of mammary tumors from hyperplastic alveolar nodules transplanted into gland-free mammary fat pads of female C3H mice. *Cancer Res.* **19**:515–520.
6. R. V. Nie and A. Dux (1971). Biological and morphological characteristics of mammary tumors in GR mice. *J. Natl. Cancer Inst.* **46**(4):885–897.
7. C. W. Daniel, K. B. DeOme, J. T. Young, P. B. Blair, and L. J. Faulkin, Jr. (1968). The *in vivo* life span of normal and preneoplastic mouse mammary glands: a serial transplantation study. *Proc. Natl. Acad. Sci. USA* **61**(1):53–60.
8. E. M. Rivera (1971). *Mammary Gland Culture*, Freeman, San Francisco.
9. M. R. Banerjee, B. G. Wood, F. K. Lin, and L. R. Crump (1976). Organ culture of the whole mammary glands of the mouse. *Tissue Culture Associ. Manual* **2**(4):457–462.
10. D. Medina (1973). Preneoplastic lesions in mouse mammary tumorigenesis. *Metho. Cancer Res.* **7**:3–53.
11. H. Nagasawa and R. Yanai (1978). *Normal and Abnormal Growth of the Mammary Gland*, Japan Scientific Societies Press, Tokyo.
12. G. H. Smith, D. Gallahan, F. Diella, C. Jhappan, G. Merlino, and R. Callahan (1995). Constitutive expression of a truncated *INT3* gene in mouse mammary epithelium impairs differentiation and functional development. *Cell Growth Differentiation* **6**:563–577.
13. D. Gallahan, C. Jhappan, G. Robinson, L. Hennighausen, R. Sharp, E. Kordon, R. Callahan, G. Merlino, and G. H. Smith (1996). Expression of a truncated *Int3* gene in developing secretory mammary epithelium specifically retards lobular differentiation resulting in tumorigenesis. *Cancer Res.* **56**:1775–1785.
14. J. K. Presnell and M. P. Schreibman (1997). *Humason's Animal Tissue Techniques*, The John Hopkins University Press, Baltimore, MD.
15. E. C. Clayden (1971). *Practical Section Cutting and Staining*, Churchill and Livingstone, London.
16. H. A. Davenport (1960). *Histological and Histochemical Technics*, W.B. Saunders Company, Philadelphia, PA.
17. L. G. Luna (ed.) (1968). *Manual of Histologic Staining Methods of the Armed Forces Institute of Pathology*, McGraw-Hill, New York.
18. J. B. Carnoy (1887). *Cellule* **3**:247–324.
19. J. M. Strum (1979). A mammary gland whole mount technique that preserves cell fine structure for electron microscopy. *J. Histochem. Cytochem.* **27**(9):1271–1274.
20. M. Heidenhain (1892). *Ueber Kern und Protoplasma*, Wilhelm Englemann, Leipsig.
21. P. Mayer (1899). Üeber haematoxylin, carmin, und verwandte materien. *Z. Wiss. Mikrosk.* **16**:196–220.
22. M. A. Hayat (1993). *Stains and Cytochemical Methods*, Plenum Press, New York.
23. K. P. Hummel, F. L. Richardson, and E. Fekete (1966). Anatomy. In E. L. Green (ed.), *Biology of the Laboratory Mouse*, McGraw Hill, New York, p. 267.

Chapter 8

Slow-Release Plastic Pellets (Elvax) for Localized *In Situ* Treatments of Mouse and Rat Mammary Tissue

Gary B. Silberstein and Charles W. Daniel

Abstract. The need to define the actions of paracrine and autocrine signaling factors against a background of systemic hormones led to the development of the slow-release implant technique. Elvax40P® is an ethylene vinyl acetate copolymer. Formed into a matrix containing test materials such as hormones or growth factors, Elvax releases metered amounts and can be used to treat small zones within the mammary gland. Importantly, Elvax is generally nondenaturing to proteins and steroids and does not elicit a tissue response. To date, Elvax experiments have been used to help define the *in vivo* roles of a variety of growth factors and hormones. Here we describe the fabrication and surgical techniques necessary to use this material.

Abbreviations. bovine serum albumin (BSA); deoxycorticosterone acetate (DCA); dichloromethane (DCM); epidermal growth factor (EGF); Elvax 40W®, ethylene vinyl acetate copolymer (Elvax); insulin-like growth factor (IGF); lobuloalveolar (LA); tetradecanoyl phorbol myristic acid (TPA); transforming growth factor (TGF).

INTRODUCTION

Plastic implants made of ethylene vinyl acetate copolymer (Elvax 40P®) are capable of the sustained release of undenatured, bioactive molecules and can be used inside living tissue, as first demonstrated by Langer and Folkman in the late 1970s, who investigated the induction of neovascularization (1, 2). In the mammary gland, Silberstein and Daniel, adapting this technique, first used Elvax implants containing either deoxycorticosterone acetate (DCA), a lobuloalveolar mammogen, or an extracellular matrix-degrading enzyme, hyaluronidase, in "proof-of-principle" experiments (3). With DCA, lobuloalveolar development was most intense close to the implant and attenuated with distance from the source, whereas the untreated, contralateral gland was unaffected. The localized degradation of extracellular matrix by implanted hyaluronidase, on the other hand, demonstrated that denaturation-sensitive proteins could be effectively delivered inside the gland. Of great importance, Elvax

Gary B. Silberstein and Charles W. Daniel   **Department of Biology, University of California, Santa Cruz, California 95065.**

Methods in Mammary Gland Biology and Breast Cancer Research, edited by Ip and Asch. Kluwer Academic/Plenum Publishers, New York, 2000.

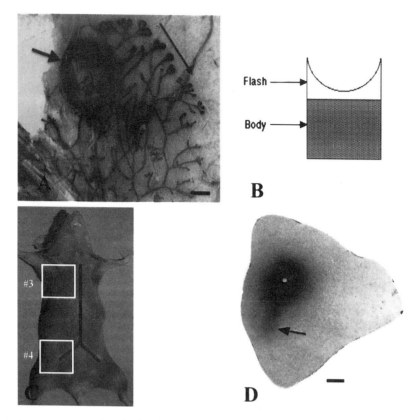

Figure 8-1. (A) Elvax implant in gland of 5-week-old mouse. Implant containing BSA (large arrow) was placed in front of the growing ducts in a 3- to 4-week-old animal (14). Ducts grew around the implant. The end bud array is normal; the largest end buds appear in the center of the gland and decrease in size toward the edge of the fat pad (small arrow). Bar = 1 mm. (B) Cartoon showing cross section of an Elvax pellet removed from its shell vial. Remove the flash and cut implant-sized pieces from the body (shaded area) of the pellet. (C) Mouse with the skin incisions (heavy, black lines) required to expose the axial (no. 3) and inguinal (no. 4) mammary glands for implantation. Skin is reflected to expose glands beneath (white boxes). (D) Zone of diffusion and glandular retention of Elvax-delivered TGFβ1. Implants contained 5×10^4 cpm iodinated ligand and were left *in situ* for 5 h. (approximately 30% of ligand released). Film exposure was for 7 days. White dot, position of implant; arrow, surgical channel. Bar = 3 mm. (*Developmental Biology* **93**:272–278, 1982).

is biologically inert in the mammary gland as evidenced by growing end buds confronting and growing around a piece of the plastic (Figure 8-1A).

In the 15 years since Elvax implants were first adapted for use in the mammary gland, they have been used successfully to investigate the local actions of mammogenic peptides and steroids (4–6). Denaturation-sensitive peptides and proteins such as EGF, IGF, and the TGFβs, as well as antibodies, have also been effectively implanted (4, 6–9). The use of Elvax implants is simple, and it is possible that in some cases they may substitute for the more laborious and expensive engineering of transgenic mice. It is also expected that the increasing availability of transgenic and knockout mice and the use of DNA microarrays will provide a new and expanded scope for the use of slow-release implants in which further insights into the effects of genetic alterations on the local responses to hormones and growth factors can be gleaned. It is the purpose of this chapter to provide the technical details to enable investigators to use the Elvax implant technique easily and quickly. The reader should be aware that other slow-release implant techniques have also been used in mammary gland investigations; these include growth-factor-containing cholesterol pellets (see Chapter 9) as well as agarose beads loaded with protein (10).

MATERIALS

- Elvax 40W® (the earlier, 40P designation has been superseded by 40W; there is no difference between these products with respect to implant preparation or release). The manufacturer, DuPont, Inc., generously supplies Elvax for research purposes. To procure a research sample, call 302-992-4318 and speak with Mr. Roger Richmond, or 800-438-7225 and ask for technical assistance.
- Dichloromethane (Fisher Chemicals, Fairlawn, NJ) (hazardous chemical: highly flammable and fumes toxic)
- Bovine serum albumin (Sigma, St. Louis, MO)
- Glass shell vials (8 × 43 mm) (Fischer Scientific, Pittsburgh, PA; cat. no. 03-340-17B)
- Scintillation vials, glass
- Sturdy, curved instrument for extracting solidified plastic from vial (gross anatomy probe; Fine Science Tools Inc., Foster City, CA; cat. no. 10088-15).
- Dissecting needle
- Forceps, two pair, fine with pointed tips, e.g., Dumont No. 5 (Fine Science Tools Inc., Foster City, CA; cat. no. 11250-20)
- Standard instruments used in mouse surgery: scissors, forceps (curved, toothed, and plain tipped)
- Wound clips (9 mm) with Autoclip applicator (Clay Adams, Parsippany, NJ)
- Cotton swabs, sterile

Note: Surgical instruments and the wound-clip device should be washed and sterilized by autoclaving or by soaking in 70% ethanol for 60 min.

METHODS

Preparation of Stock Elvax for Subsequent Implant Preparation

WASHING STOCK ELVAX 40W.   Elvax comes from DuPont coated with a talc-like substance that must be removed.

1. Place 10–20 g Elvax in 300–500 ml 95% ethanol and wash with stirring for 24 h. Drain old ethanol and replace with fresh and repeat for 3 more days, changing the ethanol each day.
2. Dry the washed Elvax on paper toweling and store in container of choice. Shelf-life: indefinite.

DISSOLVING ELVAX FOR IMPLANT PREPARATION

1. In a scintiallation vial, dissolve 1 g washed Elvax in 5 ml DCM (20% w/v), using a small stir bar to agitate the mixture.
   Note: This concentration of Elvax was arrived at empirically for use in mouse. The ratio of Elvax to incorporated material can be changed to alter the release kinetics of the implant (11, 12).

Note: DCM is extremely volatile; therefore plastic vial cap must be tightly sealed and then covered with Parafilm to maintain volume.

2. Store dissolved Elvax at 4°C. Depending on seal, this preparation may last for months. Warm vial to room temperature to reliquefy the Elvax.

Preparation of Test Material for Incorporation into Elvax Matrix

LIPID-SOLUBLE MATERIAL.   Lipid-soluble material is dissolved directly in DCM to desired concentration and requires no further preparation (2, 5, 6).

WATER-SOLUBLE MATERIALS.   If large amounts of a protein or sugar are required, these may be added dry directly to the dissolved Elvax. In the case of scarce or potent substances, e.g., growth factors, microgram amounts are typically used and a second, nonbioactive, carrier such as BSA must be added to create the plastic matrix necessary for stable release kinetics (13). Since the latter type of implant is used most commonly, in the next section we describe its preparation.

Preparing a Typical Stock Elvax Pellet from Which Implant-Sized Pieces Are Then Cut

(In this example, the stock pellet contains approximately 20 mg BSA when finished plus microgram amounts of bioactive protein X, and will weigh approximately 35 mg. This typical stock pellet weight should be distinguished from the weight of the final implant, which for mouse mammary glands is 0.5–1.5 mg, depending on desired dosage).

LYOPHILIZATION OF TEST MATERIAL

1. In a shell vial, dissolve 20 mg BSA carrier in 100 µl distilled water and add desired amount of protein X.
   Note: Lyophilized materials, i.e., peptide growth factors, should be reconstituted in water and the appropriate volume added to the dissolved BSA prior to lyophilization.
   Note: Water and DCM are not miscible; therefore do not add aqueous solutions of test material directly to dissolved Elvax.
2. Lyophilization should be carried out in the container in which you intend to make the stock pellet. This ensures quantitative incorporation and minimizes handling.
3. Tightly cover the vial with Parafilm, make a pinhole through the top, and then, on dry ice, shell-freeze the mixture onto the sides of the vial.
4. Place vial on lyophilizer overnight.

POSTLYOPHILIZATION PREPARATIONS

1. Set up an acetone–dry ice bath.
2. Label a scintillation vial with implant information and prechill on dry ice along with sturdy, curved dental-type instrument.

MANIPULATION OF THE LYOPHILATE

1. Remove vial from lyophilizer. Do not remove the Parafilm. The finely powdered lyophilate is often charged with static electricity and may fly out of the vial.

2. Using a clean dissecting needle inserted and manipulated through the pinhole, pulverize the lyophilate to a fine powder.

3. Compact the powdered lyophilate in the bottom of the vial by tapping vial on bench top.

PREPARING AND HANDLING ELVAX–LYOPHILATE SUSPENSION

1. Open the vial containing the dissolved Elvax. Place the tip of a 1-ml *borosilicate* pipette (plastic will dissolve in DCM) with a propipette bulb just below the surface of the dissolved plastic, load approximately 125 μl, cap the Elvax stock, and quickly transfer the pipette load into the shell vial on top of the powdered mixture. After the initial volume is delivered, wait a moment for retained volume to settle in the pipette tip and then deliver that as well.
   Note: Elvax is viscous, but do not worry, because exact pipetting is not critical.

2. Mixing. Thoroughly mix lyophilate and dissolved Elvax, using a clean dissecting needle. Be quick about this but do not rush so much that you neglect good dispersal. Do not be concerned if some of the mixture remains stuck to the sides of the vial.

3. Freezing. Quick-freeze the mixture for several minutes in the acetone–dry ice bath, then place vial on dry ice for an additional 10 min.

REMOVAL OF PELLET FROM VIAL AND EVAPORATION OF DCM

1. Removing the frozen pellet from the vial can be tricky. The goal is to remove it intact into the prechilled scintillation vial. The problem is that it tends to melt. To remove pellet, first grasp the vial in your fingertips for about 10 s, just enough time to warm it and release the frozen pellet from the sides. Then, using the prechilled, curved instrument, scoop the pellet free, slide it out of the vial, and drop it into the chilled scintillation vial. The pellet may be slightly damaged but ample matrix remains for implants. It is strongly recommended that you become facile with this technique, using BSA for practice before committing valuable materials.

2. Desiccation of pellet to remove DCM. Place the open scintillation vial containing the pellet in a −20°C freezer for 12–16 h. There is no need for a vacuum desiccator at this point.

WEIGH DRIED PELLET

1. Record the weight of the pellet both in your experimental records and on the side and top of the storage vial. This number is crucial because dosage is expressed on a load-to-total-pellet-weight basis, e.g., weight of incorporated test material:total weight of pellet. Also, the weight of a pellet uniquely identifies the implant and, hence, the experiment.

2. If the weight of the pellet described using the preceding protocol is substantially higher than 35 mg after freezer desiccation, the pellet should be further dried in a vacuum desiccator at room temperature for another 10–12 h.

Cutting the Elvax Pellet into Implant-Sized Fragments

The dried pellet consists of a "body" from which the fragments are cut and "flash," formed by the meniscus of the suspension, that is discarded (Figure 8-1B).

1. Under a dissecting microscope, use a clean razor blade or scalpel to remove the flash.
2. Cut implant-sized, rectangular solid pieces from the body of the pellet, using a clean razor or scalpel. Return unused material to original vial. Mouse-mammary-sized implants weigh between 0.5 and 1.5 mg.
   Note: We have not prepared implants for rat mammary gland. Implant size and load for this application must therefore be determined empirically by scaling up from mouse studies.
3. Weigh each implant and record weight prior to implantation.
   Tip: As you weigh implants, place them in a line on a clean glass slide, writing the weight next to each one. To store and protect the implants for short periods, place slide in a small box.
4. Implant shelf-life. The shelf-life of material in Elvax varies greatly. Steroid-containing implants seem to retain activity for years stored at room temperature. Proteins, on the other hand, may or may not be stable. Each must be evaluated separately. For example, TGFβ1 was stable in Elvax pellets for months stored at 4°C, whereas EGF in pellets lost activity in a week and therefore had to be used immediately after fabrication.

Surgical Implantation of Elvax

1. Anesthetize mouse or rat.
2. Lay animal on back on a small board, restraining limbs with surgical tape (Figure 8-1C).
3. Thoroughly cleanse abdomen with 70% ethanol. Although not necessary, stomach can be shaved to prevent fur from entering incision.
4. Using a pair of toothed forceps, raise the skin at the junction of the three incision lines (Figure 8-1C). With small scissors, taking care not to puncture the peritoneal wall, make an incision forward to the sternum. The axial (no. 3) and inguinal (no. 4) glands (boxes) are the most accessible and are usually used for implanting. To access the inguinal glands, make secondary cuts as indicated.
5. Use a sterile swab to gently separate the skin from the abdominal wall, exposing the mammary fat pads. Reflect and pin out the abdominal skin so that the mammary gland presents a flat surface.
6. Placing an implant in the mammary gland. While you will ultimately develop your own technique, here is one method. Two pairs of jeweler's forceps are used, one to hold the tissue in place, the other to create a pocket and place the implant. With one pair of forceps, grasp the fascia above the point where the implant is to enter. Holding a second pair of forceps nearly parallel to the surface of the gland, insert the tip into the gland several millimeters to create a pocket. While maintaining first forceps above pocket, retrieve an implant from the glass slide with the second forceps and place the implant into the pocket. The first instrument is pressed gently down to restrain the implant as you release it and withdraw the forceps tip. Practice this before trying it with valuable materials or animals. (For most experiments an implant containing the test material can be placed on one side of the animal with a carrier-only, control implant on the contralateral side.)
   Note: The implant is held in place by the tissue, so the pocket requires no suturing.

7. Close skin incisions with the wound clip applicator and place the mouse in a warm location to monitor recovery.

CRITICAL ISSUES

Reporting Dosage

In all implant dose–response studies to date, the dose has been expressed as the total amount of the test material in the implant as opposed to some estimate of actual levels in the tissue (for examples of dose–response curves see Refs. 5, 7, and 14). The rationale for this method is twofold. First, as we will discuss, the true tissue levels of a test material are in constant flux due to the open tissue milieu and the nonconstant release kinetics of the implant. These factors make any estimate of tissue levels just that. Second, not all of the material in an implant is necessarily delivered in the tissue during the course of an experiment, but the magnitude of a response always reflects the starting amount in the implant.

Tissue Levels of Test Material

While acknowledging the uncertainties of estimating tissue levels of material released by an implant, at times the question arises whether an implant is delivering a physiological versus a pharmacological dose. The true dose received from an implant is a complex function of the amount of bioactive material used to make the pellet, the concentration and molecular weight of Elvax itself (12), and the amount of carrier material (13). These factors combine to determine the characteristic release kinetics for a test material, which in turn, determine dosage.

In fact, there is no way of knowing the instantaneous concentration of a test substance at its site of action any more than the instantaneous concentration of a growth factor at a cell surface can be known. Nevertheless, attempts have been made to evaluate tissue levels of Elvax-delivered growth factors in the mammary gland. Estimating tissue levels requires that the release kinetics of the material be determined. When *in vitro* release, determined for TGFβ1 by using iodimated ligand, was compared with release *in vivo*, both curves were essentially the same and indicated, as with other peptides, that 40–50% of the loaded material was released in the first 48 h (Figure 8-2) (14). By 5 days, 80–100% of peptide test material is usually released (3, 7).

In order to estimate tissue levels of implanted material, the amount released into a hypothetical 1-ml effective volume around an implant is assumed, and the amount released at any particular time is then determined based on the *in vitro* release kinetics. When this calculation was done for an implant containing 3 μg of EGF, tissue concentrations of less than 100 ng/ml were derived. Similar concentrations, considered physiological when applied to mammary cells *in vitro*, were shown to stimulate mammary epithelial cell division (see Ref. 4 for discussion).

If tissue response to an implanted protein varies with distance from the source, it may be desirable and feasible to use radio-iodinated protein to define relative concentrations in various regions of an implanted tissue. Implants containing iodinated TGFβ1 were allowed to release their contents for a period before sandwiching the gland between pieces of clear plastic and then exposing a sheet of X-ray film (Figure 8-1D) (14). The resulting exposure gradient reflects declining TGFβ concentration with distance from the implant. Using a

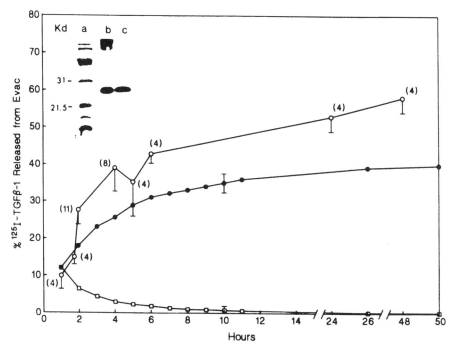

Figure 8-2. Time-course of ^{125}I-TGFβ1 release from Elvax *in vivo* and *in vitro*. The technique for preparing implants with radiolabeled test material, as well as the technique for assaying release, is described in detail in Ref. 14. Percentage released *in vivo* (open circles), *in vitro* (closed circles), and per hour *in vitro* (squares). ( ), number of glands tested. Error bars represent standard errors; a representative error bar is shown for the *in vitro* release data. Inset: Effect of Elvax on TGFβ1. Lane a. molecular weight standards. Lane b. ^{125}I-TGFβ1 released from Elvax *in vitro* (above study). Lane c. Stock iodinated ligand. (*Developmental Biology* **93**:272–282, 1982).

densitometer to scan an autoradiograph such as this, the relative levels of released material could be quantified.

Kinetics of Test Material Release

For most experiments determination of the release kinetics of a test material is not necessary if you use the described pellet fabrication scheme and use test materials, proteins, or steroids that are similar to those for which release kinetics have been determined. In these cases, and especially for experiments designed to determine if something has any effect at all, it is enough to know that mouse-mammary-sized implants (1.5 mg or smaller) have a high surface-to-volume ratio that favors rapid hydration; proteins are released in a pulse over the first 24 h, followed by a slower release rate lasting up to several days (7). In contrast, steroids are released at a slowly decelerating rate for up to several weeks. Although the release kinetics of proteins differs greatly from lipid soluble materials, with consistent pellet composition the variation is not extreme within each class of materials (5, 6). If different release kinetics are desired, then a different fabrication scheme must be developed (12, 13).

Experiments with Antibodies

Delivered *in situ*, an antibody can be a powerful tool for defining local protein function, as we demonstrated in the case of E-caherin (8). The use of antibodies targeted to structural proteins, such as the cadherins, worked quite well in this application, whereas attempts to interfere with the function(s) of soluble growth factors such as TGFβ and EGF did not (unpublished observations). The zone of tissue exposed to an antibody delivered via implant can be simply demonstrated in a single step by using the appropriate fluorochrome or chromogen-conjugated secondary antibody on the sectioned tissue.

PITFALLS

Reactions to Implanted Material: Inflammation, Toxicity, and Immunization

If the implant preparation and surgery protocols previously described are followed carefully, there should be no infection or local tissue reaction to the implant. The implantation of some test materials, however, may cause extreme irritation or toxicity. The protein kinase C activator, TPA, for example, caused local inflammation in the gland as well as irritation of the adjacent skin, and initial experiments with insulin implants caused a fatal reaction. Investigators must therefore consider possible adverse reactions from implanted materials and test for them using low doses, e.g., 10- to 100-fold lower than those used *in vitro*. Tissue irritation and inflammatory reactions are characterized by infiltrates of neutrophils and other leukocytes and will invalidate an experiment by introducing abnormal cell types, cytokines, cell death, etc. Therefore time spent avoiding this problem by careful consideration of the possible adverse effects of an implanted material followed by low-dose, range-finding experiments makes good scientific sense and spares animal suffering.

For some experiments prolonged exposure to the test material may be desirable. For systemic treatments larger, subcutaneous implants capable of sustained release may be used, whereas for the study of local effects in the mammary gland, serial implantation of smaller implants is necessary (14). If the test material is a foreign protein or glycoprotein, however, exposure over a period of weeks can lead to inactivation of the test material due to immune response. Emphasizing this fact, Elvax implants have been exploited in a novel immunization protocol (15).

Denaturation of Implant Contents

Peptide growth factors incorporated into Elvax matrices have unpredictable life spans; EGF denatured within 2 weeks, but TGFβ remained active for a month or more. In the absence of evidence that proteinaceous material contained in an implant has retained its activity, a negative result means nothing. If there is no observed response to an implant, the possibility that denaturation has occurred should be tested by using a suitable bioassay. The exception to this rule would be steroids, such as estrogen, etc., that retain activity in implants for up to a year or more.

ACKNOWLEDGMENT. This chapter was written under the support of NIH grant DK-48883.

REFERENCES

1. R. Langer, H. Brem, K. Falterman, M. Klein, and J. Folkman (1976). Isolation of a cartilage factor that inhibits tumor neovascularization. *Science* **193**:70–72.
2. R. Langer and J. Folkman (1976). Polymers for the sustained release of proteins and other macromolecules. *Nature (London)* **263**:797–800.
3. G. B. Silberstein and C. W. Daniel (1982). Elvax 40P implants: sustained, local release of bioactive molecules influencing mammary ductal development. *Dev. Biol.* **93**:272–278.
4. G. B. Silberstein and C. W. Daniel (1987). Investigation of mouse mammary ductal growth regulation using slow-release plastic implants. *J. Dairy Sci.* **70**:1981–1990.
5. G. B. Silberstein, K. Van Horn, G. S. Harris, and C. W. Daniel (1994). Essential role of endogenous estrogen in directly stimulating mammary growth demonstrated by implants containing pure antiestrogens. *Endocrinology* **134**:84–90.
6. C. W. Daniel, G. B. Silberstein, and P. Strickland (1987). Direct action of 17 beta-estradiol on mouse mammary ducts analyzed by sustained release implants and steroid autoradiography. *Cancer Res.* **47**:6052–6057.
7. S. Coleman, G. Silberstein, and C. W. Daniel (1988). Ductal morphogenesis in the mouse mammary gland: evidence supporting a role for epidermal growth factor. *Dev. Biol.* **127**:304–315.
8. C. W. Daniel, P. Strickland, and Y. Friedmann (1995). Expression and functional role of E- and P-cadherins in mouse mammary ductal morphogenesis and growth. *Dev. Biol.* **169**:511–519.
9. W. Ruan, V. Catanese, R. Wieczorek, M. Feldman, and D. Kleinberg (1995). Estradiol enhances the stimulatory effect of insulin-like growth factor I on mammary development and growth hormone-induced IGF-1 messenger ribonucleic acid. *Endocrinology* **136**:1296–1302.
10. B. K. Vonderhaar (1987). Local effects of EGF, alpha-TGF, and EGF-like growth factors on lobuloalveolar development of the mouse mammary gland *in vivo*. *J. Cell. Physiol.* **132**:581–584.
11. W. D. Rhine, S. T. Dean, D. S. T. Hsieh, and R. L. Langer (1980). Polymers for sustained macromolecule release: procedures to fabricate reproducible delivery systems and control kinetics. *J. Pharmacol. Sci.* **69**(3):265–270.
12. T. Hsu and R. Langer (1985). Polymers for the controlled release of macromolecules: effect of molecular weight of ethylene-vinyl acetate copolymer. *J. Biomed. Mater. Res.* **19**:445–460.
13. J. B. Murray, L. Brown, R. Langer, and M. Klagsburn (1983). A micro-sustained release system for epidermal growth factor. *In Vitro* **19**:743–748.
14. C. W. Daniel, G. B. Silberstein, K. Van Horn, P. Strickland, and S. Robinson (1989). TGF-beta 1-induced inhibition of mouse mammary ductal growth: developmental specificity and characterization. *Dev. Biol.* **135**:20–30.
15. R. Langer (1981). Polymers for the sustained release of macromolecules: their use in a single-step method of immunization. *Meth. Enzymol.* **73**:57–74.

Chapter 9

Intramammary Delivery of Hormones, Growth Factors, and Cytokines

Barbara K. Vonderhaar and Erika Ginsburg

Abstract. Direct delivery of hormones, growth factors, and cytokines to the mammary gland aids in assessing local versus systemically mediated effects. One of the three effective procedures utilizes cholesterol-based pellets inserted directly into the fat pad.

INTRODUCTION

The mammary gland is impacted by multiple hormones, growth factors, and cytokines. To distinguish between effects that are direct versus indirect and local versus systemically mediated, methods to deliver these agents directly to the mammary gland without changing the balance of hormones in the serum have been developed. Historically, three methods have proven effective. The first method involves Elvax pellets (1, 2) and is discussed in detail by Silberstein and Daniel in Chapter 8 in this volume. The second method involves injection of a solution of the hormone, cytokine, or growth factor through the nipple, up the teat canal, in an anesthetized animal. This method has been used in goats, cows, and rats to successfully deliver hormones and growth factors such as prolactin, somatotropin, insulin-like growth factor 1, and epidermal growth factor (3) and cytokines such as interleukin-1β or interleukin-2 (4). This infusion method, as adapted for the infusion of DNA or viral vectors, is described by Thompson and Gould in Chapter 22 in this volume. Using this method, it also is possible to transfect the mammary cells with the genes for peptide hormones (5), growth factors, or cytokines of interest and, hence, produce a local synthesis and delivery of the agent. This indirect method does not allow for control of the amount of ligand to which the gland is exposed, because there can be significant variations in the levels of the transfected gene products synthesized *in vivo*.

The third method, used in our laboratory for treating mice, utilizes a matrix-driven pellet system (6, 7). The biodegradable matrix is generally cholesterol. In some cases, fillers such as lactose, celluloses, phosphates, and stearates are included in the pellets.

Barbara K. Vonderhaar and Erika Ginsburg Laboratory of Tumor Immunology and Biology, National Cancer Institute, National Institutes of Health, Bethesda, Maryland 20892.

Methods in Mammary Gland Biology and Breast Cancer Research, edited by Ip and Asch. Kluwer Academic/Plenum Publishers, New York, 2000.

MATERIALS

Pellets

Pellets may be purchased commercially (Innovative Research of America, Sarasota, FL) or prepared in-house. To prepare pellets, the cholesterol along with the desired concentration of hormone, growth factor, or cytokine is dissolved in 100% ethanol, if possible, or physically mixed with a mortar and pestle. The solution is then dried under a stream of nitrogen gas. Individual pellets are then formed by using a pellet maker (Parr Instrument Co., Moline, IL) with an appropriately sized punch and die. Pellets as small as 1.5 mm in diameter can be obtained. The size of the pellet used will be determined by the age of the animal and size of the mammary fat pad. Pellets larger than 3 mm are not recommended for mice of any age.

Anesthesia

Avertin (2,2,2-tribromoethanol purchased from Aldrich Chemical Co., Milwaukee, WI) is prepared freshly at 25 mg/ml in distilled water and is dissolved by mixing end-over-end. Animals are injected intraperitoneally with 0.04 ml/g body weight. Alternatively, an anesthetic approved by the local IACUC (Institutional Animal Care and Use Committee) should be used.

METHODS

In order to insert the pellets, anesthetized mice are mounted on an approved surgical board, ventral side up. After liberally wiping down the fur with Wescodyne, make a small, midline incision from a point midway between the inguinal mammary glands toward the sternum; be careful to cut only the skin and not injure the abdominal musculature. Lateral incisions along the inguinal glands are then made so that the final incision resembles an inverted Y. Sterile forceps and cotton swabs are used to loosen the skin from the body wall; skin flaps are pinned back with sterile pins, thus exposing the abdominal and inguinal glands.

A pocket is prepared at the site of insertion of the pellet by holding points of sterile jeweler's forceps together and carefully inserting the points into the fat pad such that they do not rupture the surrounding connective tissue layer on the underside. Tension on the fat pad can be produced by holding the fat pad near the lymph node with another sterile forceps, thus making it easier to insert the jeweler's forceps. Remove the forceps points from the fat pad and insert the pellet into the prepared pocket, using the same forceps. As you remove the forceps, gently release the points to allow the pellet to slip fully and securely into the pocket. The pocket in the fat pad will "self-seal" and does not require suturing. Suture the skin flaps with wound clips, taking care that the abdominal wall is not attached to the skin. Align the cut edges of the skin as closely as possible to aid in healing.

COMMENTS

This cholesterol-based system is similar to that which uses Elvax. However, preparation of Elvax pellets requires exposure of the compound of interest to methylene chloride. Not all peptide hormones, growth factors, and cytokines are able to retain biological activity after exposure to organic solvents (including the 100% ethanol, which is the method of choice for preparing cholesterol-based pellets). If solvents cannot be used, thorough mechanical mixing will accomplish the same thing.

Cholesterol-based pellets have been used with small (young) mice (4 weeks old) (6, 7) where the teat canal is very small and may not readily accommodate the needle used for infusion.

An advantage of direct delivery, via pellet, into the fat pad of the mammary gland is that the contralateral gland can be used as an internal control for systemic effects. If the observed effect of the hormone, growth factor, or cytokine is also obtained in the contralateral gland, the dose must be reduced until no effect is seen therein in order to be certain that one is observing direct effects in the treated gland.

Since some commercially prepared pellets contain fillers and binders, it is important that their reactivity be taken into consideration when designing an experiment. Be sure that the placebo pellet, inserted into the contralateral gland, contains all of the appropriate ingredients except the active agent being tested.

It is important to note that cholesterol itself is not inert. Our experience has shown that local cholesterol alone increased the EGF and prolactin binding activity in mammary gland membranes [7].

CONCLUSION

Cholesterol-based slow-release pellets can be used as an acceptable alternative to Elvax pellets for local delivery of hormones, growth factors, and cytokines to the mammary gland. Care must be taken to ensure that the dose is adjusted to prevent systemic effects and that cholesterol itself does not contribute to, or interfere with, the endpoint being examined. Use of cholesterol-based pellets is helpful for studies utilizing peptides that do not retain activity after exposure to harsh organic solvents.

REFERENCES

1. S. Z. Haslam (1988). Local versus systemically mediated effects of estrogen on normal mammary epithelial cell deoxyribonucleic acid synthesis. *Endocrinology* **122**:860–867.
2. S. D. Robinson, G. B. Silberstein, A. B. Roberts, K. C. Flanders, and C. W. Daniel (1991). Regulated expression and growth inhibitory effects of transforming growth factor-beta isoforms in mouse mammary gland development. *Development* **113**:867–878.
3. R. J. Collier, M. F. McGrath, J. C. Byatt, and L. L. Zurfluh (1993). Regulation of bovine mammary growth by peptide hormones: involvement of receptors, growth factors and binding proteins. *Livestock Production Sci.* **35**:21–33.
4. J. J. Rejman, D. A. Luther, W. E. Owens, S. C. Nickerson, and S. P. Oliver (1995). Changes in bovine mammary-secretion composition during early involution following intramammary infusion of recombinant bovine cytokines. *J. Vet. Med. B* **42**:449–458.
5. J. S. Archer, W. S. Kennan, M. N. Gould, and R. D. Bremel (1994). Human growth hormone (hGH) secretion in milk of goats after direct transfer of the hGH gene into the mammary gland by using replication-defective retrovirus vectors. *Proc. Natl. Acad. Sci. USA* **91**:6840–6844.
6. B. K. Vonderhaar (1987). Local effects of EGF, αTGF, and EGF-like growth factors on lobuloalveolar development of the mouse mammary gland *in vivo*. *J. Cell. Physiol.* **132**:581–584.
7. B. K. Vonderhaar (1993). Local effects of cholesterol carrier system on binding of lactogens and epidermal growth factor to the developing mammary gland. *Endocrinology* **133**:427–429.

Hormonal Stimulation of the Mouse Mammary Gland

Daniel Medina and Frances Kittrell

Abstract. The intent of this chapter is to illustrate the use of a pituitary isograft to provide hormonal stimulation of the mammary gland. This chapter describes the procedure for implanting the pituitary gland under the kidney capsule and the consequences of the grafted pituitary for normal development of the mammary gland and for facilitating neoplastic transformation induced by chemical carcinogens.

Abbreviations. terminal end buds (TEB); mouse mammary tumor virus (MMTV); dimethylbenzanthracene (DMBA).

INTRODUCTION

The growth of the mouse mammary parenchyma occurs predominantly postpuberty and is absolutely dependent on ovarian steroids (estrogen, progesterone) and growth hormone (reviewed in Ref. 1). The increased ovarian steroid hormone levels attained with the onset of puberty bring about allometric growth of the glandular epithelium. The elongation of the mammary ducts occurs by mitotic activity in the terminal end bud (TEB) and its subtending duct (2). In mouse strains with a functional ovarian luteal phase (e.g., C3H), the development of alveoli is subsequently superimposed upon the mammary ductal tree as a result of normal estrous cycles in the virgin mouse. In mouse strains without a functional luteal phase (e.g., BALB/c), alveolar development occurs infrequently in virgin mice. Under the stimulus of pregnancy, the mammary epithelium undergoes intense proliferation activity followed by alveolar differentiation driven by increased levels of estrogen, progesterone, adrenal steroids, and growth hormone; secondarily, increases of the lactogenic hormones, prolactin and placental lactogen, occur. This exquisite and precise control of mammary epithelial growth impacts subsequent tumorigenesis. In the absence of appropriate hormones at critical stages of development, tumorigenesis is blocked or delayed (reviewed in Ref. 3). Conversely, increased hormonal stimulation of the mammary epithelium enhances tumorigenesis induced by chemical carcinogens or mammary tumor viruses (4). Chapters 8 and 9 in this volume

Daniel Medina and Frances Kittrell   Department of Molecular and Cell Biology, Baylor College of Medicine, Houston, Texas 77030.

Methods in Mammary Gland Biology and Breast Cancer Research, edited by Ip and Asch. Kluwer Academic/Plenum Publishers, New York, 2000.

discuss alternative means of hormonally stimulating the mammary gland. This chapter describes the use of pituitary isografts to provide an enhanced hormonal environment and ovariectomy to provide a hormone-deficient environment.

PITUITARY ISOGRAFTS: TUMORIGENESIS

A single pituitary isograft transplanted under the kidney capsule of syngeneic female mice provides a continuous source of prolactin (Prl) that acts on the ovary, to stimulate estrogen and progesterone synthesis and secretion, and on the gland, to stimulate functional differentiation and DNA synthesis (3, 5). A pituitary isograft in place for 3–5 weeks increases circulating blood prolactin levels five times, progesterone levels seven times, and estrogen levels two times. The proliferation index, as measured by BrdU labeling, increased to 5% and 8% in ductal and alveolar cells, respectively, compared to 1% in ductal cells of age-matched virgins. As a consequence of this hormonal stimulation, the gland resembles that seen in a late pregnant mouse (Figure 10-1).

The effects of hormonal stimulation on mammary tumorigenesis are profound and are illustrated for BALB/c mice in Figure 10-2; these findings apply to most strains. Hormonal stimulation, whether achieved by pregnancy or a pituitary isograft, markedly enhances MMTV- and DMBA-induced mammary tumorigenesis. In the absence of viral or chemical carcinogens, hormonal stimulation of the mammary gland acts as a very weak carcinogen (3, 6); most likely, hormones are acting as promoters for DNA damage induced by endogenous sources.

The principal advantage of using a pituitary isograft compared to other means of hormonally stimulating the mammary gland is that it achieves a consistent and long-lasting stimulation of the mammary epithelium and requires only a single surgical intervention (at the time of implantation). In chemical carcinogenesis, the hormonal stimulation is required for a high frequency of initiation and for facilitating expression of the initiated cells (7). If the pituitary isograft is removed after DMBA treatment is finished, the mammary tumor incidence decreases by 50% (see Figure 1-2 in Chapter 1). If the pituitary isograft is implanted 6 weeks after carcinogen treatment, there is no significant enhancement in tumor incidence. The

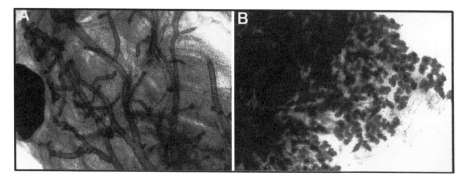

Figure 10-1. (A) Effect of a pituitary isograft on mammary development in the virgin mouse. Mammary gland from a mature virgin BALB/c female mouse. The gland is composed of mammary epithelial cells organized as ducts that ramify throughout the fat pad. (B) Mammary gland from a BALB/c female mouse 5 weeks after a pituitary isograft was transplanted under the kidney capsule. The gland is composed of mammary epithelial cells that have differentiated into alveolar cells and are organized in clusters of lobules. The density of the alveoli obscures the underlying ducts.

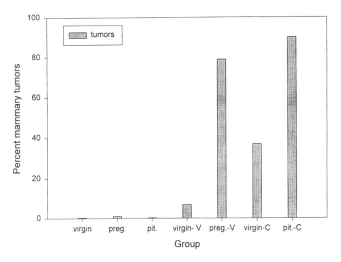

Figure 10-2. Mammary tumorigenesis in BALB/c mice. The mice arose from a breeding pair of BALB/cCrl mice and have been maintained as a separate inbred strain since 1970. The different groups are virgin, multiparous (preg.), and pituitary isograft containing (pit.). V = mice carrying exogenous MMTV; C = mice treated with 7,12-dimethylbenzanthracene. The tumor incidences in virgin, multiparous, and pituitary-isograft-containing BALB/c mice were obtained from mice 18–24 months of age. The tumor incidences in the mice carrying exogenous MMTV were observed at 12–15 months of age, and in mice treated with chemical carcinogen were observed at 12 months of age.

critical hormone appears to be progesterone, as is demonstrated in the original experiments by Jull (8), who showed that progesterone and estrogen, but not estrogen alone, were required for chemical-carcinogen-induced mammary tumorigenesis in ovariectomized mice. More recently, Lydon (4) demonstrated that DMBA-induced mammary tumorigenesis was significantly reduced in progesterone receptor knockout (PRKO) mice.

Materials

ISOLATION OF PITUITARY
- 11.5-cm and 14.5-cm scissors [Fine Science Tools (FST), Foster City, CA; 14060-11, 14001-14]
- $3\frac{1}{2}$ inch fine forceps (FST, 11063-07)
- Broad forceps (FST, 1030-12)
- Petri dish
- Phosphate-buffered saline

GRAFTING OF PITUITARY
- Anesthetic (Nembutal Sodium, Abbott Cabs)
- Shaver (Oster small animal clipper, No. 40 blade)
- 70% ethanol
- Trocar (18 gauge, $1\frac{1}{2}$ inch, BD1296)
- Antibiotic solution (AKSPORE, Bausch and Lomb Pharmaceuticals)
- Suture silk, size 4-0
- Autoclips 9 mm with applicator
- Dissecting scope

PITUITARY ISOGRAFT: METHOD (FIGURE 10-3). The procedure was originally established and publicized by Muhlbock and his laboratory (6) and has been used extensively (3, 5). It is easy to learn and, with practice, one can become proficient with it. We routinely perform the procedure as follows:

1. To remove donor pituitary (Figure 10-3A)
   a. Kill donor mouse, using cervical dislocation or CO_2. Donors may be male or female.
   b. Sever head from body, using a sharp pair of scissors to cut spinal cord at the base of the skull.
   c. Pull skin toward front of skull to expose top of the cranium.
   d. From the rear of the skull, cut along cranial suture lines and remove the inter-parietal, parietal, and frontal portions of the skull to expose the brain.
   e. Using broad forceps, gently grasp both cerebral hemispheres and remove the brain. This will empty the cranial cavity and visually expose the pituitary beneath.
   f. With very fine forceps, trace along the right and left edges of the pituitary gland to disrupt the membrane that holds the pituitary in place.
   g. Gently slip the ends of the forceps under the pituitary. Use the forceps tips to cradle the pituitary; do not try to use the tips to pick up the pituitary because the tissue is too soft and fragile to grasp.
   h. Place the pituitary in a petri dish containing PBS. You can collect up to 10 pituitary glands before starting implantation procedure.
2. Implantation of the pituitary under the kidney capsule of the host (Figure 10-3B–D)
   a. Anesthetize recipient mouse.
   b. Shave hair from one side of back.
   c. Swab with 70% ethanol or betadine.
   d. Make a posterior to anterior incision approximately 1.5 cm in length through the skin over the area of the kidney.
   e. Make a small (about 7–8 mm) incision in the abdominal wall over the kidney. The kidney should be visible through the body wall; the spleen is readily visible on the left side.
   f. Load the pituitary in the trocar (18 gauge, $1\frac{1}{2}$ inch BD1296), being careful to keep everything wet with PBS. (One or two pituitary glands may be loaded in the trocar.)
   g. Using a cotton swab, carefully roll the kidney out through the incision in the abdominal wall, and gently hold it in place between the cotton swab and your index finger (Figure 10-3B).
   h. Viewing through a dissecting scope or magnifier, use the point of a very sharp pair of forceps to make a small (1 mm or less) hole in the kidney capsule. A left-handed person will probably be most comfortable inserting the pituitary from the anterior end of the kidney, whereas a right-handed person will find the posterior end of the kidney most convenient.
   i. With care, insert the trocar containing the pituitary under the kidney capsule through the small hole you have made. The bevel of the trocar should be facing up. Insert the trocar far enough for the entire bevel surface to be within the capsule (Figure 10-3C). Hold the trocar level to avoid damaging the kidney or the capsule. Push the plunger of the trocar, to expel the pituitary

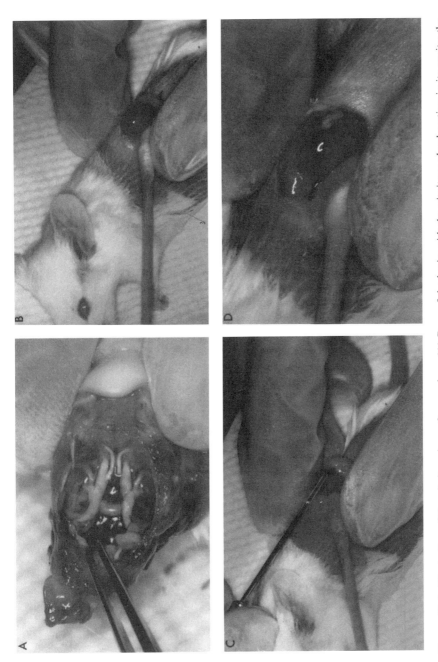

Figure 10-3. Illustration of the pituitary isograft procedure. (A) Base of the brain with the pituitary gland resting in its cavity, the sella turcica. The tip of the forceps point to the pituitary gland. (B) The kidney of the anesthetized mouse is exposed and ready to receive the trocar. (C) The trocar is shown with the beveled end completely under the kidney capsule. (D) The trocar has been withdrawn leaving the pituitary gland (the white body at tip of arrowhead) under the kidney capsule. (For a color representation of this, see figure facing page 106.)

under the capsule. Carefully extract the trocar, leaving the pituitary in place under the kidney capsule (Figure 10-3D).

j. Allow the kidney to roll back into the abdominal cavity. Deliver two drops of antibiotic solution (AKSPORE, Bausch & Lomb Pharmaceuticals, Inc.) into the abdomen. Sew one or two stitches to close the abdominal opening. Use two wound clips to close the transdermal incision.

k. The pituitary can remain in place for the lifetime of the animal. Over a period of months, the pituitary gland will exhibit hyperplastic, but not neoplastic, growth. The pituitary gland can be effectively removed at any time by cauterization of the implant.

PSEUDOPREGNANCY

An alternative method of hormonally stimulating the mammary gland to a state equivalent to midpregnancy is to induce pseudopregnancy by housing sexually mature females with an adult vasectomized male, who is allowed to remain in the cage throughout the experiment. With successful pseudopregnancy, the mammary glands, ovary, and uteri will appear histologically equivalent to pregnancy in the absence of embryo implantation and fetal development. The mammary glands exhibit extensive alveolar development, the ovaries show large corpora lutea, and the uteri show increased surface epithelium with numerous tortuous glands. Mammary tumor incidence in chemical-carcinogen-treated mice is significantly increased under the influence of pseudopregnancy (9).

OVARIECTOMY

Bilateral ovariectomy can be performed at almost any time postpuberty. At 5 weeks of age, the mammary epithelium has occupied approximately 50% of the mammary fat pad and is characterized by ducts capped by terminal end buds. Bilateral ovariectomy removes the source of estrogen and progesterone, resulting in a quiescent epithelium without terminal end buds. Depending on the age of ovariectomy, MMTV-induced mammary tumorigenesis is delayed significantly (3, 10). In addition, growth of some preneoplastic cell populations is significantly reduced (3).

The procedure is relatively straightforward:

1. Anesthetize mouse.
2. Shave hair from the back of the mouse; swab area with 70% alcohol.
3. Make a dorsal, posterior to anterior, midline incision through the skin (1.5 cm in length).
4. Make a 2- to 3-mm incision through the abdominal wall over the left kidney. The fat surrounding the kidney should be visible from outside the abdominal cavity.
5. With forceps, grasp the ovary and bring it outside the abdominal cavity. Cauterize through the left horn of the uterus just below the fallopian tube and allow the left horn of the uterus to slip back into the abdominal cavity. Use one stitch to close the interior incision.

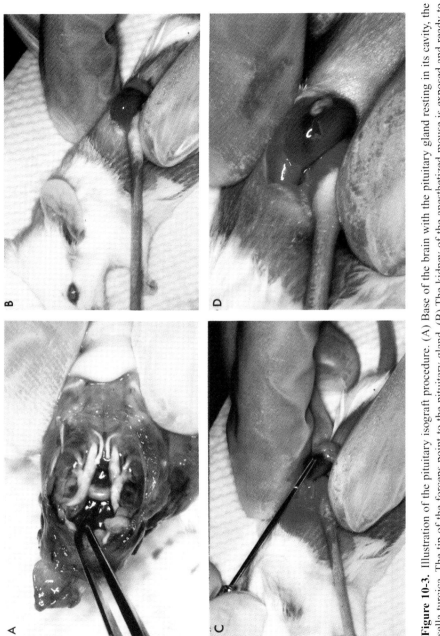

Figure 10-3. Illustration of the pituitary isograft procedure. (A) Base of the brain with the pituitary gland resting in its cavity, the sella turcica. The tip of the forceps point to the pituitary gland. (B) The kidney of the anesthetized mouse is exposed and ready to receive the trocar. (C) The trocar is shown with the beveled end completely under the kidney capsule. (D) The trocar has been withdrawn leaving behind the pituitary gland (the white body at tip of arrowhead) under the kidney capsule.

6. Repeat steps 4 and 5 to remove the right ovary. Add 2 drops of antibiotic solution before sewing the right abdominal incision.
7. Close external incision using two wound clips.

SUMMARY

All aspects of mammary development and tumorigenesis are affected by the absence or presence of hormones. The use of pituitary isografts to provide a prolonged hormonal stimulation of the mammary epithelium is easy, efficacious, and economical. Hormonal stimulation resulting from a pituitary isograft markedly enhances the susceptibility of the mammary epithelium to low doses of chemical carcinogens. With this system, factors that enhance or inhibit (e.g., p53 mutations) carcinogen-induced tumorigenesis can be readily studied in a single model system.

REFERENCES

1. W. Imagawa, J. Yang, R. Guzman, and S. Nandi (1994). Control of mammary gland development. In E. Knobil and J. D. Neill (eds.), *The Physiology of Reproduction*, Vol. 2, 2nd ed., Raven Press, New York, pp. 1033–1065.
2. J. M. Williams and C. W. Daniel (1983). Mammary ductal elongation: Differentiation of myoepithelium and basal lamina during branching morphogenesis. *Dev. Biol.* **97**:274–290.
3. D. Medina (1982). Mammary tumors. In H. L. Foster, J. D. Small, and J. G. Fox (eds.), *The Mouse in Biomedical Research*, Vol. IV, Academic Press, New York, pp. 373–396.
4. J. Lydon, G. Guoging, F. S. Kittrell, D. Medina, and B. W. O'Malley (1999). Murine mammary gland carcinogenesis is critically dependent on progesterone receptor function. *Cancer Res.* **59**:4276–4284.
5. K. Christov, S. M. Swanson, R. C. Guzman, G. Thordarson, E. Jin, F. Talamantes, and S. Nandi (1993). Kinetics of mammary epithelial cell proliferation in pituitary isografted BALB/c mice. *Carcinogenesis* **14**:2019–2025.
6. O. Muhlbock and L. M. Boot (1959). Induction of mammary cancer in mice without the mammary tumor agent by isografts of hypophyses. *Cancer Res.* **19**:402–412.
7. D. Medina (1974). Mammary tumorigenesis in chemical carcinogen-treated mice. II. Dependence on hormone stimulation for tumorigenesis. *J. Natl. Cancer Inst.* **53**:223–226.
8. J. W. Jull (1954). The effects of estrogens and progesterone on the chemical induction of mammary cancer in mice of the IF strain. *J. Path. Bacteriol.* **68**:547–559.
9. C. Biancifiori and F. Caschera (1962). The relation between pseudopregnancy and the chemical induction by four carcinogens of mammary and ovarian tumors in BALB/c mice. *Br. J. Cancer* **16**:722–730.
10. H. I. Pilgrim (1957). A method for evaluating tumor morbidity as applied to the effect of ovariectomy at different ages on the development of mammary tumors in C3H mice. *Cancer Res.* **17**:405–408.

Part III

In Vitro Model Systems

Chapter 11

Collagen Gel Method for the Primary Culture of Mouse Mammary Epithelium

Walter Imagawa, Jason Yang, Raphael C. Guzman,
and Satyabrata Nandi

Abstract. A method for culturing mouse mammary epithelial cells (MECs) within Type I collagen gels is described. This method is permissive for multifold growth, "ductlike" morphogenesis, and hormonal responsiveness. Subcutaneous mouse mammary glands are harvested, digested with collagenase, and epithelial cells obtained after Percoll gradient centrifugation. MECs are then mixed with neutralized, isosmotic collagen, which is pipetted into culture dishes and overlaid with culture medium after gel formation. Preparation of all serum-free medium and stocks required for the procedure and termination of cultures are described, and comments concerning critical procedural steps are given.

Abbreviations. mammary epithelial cells (MECs); medium 199 (M199); penicillin/streptomycin (pen/strep); Amphotericin B (Amp B); N-(2-hydroxyethyl)piperazine-N'-(2-ethanesulfonic acid) (HEPES); Dulbecco's modified Eagle's medium (DMEM); bovine serum albumin (BSA); Hanks' balanced salt solution (HBSS).

INTRODUCTION

Matrix-based primary culture of mammary gland epithelium is the *in vitro* method that best preserves *in vivo* responses in an *in vitro* setting. Although no *in vitro* system perfectly replicates the as-yet-undefined *in vivo* environment, collagen gel culture systems utilizing Type I collagen or a more complex biomatrix isolated from the EHS sarcoma (commercially available as Matrigel) are permissive for hormone-responsive cell proliferation, milk product synthesis, and three-dimensional morphogenesis (recently reviewed in Refs. 1 and 2). The use of Type I collagen gels for the culture of mammary epithelium was begun by Emerman *et al.* (3, 4), who observed that cells cultured on the top of floating collagen gels underwent morphological and functional differentiation in the presence of mammogenic hormones. Type I collagen gels provide two major functions: (1) the stabilization of epithelial-derived matrix molecules such as Type IV collagen, laminin, and fibronectin at the cell surface; and (2) a three-dimensional matrix for cell attachment and morphogenesis. Mouse MECs cultured within Type

Walter Imagawa   Department of Molecular and Integrative Physiology, University of Kansas Medical Center, Kansas City, Kansas 66160.   Jason Yang, Raphael C. Guzman, and Satyabrata Nandi   Department of Molecular and Cell Biology, Cancer Research Laboratory, University of California, Berkeley, California 94720.

Methods in Mammary Gland Biology and Breast Cancer Research, edited by Ip and Asch. Kluwer Academic/Plenum Publishers, New York, 2000.

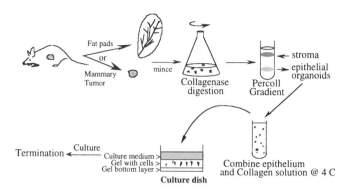

Figure 11-1. Overall scheme for the isolation and culture of normal and tumor mouse MECs within collagen gels. MECs obtained after the tissue dissociation procedure and Percoll gradient centrifugation are mixed with cold neutralized, isoosmotic collagen gel solution (kept on ice) at the desired cell density. The appropriate amount of collagen solution containing the cells is then pipetted into culture dishes containing preformed collagen gel bottom layers and allowed to gel at room temperature. After gelation, the gels are overlayed with culture medium. It takes 1 day to perform a dissociation and another 7–12 days of culture to assess proliferative responses to mitogens. Morphology is apparent after growth occurs, which is usually by 3 days of culture, depending on the growth conditions.

I collagen gels (5–8) undergo multifold growth, form three-dimensional colonies surrounded by basement membrane proteins, and are composed of cells joined by tight junctions arranged around a central lumen (9). Mouse MECs from virgin mice grown in the presence of a variety of mitogens will generate whole mammary glands when transplanted into cleared fat mammary pads *in vivo* and can be induced to synthesize milk proteins *in vitro* (10), indicating that stem cells and the luminal epithelial cell phenotype are preserved in collagen gel culture.

The intent of this chapter is to describe the enzymatic dissociation of mouse mammary glands and the culture of isolated epithelium within collagen gels as summarized schematically in Figure 11-1. The collagen gel system has been successfully used for the primary culture of mouse, rat (11, 12), and human breast epithelium (8). This protocol is optimized for mouse but is generally similar for other species. Previous accounts of this procedure (13, 14) as well as alternative descriptions of the isolation of mouse mammary epithelium have been published (15).

MATERIALS AND INSTRUMENTATION

1. Equipment
   a. Rotary-shaking water bath or environmental shaker with platforms containing holders for flasks (125–500 ml)
   b. Benchtop centrifuge (up to 3000 × g maximum) with swinging bucket rotor and holders for 50-ml conical and 5–30 ml round-bottom tubes
   c. High-speed centrifuge (up to 20,000 × g) with rotor for centrifuging bottles (at least 250 ml)
   d. Binocular, inverted stage, phase microscope with 4×, 10×, and 30× objectives

      e.   Laminar flow culture hood with 2-L vacuum flask and tubing for attachment of Pasteur pipettes

      f.   Lab counter (cell counts), hemocytometer

      g.   Cell culture incubator and carbon dioxide cylinder

2. For collagen preparation: rat tails, pliers, single-edge razor blades

3. Glassware and plasticware

      a.   Plasticware: sterile, disposable culture dishes (multiwell plates, petri dishes, flasks), media bottles, pipettes (1–25 ml), round-bottom snap-cap polystyrene test tubes (Falcon 5 ml, 12 ml), 50-ml screw cap, polypropylene conical centrifuge tubes (e.g., Falcon, Blue Max). For Percoll gradients: 30-ml round-bottom, screw-cap polycarbonate centrifuge tubes. These tubes are sterilized by soaking in 70% ethanol, the excess ethanol is removed by aspiration, and the tubes rinsed with M199 before use.

      b.   Glassware: All glassware is baked or autoclaved for sterilization. Trypsinization flasks (125–500 ml, Wheaton or Pyrex) sealed with heavy tin foil, screw-cap glass bottles (200 ml, 500 ml), 1-L volumetric flasks, beakers, 100-ml graduated cylinders, 4-L flask, small-bore 5 3/4-inch Pasteur pipettes.

4. Reagents and chemicals: All reagents are prepared with deionized, double-distilled water of the highest available quality.

      a.   Ethanol (70%), glacial acetic acid (0.017 M prepared from sterile water, and 4.3 M prepared as a nonsterile stock), sodium hydroxide (0.34 N and 1 N), HEPES, sodium bicarbonate, crystal violet, citric acid monohydrate

      b.   Percoll (Amersham Pharmacia Biotech, provided as a sterile solution, stored at 4°C)

      c.   Culture media and salt solutions (all powdered culture media are from GIBCO/BRL): Medium 199 (M199, Hanks' salts), Dulbecco's modified Eagle's medium (DMEM) containing 1 g/L glucose, Ham's F-12 medium, 10× Hanks' balanced salt solution (HBSS, Sigma H6136),

      d.   Antibiotics (all from Sigma Chemical Co.): Amphotericin B (solubilized no. A9528), streptomycin sulfate (no. S6501), penicillin G (no. P3032). Alternatively, premixed penicillin–streptomycin is available from Sigma and GIBCO/BRL.

      e.   Fraction V bovine serum albumin (Sigma Chemical Co., no. A-4503)

      f.   Enzymes: collagenase (Worthington Biochemical Corp. or Boehringer Mannheim and batch pretested), bovine pancreas deoxyribonuclease I (Sigma D-0876), pronase (Calbiochem, #53702)

METHODS

Reagent Preparation

1. Medium and collagen neutralizing mix

      a.   Medium 199 with HEPES buffer: To prepare 10 L of medium, combine powdered M199 (109.7 g), HEPES (23.8 g), and sodium bicarbonate (3.5 g) in 9.9 L of water. Add, while stirring, 1 N NaOH (approximately 65 ml) to pH 7.3. Adjust volume to 10 L and filter sterilize.

      b.   Serum-free culture medium: This medium is a 1 : 1 (v : v) ratio of Ham's F-12 and DMEM. For 10 L of medium combine in sequence while stirring F-12

(53.1 g), DMEM (49.9 g), HEPES (47.6 g), and NaCl (2.9 g) in 9.8 L of water. Add 100 ml of NaOH (1 N) and sodium bicarbonate (6.72 g) and adjust the pH to 7.4. Bring total volume to 10 L and filter-sterilize. This medium contains 20 mM HEPES buffer with a reduction in bicarbonate and is formulated for a 2% CO_2 atmosphere. Growth-promoting agents for MEC including hormones, growth factors, and lipids are enumerated and discussed in published studies (16–19).

    c. Neutralization mix for collagen gels: 10× HBSS with 200 mM HEPES. For 1 L, dissolve enough HBSS for 1 L of 10× and add 47.6 g HEPES while stirring. No bicarbonate is added. Add antibiotics, stir, and filter-sterilize. Aliquot and store at 4°C for immediate use or freeze at −20°C for longer storage. This solution can also be used for Percoll gradients, but a standard 10× HBSS buffered with bicarbonate is also suitable for this purpose.

2. Medium additives

    a. Antibiotics: pen–strep (respectively, 30 and 50 µg/ml final concentration) and Amp B (2 µg/ml final concentration). Dissolve one vial of Amp B in 100 ml of water for a 1 mg/ml, 500× stock. To make 100 ml of a pen (30 mg/ml)–strep (50 mg/ml) 1000× stock solution in M199, dissolve, in order, 5 g strep sulfate at 37°C, then add 3 g pen. Filter (0.4 µ) sterilize. All antibiotics are aliquoted and stored at −20°C.

    b. BSA stock (0.1 g/ml): To prepare 1 L of stock, 100 g of BSA is added to 900 ml of DME:F12 culture medium containing antibiotics and stirred gently at room temperature until the BSA dissolves. Titrate to pH 7.4 with 1 N NaOH (approximately 28 ml), adjust volume to 1 L, and spin at about *15,000 × g* (9000–10,000 rpm in GSA rotor of Sorvall RC-5B or equivalent) for 45 min. Recover the supernatant, filter-sterilize, aliquot, and store at 4°C.

3. Enzymes

    a. Collagenase is dissolved at a final concentration of 1% (10 g/L) in M199, aliquoted, and stored at −80°C. It is diluted to 0.05–0.1% for use. No centrifugation or sterile filtration is necessary.

    b. DNAse stock (0.40 g/L). Dissolve 0.12 g of DNAse in 300 ml M199 containing antibiotics. Filter-sterilize, aliquot, and store at −20°C. It is best to thaw immediately before use and not refreeze, to minimize loss of enzyme activity.

    c. Pronase stock (1250 U/ml, approximately 2.5%): Dissolve contents of one vial (50,000 U) in 40 ml M199 at 37°C. Filter-sterilize, aliquot, and store at −80°C.

4. Crystal violet solution (0.04%) for cell counting: Dissolve 2.1 g citric acid in 100 ml of water. Make a paste of 0.04 g of crystal violet with a few drops of 70% ethanol and combine with the citric acid. This solution can be stored for long periods at room temperature.

Preparation of Rat-Tail Collagen

We describe the preparation of Type I collagen from rat tails. If only a small amount of collagen is desired, it is also commercially available from Sigma (catalogue no. C-7661) and Upstate Biologicals Incorporated (catalogue no. 08-115).

1. Rat-Tail Collagen Preparation

    a. Rat tails are stored frozen (−20°C), then thawed and cleaned by soaking in 70% ethanol for approximately 30 min.

    b.   Beginning from the base of the tail, the tendons are collected with pliers being used to break off about a 0.5- to 1.0-inch section of the tail. As the tail breaks off, tendons from the removed segment will remain attached to the remainder of the tail. Using a razor blade, cut the trailing fibers from the tail into a preweighed petri dish. Repeat this procedure, working down the tail as far as possible.

    c.   Weigh the dish to obtain the weight of the tail tendons. The collected fibers can be stored frozen (−20°C) until use.

    d.   Sterilize the tendons by soaking in 70% ethanol for 15 min; do not store them in ethanol. Remove from ethanol and rinse in sterile water. If the fibers are knotted together, untangle and tease apart with fine forceps. This aids in solubilization in acetic acid.

    e.   Stir tendons in 0.017 M acetic acid (5 g tendons/L) in a sterile flask at 4°C for at least 48 h.

    f.   Centrifuge the collagen at 16,000 × g (ex. Sorvall GSA rotor, 10,000 rpm) for 1 h at 4°C to remove undissolved material. Decant the supernatant into sterile bottles and store in the refrigerator. The final collagen suspension should be a clear, viscous fluid.

2. Collagen dilution: The initial preparation of solubilized collagen needs to be diluted before use. The desired endpoint is the maximum dilution capable of forming a firm gel within several minutes at room temperature. This dilution is then used to prepare a working collagen solution.

    a.   Collagen dissolved in acetic acid will self-assemble, forming a hydrated gel when the pH is raised (20). A neutralizing solution is prepared to initiate gelation and adjust osmolarity. Working under sterile conditions, have the following solutions and test tubes on ice: 0.34 N NaOH, 10× HBSS (containing 200 mM HEPES). Prepare neutralizing solution by combining NaOH and 10× HBSS in the ratio of 0.9 part NaOH to 1.0 part HBSS and keep on ice. A previous protocol used 10× Waymouth's instead of HBSS (13). Waymouth's can be used; however, it forms a cloudy solution at 10×.

    b.   To start, prepare 1 : 1, 1 : 2, and 1 : 3 dilutions of collagen in 0.017 M glacial acetic acid and keep on ice. Collagen concentrations are, respectively, 50%, 33%, and 25%. On ice, combine 8.5 parts of each collagen dilution with 1.5 parts neutralizing solution and mix. The neutralized collagen solution should be red–violet, not yellow or dark purple. Pipette about 1 ml of each into a 12- or 24-well plate and leave at room temperature to gel. The neutralized collagen should gel within about 5 min at room temperature, yet remain ungelled when kept on ice for up to at least 10 min. The collagen gels should be firm enough for the plate to be inverted and tapped gently without disturbing the gel. It should be possible to pick up the released gel intact with flat-bladed forceps. The final pH of the gel is about 7.6–7.7, which is not detrimental to the viability or growth of the cells. Final osmolarity is about 300 mOsM. Choose the appropriate collagen dilution for use or prepare more dilutions to test.

Mouse Mammary Gland Dissociation Procedure

    See Figure 11-1 for an overview of the procedure. One can expect to recover about 3–5 million cells from all 10 mammary glands from a single virgin mouse. Cell yield from midpregnant mice is at least two- to three-fold higher.

1. Euthanize mouse by cervical dislocation. Place on back on a cork board and pin in place through feet.

2. Wet hair with 70% ethanol and expose all 5 pairs of subcutaneous mammary glands by performing a midline ventral incision through the skin. Additional incisions from the midline down each rear leg and below each ear facilitate the removal of the no. 4 and no. 1 fat pads, respectively. Pull the skin away from the body, exposing the attached mammary fat pads and pin in place.

3. Excise mammary glands, leaving lymph nodes and muscle (between the no. 2 and no. 3 thoracic glands) behind if possible. When excising the no. 1 pair of fat pads be careful not to include salivary gland tissue, which is darker in color than the mammary tissue.

4. Place tissue (5–7 gram lots) in a 10-cm sterile plastic petri dish and mince with a single-sided razor blade mounted in a paint scraper (sterilized by soaking in 70% ethanol and flaming). This is the easiest and most efficient way to mince the tissue. Chop tissue until it is uniform and oily in appearance. Approximately 0.5–1 mm pieces are desirable; uniformity in size is important and will give a more even digestion.

5. Transfer the minced tissue to a fluted flask containing M199 (10 ml/g tissue) containing BSA V (1–2.5 mg/ml) and antibiotics. To obtain adequate agitation during shaking, medium volume should not exceed about one third of the flask volume; e.g., for volumes >50 ml use a 250–500 ml flask.

6. Add the appropriate volume of 1% collagenase stock (or directly add lyophilized enzyme stored at −80°C) to achieve a final collagenase concentration of 0.05–0.1%, depending on the activity of the preparation determined during pretesting (see Comment 4).

7. Mix and shake in a gyratory water bath or environmental shaker at 37°C. Lower temperatures will inhibit enzyme activity and prolong the digestion time. Shaking speed will vary depending on flask size and digestion volume. The speed should be fast enough to cause thorough mixing yet not produce splashing of medium and tissue onto flask walls.

8. Check the completeness of digestion starting at 1 h by removing a 0.5-ml aliquot under sterile conditions for low-power (40× total magnification) microscopic examination, by using an inverted stage, phase microscope. At this time, the speed of shaking can be increased if digestion is very incomplete.

    a. The length of the dissociation depends on the "activity" of the collagenase and can vary from 1 to 3 h. In the digestate one will observe muscle (smooth translucent in appearance), nerve, blood vessels, and mammary epithelial tissue, which appear as grapelike cell clumps (midpregnant mouse) or pieces of duct (virgin mouse).

    b. The desired endpoint is an epithelial preparation in which more than 80% of epithelial organoids are free (appearing smooth bordered) of adhering stromal tissue including fat cells (Figure 11-2 and Ref. 13). No visible tissue pieces should remain. As a rule of thumb, if numerous smooth-bordered, stroma-free organoids are not visible when an aliquot of digestate is examined, then the digestion needs to continue.

9. When the digestion is satisfactory, transfer the tissue digest to 50-ml screw-cap, conical polypropylene centrifuge tube(s) and centrifuge for 3–5 min at 100 × g to pellet the epithelial organoids.

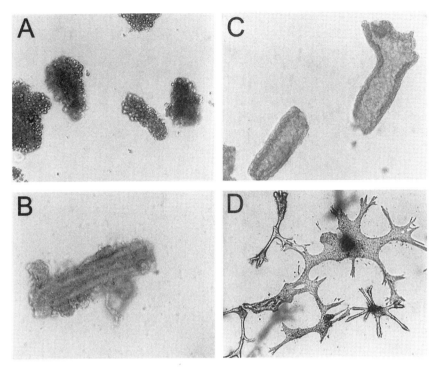

Figure 11-2. Phase contrast photographs of organoids obtained after collagenase dissociation of mammary glands from midpregnant (panel A) or virgin mice (panel B, C) (40× magnification). Panel B shows an epithelial organoid with associated stroma; panel C shows organoids freed of stroma. Notice the difference in morphology, ductal versus alveolar, respectively. If digestion is too long then the epithelial organoids will be reduced in size and damaged cells will degenerate during the initial culture period. Panel D is a phase contrast photograph of epithelial colonies growing within a collagen gel (19× magnification). Note the "ductlike" branching; the colonies contain a lumen around which the epithelial cells assume an apical–basal polarity.

10. Aspirate the collagenase solution and resuspend the pellet in the appropriate volume of M199; about 1–2 ml of M199 per Percoll gradient to be used in the following purification step. In general, 4 gradients are used for cell dissociations yielding 4–6×10^7 cells. If large organoids are present, then vigorous vortexing in a small volume (10 ml/50 ml conical centrifuge tube) for 10 s can be tried at this stage to break them into smaller pieces. No clumping of cells should be present; if cells have lysed and released DNA to produce a "stringy" clumping of organoids, then add sufficient DNase stock solution (0.1–0.5 ml) until all clumping disappears. This must be done prior to Percoll gradient purification to obtain proper banding of epithelial cells.

Percoll Gradient Enrichment of Epithelial Cells

Percoll, a colloidal silica solution coated with polyvinylpyrolidone, is used to generate density gradients for the purification of epithelial cells by isopycnic banding. It is adjusted to the proper osmolarity and diluted to the appropriate percentage Percoll before centrifugation to form the gradient.

1. Percoll gradients are prepared in 30-ml screw-cap, round-bottom polycarbonate centrifuge tubes. To each tube add 10.8 ml Percoll, 1.2 ml 10× HBSS, 16 ml of M199 and shake to mix thoroughly.
2. Centrifuge in a fixed angle rotor at *20,000 × g* for 60 min at room temperature. The midpoint density is about 1.055 g/ml. There should be about a 1–1.5 cm clear zone at the top of the gradient where Percoll has been essentially removed by sedimentation and about a 1.0-cm-diameter translucent plug of Percoll at the bottom of the tube. Gradients can be prepared and stored in advance if desirable. The manufacturer indicates that the preformed gradients are stable for months if the tubes are left undisturbed.
3. Layer a cell aliquot (in 1–2 ml, not exceeding 3×10^7 cells for best results) over premade Percoll gradients and centrifuge in a swinging bucket rotor at *800 × g* for 20 min at room temperature. When pipetting cells it is advisable to coat the pipette with BSA stock solution to reduce the sticking of organoids to the inner wall of the pipette.
4. After centrifugation, the muscle and stromal cells will remain near the top of the gradient while the epithelial cell organoids will band at a higher density of 1.05–1.07 g/ml near the bottom of the gradient, about 3/4 of the distance below the top of the Percoll solution. Below the epithelial band there will be a band of red blood cells and a band of lymph node fragments, if present.
5. Aspirate carefully the Percoll solution to the top of the epithelial band. With a 5-ml pipette precoated with BSA solution, collect the epithelial cells from one or more gradients and place in a 50-ml conical centrifuge tube. Dilute cells and Percoll to 50 ml with M199 and pellet the cells by centrifuging for 5 min at *100 × g*. Dilution of the Percoll by M199 needs to be sufficient to allow sedimentation of the cells at 100 × g.
6. Resuspend pellet in 10 ml of M199 and transfer to a 12-ml snap-cap, round-bottom, polystyrene tube (Falcon No. 2051) precoated with BSA to reduce sticking of cell organoids to the walls of the tube. Allow epithelial cell clumps to settle to the bottom of the tube by supporting the tube in a vertical position in a test tube rack. Collect the supernatant containing contaminating blood vessels, single cells, and very small epithelial cells clumps and discard. The settling procedure can be monitored by examining the tube through an inverted, phase microscope and varying the time of settling to achieve optimal results. Repeat this settling procedure several times if necessary.
7. Suspend the cells in M199 of sufficient volume to give at least 5×10^6 cells per milliliter. Count the cells and plate in ol on collagen gels or on collagen-coated plates.

Cell Counting

Epithelial cell organoids must be disrupted in order to perform a cell count. This is done by vortexing in citric acid containing crystal violet to stain the nuclei. The stained nuclei are then counted in a hemocytometer.

1. In a 10 × 75 mm round-bottom, polystyrene tube mix 0.05 ml of the cell suspension with 0.45 ml of crystal violet solution (1/10 dilution) and vortex at maximum

speed for 20 s. Examine the cell suspension using the low-power objective of an inverted binocular microscope to assess the degree of organoid disruption. Repeat as necessary, but be careful not to overdo the vortexing or nuclei may be disrupted and the cell number underestimated.

2. An aliquot of the nuclear suspension is then counted in a hemocytometer, and the cell count is corrected for the dilution factor (1/10).

Collagen Gel Culture

1. Prepare and keep on ice a neutralizing solution composed of a mixture of 0.34 N NaOH and 10× HBSS containing 200 mM HEPES in a ratio of 0.9/1.0 as done for the collagen titration. Enough mix is prepared to neutralize the required amount of collagen.

2. The surface of the culture dish is first covered with a "bottom" layer of collagen gel, which serves to prevent cell attachment to the surface of the dish when gel containing cells is added. Mix the appropriate volume of collagen with neutralizing solution in the standard ratio of 0.85 volume of collagen to 0.15 volume of neutralizing mix. This ratio may be slightly different (relative increase in amount of neutralizing mix to 0.17 volumes) if some lots of collagen do not form firm gels at the standard ratio.

3. Pipette the collagen solution into the desired culture plate at room temperature. For 24- or 12-well plates, 0.25–0.3 ml is sufficient, for 35-mm and 100-mm dishes, respectively, 2.0-ml and 5.0-ml bottom layers are sufficient.

4. Prepare the top layer containing cell organoids by adding cells to the desired volume of neutralized collagen and mix quickly by inverting the tube. The chosen cell density depends on the type of experiment being performed; e.g., we have used the following cell densities and cell numbers: for proliferation assays, 0.5 ml of collagen containing $1.5–2 \times 10^5$ cells (density of $3–4 \times 10^5$ cells/ml) is pipetted into each well of a 24- or 12-well plate. For experiments involving the examination of mRNA levels, up to 2×10^6 cells/ml and 5-ml total volume (total cell number of 1×10^7 cells) can be pipetted into a 100-mm dish.

5. After gelation is complete the gels are overlayed with culture medium: 0.5 ml for 24- or 12-well plates, and 10 ml for 100-mm plates containing cells at high density. Medium is changed every two days or more often if needed.

6. If it is desirable to plate cells on top of collagen gels, then a single layer of collagen gel is cast as described before. After gelation, the gels are overlayed with culture medium, and the desired number of cells is aliquoted into the culture vessel. Care should be taken to disperse the cells evenly over the surface of the collagen by shaking the dish in order to achieve optimum growth and spreading of the cells. If milk protein gene expression is of interest, the gels can be released after a period of growth by rimming the gel with sterile flat-bladed forceps. The cells will contract the gel. Original work describing this culture system can be found in publications by Emerman *et al.* (3, 4).

Recovering Cells from Collagen Gels

1. For DNA assay
   a. Transfer gels to 12×75 mm disposable round-bottom glass tubes with flat-bladed forceps (Millipore filter forceps are suitable).

b.   Add acetic acid (4.3 M) at a ratio of about 0.05 ml per 0.5 ml gel, mix, and incubate at 37°C. The gels will usually dissolve well within 20 min (time is not critical but needs to be sufficient).

c.   Pellet the cells (5 min at $100 \times g$), aspirate the medium, and resuspend the cells in about about 2 ml of 70% ethanol. After at least 2 h (it is convenient to leave them overnight) in ethanol the cells are pelleted and the ethanol aspirated.

d.   The cell pellet is dried and used directly for DNA assay by the fluorometric method of Hinegardner (21), using cells for standard curves.

2.   For recovery of viable cells

a.   Transfer cells to sterile tubes and add collagenase to 0.05% final concentration. If proteases are a concern, then Worthington has available a semipurified collagenase greatly reduced in protease activity.

b.   Shake at 37°C until the collagen is digested and pellet cells or colonies. The collagenase digestate is aspirated and the cells washed with M199 to remove the bulk of the residual collagenase.

c.   If subculture in collagen gels is planned, then the cells must be washed by sedimentation through Percoll in order to remove all traces of collagenase. This can be done by using smaller (10 ml) step Percoll systems consisting of a 27% neutralized, isosmotic Percoll solution (5 ml) layered over a smaller volume (3 ml) of a similarly prepared cushion of 38.5% Percoll in a 12-ml round-bottom polystyrene tube. Spin at $800 \times g$ for 20 min, during which the epithelial cells will migrate to the surface of the Percoll cushion with aqueous media remaining at the top of the gradient. Percoll above the epithelial cell band is then aspirated and the cells recovered and washed by resuspension in M199.

d.   Since the majority of recovered cells may be in the form of colonies it may be desirable to break up these colonies for passage or for injection into cleared mammary fat pads. This can be done in two ways. The cells (colonies) can be plated on plastic in serum-containing culture medium (or in an enriched serum-free medium) to cause monolayer formation before recovery of the cells by trypsinization in EDTA (22), or the colonies can be broken up by mild pronase digestion. The latter procedure is potentially more damaging to the cells if overdone.

COMMENTS

1.   Acid-solubilized collagen solutions will differ in concentration depending on the extent of solubilization of the tendons. This parameter is influenced by the age of the rats, which will vary; tendons from younger rats will solubilize more readily. The morphology and growth of cells are affected by collagen concentration or, more precisely, gel strength, which is a function of the extent of cross-linking in the polymerized collagen gel (23). The maximum growth response occurs at about 1–2 mg/ml collagen. Lesser concentrations cause very weak gels, higher concentrations (4–5 mg/ml) a stiff gel that impedes morphogenesis or the extension of "ductlike" structures and proliferation (23, 24). Prepare sufficient diluted collagen stock solution for use over at most a few months. This solution is advisable because storage of collagen over time in the refrigerator may result in some loss of

gelation potential; i.e., the collagen will form a looser gel than expected after performing the predetermined dilution and neutralization. If this occurs, retitrate the collagen and use a lower dilution and, if necessary, proportionately more neutralizing mix relative to collagen volume.

2. For isolating stromal cells the collagenase digestion can be stopped after about 30 min and the epithelial cells pelleted by gentle centrifugation. The stromal cells are recovered in the supernatant and pelleted by higher-speed centrifugation. The collagenase solution supernatant is then recombined with the partially digested epithelial organoids and the digestion is continued. The stromal pellet (containing fibroblasts, adipocytes, blood vessels, muscle, nerve) is washed twice with M199 containing 2 mg/ml BSA, to remove most of the residual collagenase, and plated on 10-cm culture dishes in F12/DME medium supplemented with serum. Step Percoll gradients prior to culture or differential plating can be used to remove contaminating epithelial cells. The upper band from Percoll gradients can also be recovered, washed, and plated in serum. However, the recovery of stromal, fibroblast-like cells can be low with this method. Nonadherent cells can be removed and the cells passaged. Verification of the nature of the stromal cell type and culture conditions affecting proliferation and differentiation need to be determined for each preparation.

3. Mammary tumors can be dissociated with collagenase, but more vigorous shaking is performed to physically enhance the breakup of the tissue. Usually a tumor is minced finely, centrifuged at $100 \times g$ very briefly, and the supernatant containing the blood cells is aspirated (17). The tissue is digested in 50 ml of M199 collagenase solution containing 5 ml of DNase stock solution. The progress of digestion is monitored by examining aliquots of the digest under a phase microscope. If after 2 h there are very large pieces of tissue, the cells can be pelleted and vortexed to break up the larger pieces of tissue. If this does not help then the organoids can be digested gently with pronase (0.05%) by shaking for 30 min at 37°C at a speed that just causes a gentle swirling motion.

4. The most important element of the whole procedure is the collagenase digestion. Collagenase lots are tested prior to purchase. Samples are tested for time of dissociation, quality of dissociation (bands on Percoll gradients), cell viability in culture, and proliferative response to a panel of growth-stimulating factors, including mammogenic hormones and growth factors. Most companies (Worthington Biochemical Corp., Boehringer Mannheim) have testing programs in which samples from current lots are made available. The desired collagenase activity is usually the highest available >250 U/mg with low tryptic activity <1 U/mg. In our experience it has not been possible to predict reliably the effectiveness of a collagenase based solely on predetermined proteolytic and collagenolytic activities. Both activities are required for tissue dissociation, and it is the balance between the activities of all of the digestive enzymes present in a crude collagenase preparation that determines its final usefulness for dissociating mammary gland tissue. If the collagenase contains damaging enzymatic activity, then there will be a halo of degenerating cells surrounding the cultured organoids within 24 h of culture and a noticeable lack of small cell projections emanating from the organoids that are a manifestation of cell attachment to the collagen. The inclusion of soybean trypsin inhibitor (10 μg/ml) in the culture medium can ameliorate this. Collagenase activity will change over time during storage (variable from lot to lot) probably due to

autodigestion. If this is significant, the amount of enzyme added to the dissociation as well as the time of the dissociation may have to be increased.

5. Banding of cells in Percoll gradients will depend on the completeness of the collagenase digestion. If the digestion is incomplete, then there will appear to be a "smear" of organoids, many with attached stroma, and contaminating cells from below the upper band to the lower band. Usually there is some smearing present consisting mostly of small pieces of blood vessels, single cells, and very small epithelial organoids present in the zone between the upper and lower bands. Some collagenase preparations leave an abundance of small blood vessels that can migrate into the epithelial band in the gradient. These contaminants will be recovered with the epithelial cells but can be removed by gravity settling of the organoids as described. In the worst case, underdigestion will result in only a faint lower band and a low yield of epithelial cells. If DNase pretreatment of the cell suspension is not done when necessary or cell lysis occurs during loading and running of the gradients, then a significant epithelial band will be prevented from forming. Instead, a clumping of organoids within the gradient will be observed. If this happens, the cells can be recovered, treated with DNase, and reloaded on new gradients.

6. The relative advantages and disadvantages of various *in vivo* and culture systems used for mammary gland studies, including the collagen gel system, have been discussed previously (25). In general, primary cell culture is more expensive, time-consuming, and subject to unknown variables introduced during tissue dissociation, and primary cells are more heterogeneous than cell lines. These difficulties must be weighed against the advantages of examining cells obtained directly from *in vivo* and cultured in an environment that is permissive for morphogenesis and hormonal regulation.

7. MECs from late pregnant or lactating mice are difficult to obtain and culture due to their advanced state of lactational differentiation and fragility. More MECs can be obtained from pregnant mice, but alveolar cells tend to degenerate more readily in serum-free, primary culture than ductal cells without adequate support from lipids and mitogens. The use of MECs from pregnant or virgin mice depends on the experimental purpose. Alveolar MECs derived from midpregnant mice differ from the predominantly ductal MECs from virgin mice in their mitogenic response to growth factors and hormones. One advantage of the collagen gel system is that the alveolar and ductal phenotypes are not completely lost *in vitro*, allowing the experimental manipulation of these distinct cell populations.

REFERENCES

1. C. Streuli and G. Edwards (1998). Control of normal mammary epithelial phenotype by integrins. *J. Mammary Gland Biol. Neo.* **3**:151–163.
2. T. Woodward, J. Xie, and S. Haslam (1998). The role of mammary stroma in modulating the proliferative response to ovarian hormones in the normal mammary gland. *J. Mammary Gland Biol. Neo.* **3**:117–131.
3. J. T. Emerman, J. Enami, D. R. Pitelka, and S. Nandi (1977). Hormonal effects on intracellular and secreted casein in cultures of mouse mammary epithelial cells on floating collagen membranes. *Proc. Natl. Acad. Sci. USA* **74**:4466–4470.
4. J. T. Emerman and D. R. Pitelka (1977). Maintenance and induction of morphological differentiation in dissociated mammary epithelium on floating collagen membranes. *In Vitro* **13**:316–328.
5. J. Yang, J. Richards, R. Guzman, W. Imagawa, and S. Nandi (1980). Sustained growth in primary culture of normal mammary epithelial cells embedded in collagen gels. *Proc. Natl. Acad. Sci. USA* **77**:2088–2092.

6. J. Yang, R. Guzman, J. Richards, and S. Nandi (1980). Primary culture of mouse mammary tumor epithelial cells embedded in collagen gels. *In Vitro* **16**:502–506.

7. J. Yang and S. Nandi (1983) Growth of cultured cells using collagen as substrate. In G. H. Bourne, J. F. Danielli, and K. W. Jeon (eds.), *International Review of Cytology*, Academic Press, New York, vol. 81, pp. 249–286.

8. J. Yang, A. Balakrishnan, S. Hamamoto, J. J. Elias, S. Rosenau, C. W. Beattie, T. K. D. Gupta, S. R. Wellings, and S. Nandi (1987). Human breast epithelial cells in serum-free collagen gel primary culture: Growth, morphological, and immunocytochemical analysis. *J. Cell. Physiol.* **133**:228–234.

9. S. Hamamoto, W. Imagawa, J. Yang, and S. Nandi (1987). Morphogenesis of mammary epithelial cells from virgin mice growing within collagen gels: Ultrastructural and immunocytochemical characterization. *Cell Differen.* **22**:191–202.

10. B. K. Levay-Young, S. Hamamoto, W. Imagawa, and S. Nandi (1990). Casein accumulation in mouse mammary epithelial cells after growth stimulated by different hormonal and nonhormonal agents. *Endocrinology* **126**:1173–1182.

11. J. Richards, S. Hamamoto, S. Smith, D. Pasco, R. Guzman, and S. Nandi (1983). Response of end bud cells from immature rat mammary gland to hormones when cultured in collagen gel. *Exp.Cell Res.* **147**:95–109.

12. M. McGrath, S. Palmer, and S. Nandi (1985). Differential response of normal rat mammary epithelial cells to mammogenic hormones and EGF. *J. Cell. Physiol.* **125**:1182–1191.

13. J. Richards, L. Larson, J. Yang, R. Guzman, Y. Tomooka, R. Osborn, W. Imagawa, and S. Nandi (1983). Method for culturing mammary epithelial cells in rat tail collagen matrix. *J. Tissue Cult. Meth.* **8**:31–36.

14. W. Imagawa, Y. Tomooka, J. Yang, R. Guzman, J. Richards, and S. Nandi (1984) Isolation and serum-free cultivation of mammary epithelial cells within a collagen gel matrix. In G. Sato, D. Sirbasku and D. Barnes (eds.), *Methods for Serum-Free Culture of Cells of the Endocrine System*, Alan R. Liss, New York, vol. 2, pp. 127–141.

15. W. Jones, R. Hallowes, N. Choongkittaworn, H. Hosick, and R. Dils (1983). Isolation of the epithelial subcomponents of the mouse mammary gland for tissue-level culture studies. *J. Tissue Cult. Meth.* **8**:17–25.

16. W. Imagawa, Y. Tomooka, and S. Nandi (1982). Serum-free growth of normal and tumor mouse mammary epithelial cells in primary culture. *Proc. Natl. Acad. Sci. USA* **79**:4074–4077.

17. W. Imagawa, G. Bandyopadhyay, M. Garcia, A. Matsuzawa, and S. Nandi (1992). Pregnancy-dependent to ovarian-independent progression in mammary tumors delineated in primary culture: Changes in signal transduction, growth factor regulation, and matrix interaction. *Cancer Res.* **52**:6531–6538.

18. W. Imagawa, G. K. Bandyopadhyay, and S. Nandi (1990). Regulation of mammary epithelial cell growth in mice and rats. *Endocrine Rev.* **11**:494–523.

19. W. Imagawa, G. Bandyopadhyay, and S. Nandi (1995). Analysis of the proliferative response to lysophosphatidic acid in primary cultures of mammary epithelium: Differences among normal and tumor cells. *Exp. Cell Res.* **216**:178–186.

20. B. Williams, R. Gelman, D. Poppke, and K. Piez (1978). Collagen fibril formation. *J. Biol. Chem.* **253**:6578–6585.

21. R. Hinegardner (1971). An improved fluorometric assay for DNA. *Anal. Biochem.* **41**:477–487.

22. R. Guzman, R. Osborn, J. Bartley, W. Imagawa, B. Asch, and S. Nandi (1987). In vitro transformation of mouse mammary epithelial cells grown serum-free inside collagen gels. *Cancer Res.* **47**:275–280.

23. J. Enami, M. Koezuka, and M. Hata (1985). Gel strength-dependent branching morphogenesis of mouse mammary tumor cells in collagen gel matrix culture. *Dokkyo J. Med. Sci.* **12**:25–30.

24. W. Jones and H. Hosick (1986). Collagen concentration as a significant variable for growth and morphology of mouse mammary parenchyma in collagen matrix culture. *Cell Biol. Int. Rep.* **10**:277–286.

25. B. K. Levay-Young, W. Imagawa, J. Yang, J. E. Richards, R. C. Guzman, and S. Nandi (1987). Primary culture systems for mammary biology studies. In D. Medina, W. Kidwell, G. Heppner, and E. Anderson (eds.), *Cellular and Molecular Biology of Mammary Cancer*, Plenum, New York, pp. 181–203.

Chapter 12

Chemical-Carcinogen-Induced Transformation of Primary Cultures of Mouse Mammary Epithelial Cells Grown inside Collagen Gels

Raphael C. Guzman, Walter Imagawa, Jason Yang, Shigeki Miyamoto, and Satyabrata Nandi

Abstract. A method is described for the chemical carcinogen induced transformation of mouse mammary epithelial cells cultured in three-dimensional collagen gels with defined mitogens. Transformation is assayed in this system by the transplantation of the carcinogen treated cells to the parenchyma free mammary fat pads of syngeneic female mice. Resultant mammary outgrowths are scored as to the development of morphologically distinct preneoplastic and neoplastic lesions. The phenotype and the nature of genetic lesions is greatly dependent on the mitogen used at the time of carcinogen exposure.

Abbreviations. epidermal growth factor (EGF); ductal hyperplasia (DH); hyperplastic alveolar nodule (HAN); hyperplastic outgrowth (HOG); lithium chloride (Li), mammary carcinoma (MCa); mammary epithelial cells (MEC); *N*-methyl-*N*-nitrosourea (MNU); progesterone (P); prolactin (PRL).

INTRODUCTION

A complex of hormones, growth factors, and diffusible signaling molecules regulate the growth, differentiation, and carcinogenesis of mammary epithelial cells (1). An area of major interest in mammary cancer research is the analysis of the role of these different mitogenic factors in the normal to neoplastic transformation (2, 3). Such analyses are difficult to perform in the animal because of the complex *in vivo* environment. In an attempt to understand the role of mammogenic hormones and growth factors in influencing the induction of mammary neoplasias of different phenotypes and genotypes, we have developed a defined serum-free cell culture system in which mouse mammary epithelial cells (MECs) can be grown, induced to differentiate and be neoplastically transformed with chemical carcinogens (4–7).

Raphael C. Guzman, Jason Yang, and Satyabrata Nandi   Department of Molecular and Cell Biology, Cancer Research Laboratory, University of California, Berkeley, California 94720.   Walter Imagawa   Department of Molecular and Integrative Physiology, University of Kansas Medical Center, Kansas City, Kansas 66160.   Shigeki Miyamoto   Department of Pharmacology, University of Wisconsin Clinical Science Center, Madison, Wisconsin 53792.

Methods in Mammary Gland Biology and Breast Cancer Research, edited by Ip and Asch. Kluwer Academic/Plenum Publishers, New York, 2000.

The elegant experiments of Emerman, demonstrating that mouse MECs cultured on top of collagen gels could be induced to undergo morphological and biochemical differentiation (8, 9) provided the impetus for the development of a system for the growth of MECs inside collagen gels. Yang, Enami, and collaborators first cultured mammary tumor cells (10) and later normal MECs (11) inside collagen gels. Imagawa developed serum free condition in which MECs could be demonstrated to grow in response to mammogenic hormones, growth factors, and diffusible signaling molecules (5).

By using the appropriate medium additives the MECs cultured inside collagen gels could also be induced to differentiate (6). Taken together, this series of findings provided evidence that it was luminal MECs that were being grown and differentiated and it could be demonstrated by transplantation to the gland-free mammary fat pad that the cells retained their original phenotype, either cancer or normal (12, 13).

DeOme and co-workers developed a method for the surgical removal of the mammary parenchyma in immature mice, providing a natural site for the transplantation of mammary tissues. They demonstrated by direct transplantation that a variety of hyperplasias had the potential to progress to neoplasias. They established criteria for the biological behavior of preneoplastic and neoplastic mammary tissues (14, 15). Subsequently, they found that enzymatic dissociation of mammary epithelial cells from mice either infected with the mammary tumor virus (16, 17) or treated with a chemical carcinogen (18) and transplanted to the gland-free mammary fat pad of syngeneic mice provided a means of detecting preneoplasias prior to the time they were morphologically apparent in the original mammary gland. Medina *et al.* (19) found that enzymatic dissociation of hyperplastic outgrowths and transplantation to the gland-free mammary fat pad enhanced tumorigenicity of the preneoplastic outgrowths. The development of these methods for the detection of preneoplasias or neoplasias in the relatively short period of two to three months, made it feasible to detect tranformants induced by chemical carcinogens in cultured MECs.

We have used the collagen gel culture system to transform MECs to preneoplastic and neoplastic states with either the direct acting chemical carcinogen N-methyl-N-nitrosourea (MNU) or the polycyclic hydrocarbon 7,12-dimethylbenz(a)anthracene (7, 13, 20). Transformation is assayed in this system by transplanting the control untreated MECs or the carcinogen-treated MECs to the parenchyma free mammary fat pads of syngeneic female mice. Resultant outgrowths are scored as to the development of morphologically distinct preneoplastic and neoplastic lesions (Figure 12-1).

We cultured mouse MECs in a collagen gel matrix with three different media containing mitogenic combinations of either progesterone plus prolactin (PPRL), epidermal growth factor (EGF), or lithium chloride (Li). Proliferation of MECs was approximately equivalent in all media. The MECs were treated with MNU and transplanted to the parenchyma free mammary fat pads of syngeneic female hosts. Ductal hyperplasia (DH), hyperplastic alveolar nodules (HAN), and mammary carcinomas (MCa), morphologically similar to those found in *in vivo* carcinogenesis studies, were observed following exposure of MECs *in vitro* to MNU and transplantation of host mice. The incidence of hyperplastic mammary lesions was high in the PPRL and Li groups compared to the EGF treated group. Predominantly HANs and primary MCa were induced in MECs cultured in PPRL or Li. The predominant lesions in the MECs cultured with EGF were DHs. Both HANs and DHs gave rise to MCa upon secondary transplantation. The morphology of the MCa arising from the hyperplastic outgrowths (HOG) from DHs or HANs was also different among the three groups. MCa from the EGF group were predominantly type A (mainly acinar structures), MCa from the Li group were predominantly type B (polymorphic, with solid cords of epithelia), and the PPRL group produced cystic adenocarcinomas with squamous metaplasia (2, 20). The activation of

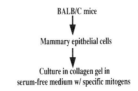

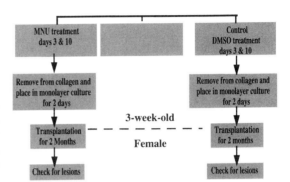

Figure 12-1. Diagram of the components used in the neoplastic transformation with chemical carcinogens of mouse mammary epithelial cells cultured inside collagen gels and transplanted to the gland-free mammary fat pads of host mice.

protooncogenes was dependent on the mitogens used during culture. Eighty percent of the HANs and MCas in the PPR1 group had an activation of c-Ki-*ras* by a G35 → A35 point mutation at codon 12. This mutation was detected in the preneoplasias and was considered to be an early event in carcinogenesis (21). Activation of c-Ki-*ras* was not detected in preneoplasias or MCas from the EGF or Li groups. However, MCas in the Li group were found to have an overexpressed novel transforming gene, MAT-1 (22). These results led us to postulate that the mitogenic environment around the time of carcinogen exposure determines the incidence and the phenotype of the resultant lesions as well as the molecular event associated with mammary carcinogenesis.

METHODS

Animals

Mice are BALB/cCrgl strain. The BALB/cCrgl strain does not express mouse mammary tumor virus and has a low spontaneous incidence of mammary hyperplasias and MCa (17). Three- to 4-month-old virgin female mice are sacrificed for mammary tissues. We estimate a yield of $3–5 \times 10^6$ MECs per donor mouse. Three-week-old female mice are utilized as transplantation hosts (10^6 MECs/host).

Mammary Gland Dissociation

See Imagawa *et al.*, Chapter 11 this volume (4) for a detailed description of the dissociation procedure and culture in collagen gels.

Materials: 0.1% collagenase (Worthington, CLS II, Freehold, NJ) in medium 199 (Gibco, Grand Island, NY); DNAase stock (0.4 g/L, Bovine pancreas deoxyribonuclease I, Sigma D-0876), Super-Mixer (Lab-Line Instruments, Melrose Park, IL); Percoll gradient (Pharmacia); 0.02% crystal violet (Sigma) in 0.1 M citric acid.

Remove all 10 mammary glands from mice, mince finely, and digest in collagenase for 2–3 h until the mammary organoids appear free of stromal components when examined at 25× magnification under an inverted microscope. Centrifuge the preparation at *200 × g* for 5 min, and resuspend the cells in medium 199 and centrifuge again. Aspirate the media, leaving approximately 5 ml including the cell pellet. Add a few drops of DNAase and resuspend the pellet in the medium by rapidly tapping the tube on the culture hood table. Mix the cells at fast setting for 5 s with a Super mixer in order to break up the larger clumps. The mechanical disruption of larger clumps is less harmful to cells than treating with proteolytic enzymes or pipetting. Purify the MECs by centrifugation through a Percoll gradient. Count the MECs by mixing 1 vol of cell suspension (50 μl) with 9 vol (450 μl) of crystal violet and counting stained nuclei in a hemocytometer.

Culture Media

Materials: 1 : 1 (vol/vol) of Ham's F-12 and Dulbecco's Eagle's medium (low glucose, Gibco/BRL); bovine insulin, bovine serum albumin fraction V, progesterone, linoleic acid, and lithium chloride (Sigma); EGF (Becton Dickinson); ovine prolactin (a gift from the National Institute of Diabetes, Digestive and Kidney Diseases, Bethesda, MD; order forms can be found in the back pages of the January issue of *Endocrinology*).

Supplement the basal medium with 10 μg/ml of insulin and 5 mg/ml bovine serum albumin fraction V. The medium is further supplemented with either 10 ng/ml EGF, a combination of 5 ng/ml progesterone plus 1 μg/ml prolactin plus 10 μg/ml linoleic acid, or 5 mM lithium chloride.

Culture

Materials: Collagen solution; 75 cm^2 Corning tissue culture flask (Corning Glass Works)

Place 4 ml of isosmotic neutralized collage in the bottom of the flasks and allow to gel. Mix MECs (10^7/flask) with 6 ml isosmotic neutralized collagen mixture and overlay on the gelled collagen bottom layer and allow to gel. Feed the cultures with 10 ml of the prepared medium every 2 days.

Carcinogen Treatment

Materials: MNU and dimethylsulfoxide (Sigma); medium 199 (pH 6).

Aliquot the MNU into tared glass vials with caps and weigh and keep on ice in the dark. Dissolve the MNU in dimethylsulfoxide at 10 mg/ml and add to medium 199 containing no additives, to a final concentration of 100 μg/ml. A concentration of 100 μg/ml MNU is slightly cytotoxic in this culture system; cytotoxicity should first be determined for other culture systems. All procedures are performed in a dark tissue culture hood. Aspirate media from the cultures and treat with 10 ml of MNU in media within 5 min of preparation. Incubate the cultures with the MNU media in the CO_2 incubator at 37°C for 1 h and then replace the media with the growth media. Optimal results have been obtained by treatment with MNU-both on day 3 and on day 10 of culture (7). Treat control cell with dimethylsulfoxide only in medium 199 and maintain for the same period as MNU treated cultures. MNU-containing media can be decontaminated by the slow addition of 0.1 N NaOH. MNU decomposes at alkaline pH resulting in an exothermic reaction.

Recovery of MECs from Collagen Gels

Materials: 10% porcine serum (Sterile Systems, Ogden, UT); 0.1% collagenase; 0.04% DNAase; 100-mm tissue culture plates (Corning); 0.05% trypsin (Worthington) and 0.025% versene (Sigma) in Puck's Saline A.

Seven to 10 days after the second MNU treatment feed the cultures with basal medium supplemented with 10% porcine serum One day later remove the entire collagen gel containing MEC colonies from the flask by means of a 9-inch Pasteur pipette with a bent tip. Place the gels in 10 ml of collagenase per 75 cm^2 gel. Dissolve the collagen gels by gentle shaking at 37°C for approximately 30 min. Colonies of MECs remain nearly intact after this treatment. To prepare MECs suitable for transplantation, wash the colonies and centrifuge twice in medium 199 containing a few drops of DNAase. Resuspend the cell pellet in 10 ml of basal medium supplemented with 10% porcine serum per collagen gel and plate in tissue culture plates. Within 2 days after plating, the cells attach and spread, forming a monolayer. Remove the MECs from the monolayer by aspirating the media and treating with trypsin–versene for 10–15 min at 37°C. Wash the detached single cells and small clumps of cells twice in medium 199 containing a few drops of DNAase and collect by centrifugation. Suspend an aliquot of MECs in 0.02% crystal violet and count nuclei in a hemocytometer. Suspend the MECs in medium 199 with a few drops of added DNAase at a concentration of 5×10^7 MEC/ml so that 10 μl containing 5×10^5 MECs can be injected into each parenchyma-free mammary fat pad.

Transplantation Assay for Transformation

See Young, Chapter 6 in this volume (23) for details of surgical removal of the mammary parenchyma.

Materials: Cautery (1 ELE 8-2 low-power transformer, 1 ELE 8-4 cautery pencil handle, and ELE 9-1 eye platinum tip 1-inch shank, Arista Surgical Supply Co., NY); 100 μl Hamilton No. 710SN (Hamilton Co. Reno, NV) syringe fitted with a 30-gauge needle 0.5 inch long; 0.04% DNAase; 0.5% trypan blue (Sigma) in 0.9% NaCl; (fine microdissecting scissors RS-5802, microdissecting tweezers RS-4980, Roboz Surgical Instrument Co., Rockville, MD).

The host animals are 3-week-old BALB/cCrgl female mice. The mammary gland rudiments are removed from the inguinal mammary fat pads by means of cautery. The injections of MECs are made by means of a Hamilton syringe. Prior to use sharpen the edges of the tip of the needle on a hard whetstone to make the tip more pointed. Rinse the syringe with DNAase and fill with 10 μl of the MEC suspension. Insert the needle near the cut edge of the mammary fat pad and push into the fat pad until it reaches the approximate middle of the fat pad and inject the MECs. Eight to 10 weeks after transplantation, inject the host mice with 0.75 ml of trypan blue i.p. and the following day examine the outgrowths in an anesthetized host under a dissecting microscope at 5–10× magnification. This procedure improves the contrast between stromal and epithelial elements and permits the tentative identification and classification of mammary outgrowths as to normal ducts, hyperplasias, or tumors. If hyperplastic or tumorous outgrowths are not visible the mice can be returned to their cages and examined again in several weeks. We have not observed any toxicity of the trypan blue at the concentration used. MECs grown inside collagen gels with any of the media used and treated only with dimethylsulfoxide produce only ductal outgrowths that are morphologically identical to the pattern of normal ducts seen in the host's own mammary glands. MECs grown inside

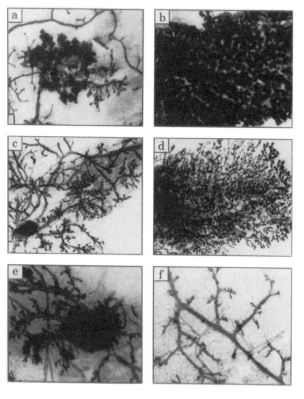

Figure 12-2. Wholemounts of mammary lesions induced in culture with MNU. (a) A primary hyperplastic alveolar nodule, 10×. (b) a secondary hyperplastic outgrowth resulting from the transplantation of a hyperplastic alveolar nodule, 10×. (c) A primary ductal hyperplastic outgrowth at the center of the mammary fat pad, 7×. (d) A secondary ductal hyperplastic outgrowth resulting from the transplantation of a ductal hyperplasia, 7×. (e) A subgross mammary carcinoma at the center of the fat pad, 15×. (f) Normal ductal outgrowth, 15×. Note the presence of both hyperplastic preneoplasias and normal ducts in the primary transplants.

collagen gels and treated with MNU produce a variety of outgrowths that are morphologically distinct from the pattern of outgrowths from control MECs or from the host's mammary glands. The primary outgrowths following the injection of MNU treated MECs contained mixed outgrowths containing areas of ducts that were morphologically identical to those from untreated MECs, areas of ductal hyperplasia, lobuloalveolar hyperplasias or HANs, and MCa (Figure 12-2). When culture conditions and transplantation is optimal from 10% to 100% of the mammary epithelial cells from carcinogen treated cultures will contain areas of hyperplasia and/or Mca.

To test for their neoplastic potential ~1-mm³ pieces of selected hyperplasias or tumors can be cut with fine scissors and forceps and secondarily transplanted to the parenchyma free mammary fat pads of host mice. Transplantation of primary preneoplastic outgrowths result in the production of a HOG which can completely fill the mammary fat pad and in which MCa will occur (Figure 12-3). The MCa producing capabilities of outgrowths can be expressed as the number of weeks required to attain the 50% MCa endpoint or as the percentage of outgrowths that develop MCa within a given time period.

Preparation of Mammary Whole Mounts

See S. B. Rasmussen *et al.*, Chapter 7 this volume (24).

Materials: Tissue-Tek Capsules (Miles); methacarn (60% methanol, 30% chloroform, 10% acetic acid); acetone, 100%, 95% and 70% ethanol; iron hematoxylin (4 L 95% ethanol,

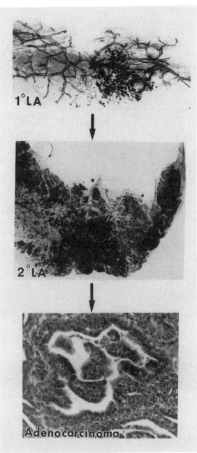

Figure 12-3. Photograph illustrating the progression of a primary hyperplastic alveolar nodule to a mammary carcinoma. The top panel (7×) shows an hyperplastic outgrowth containing morphologically normal ducts with an area of lobuloalveolar hyperplastic outgrowth (1° LA) in the lower right quadrant. Pieces of the primary hyperplastic nodule are secondarily transplanted to the parenchyma free mammary fat pad of a secondary host. The middle panel (7×) shows that the transplanted piece of primary hyperplasia completely fills the mammary fat with hyperplastic outgrowth (2° LA). Within the hyperplastic outgrowth a focal area of increased density occurs (arrow). The bottom panel is a histological section (200×) of the dense area (200×) showing that within the hyperplastic outgrowth a mammary carcinoma formed, demonstrating the preneoplastic nature of the primary hyperplasia.

2.6 g FeCl₃ in 270 ml H₂O 682.5 ml 1 N HCl, 4.4 g hematoxylin, EM Science, Cherry Hill, NJ); Histo-clear (National Diagnostics, Manville, NJ)

At termination, remove the injected inguinal mammary fat pads and a part of the host's thoracic mammary gland and spread as flat as possible in Tissue-Tek capsules, fix in methacarn for 12 h, defat in acetone for 12 h, wash in 95% and 70% ethanol for 1 h each, stain in two changes of iron hematoxylin, wash in running water for 1 h, dehydrate in 95% ethanol followed by two changes in 100% ethanol for 1 h each, and place in Histo-clear for 1 h and store in fresh Histo-clear. To confirm the identification and classification of outgrowths, examine the wholemounts, clean of extraneous tissues and photograph under a dissecting microscope with diffuse lighting from beneath the specimen. Place the whole mount on a cover slip and immerse the cover slip and whole mount in methylsalicylate in a glass dish. Methylsalicylate has a better refractive index for photography. Pieces of outgrowths can be cut out of the whole mount for preparation of histological slides or for analysis of genetic changes.

Analysis of DNA from Mammary Whole Mounts

Materials: 100%, 70%, and 50% ethanol; digestion buffer (100 mM Tris pH 8.0, 40 mM EDTA, 10 mM NaCL, 1% sodium dodecyl sulfate (Sigma), 500 µg/ml proteinase K (Gibco);

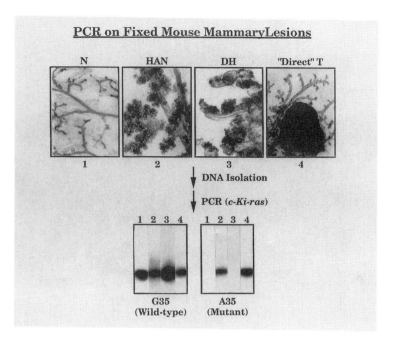

Figure 12-4. Photograph showing the results of the polymerase chain reaction analysis of DNA extracted from fixed and stained mammary wholemounts for the presence of a G35 to A35 transitional mutation in *c*-Ki-*ras*. Lane 1 contains DNA from normal ducts (N), Lane 2 contains DNA from hyperplastic alveolar nodules (HAN), Lane 3 contains DNA from a ductal hyperplasia (DH), and Lane 4 contains DNA from a subgross mammary carcinoma (Direct T). Note that only the HAN and the mammary carcinoma have the A35 mutation.

sodium acetate; phenol; phenol: chloroform: isoamylalcohol (25 : 24 : 1); chloroform: isoamylalcohol (24 : 1); TE buffer (10 mM Tris, pH 8.0 and 1 mM EDTA).

Extract DNA from preneoplasias or MCa in whole mounts by cutting out the lesions with fine scissors, mince the tissues with a razor blade, weigh the tissue, and wash twice with sterile distilled water to remove fixative (25). Rehydrate approximately 1 mg tissue pieces in serial changes of 100%, 70%, and 50% ethanol and wash once with sterile distilled water. Digest the tissue in 0.3 ml digestion buffer at 48°C for 24 h with occasional mixing. Increase the SDS and proteinase concentrations to a final concentration of 2% and 1 mg/ml respectively and incubate for another 48 h. Add sodium acetate to a final concentration of 0.25 M and extract the mixture twice with phenol, once with phenol: chloroform: isoamylalcohol and once with chloroform: isoamylalcohol. Precipitate the high molecular weight DNA with two volumes of ice cold 100% ethanol, wash with 70% ethanol, driy and resuspend in TE buffer. Figure 12-4 illustrates the result of DNA extracted from different hyperplasias in mammary whole mounts and subjected to polymerase chain reaction amplification and allele specific oligonucleotide hybridization for the analysis of mutations in *c*-Ki-*ras*.

CONCLUSION AND FUTURE DIRECTIONS

The collagen gel culture system for the transformation of mouse mammary epithelial cells provides a distinct opportunity to study the events of carcinogenesis. In this system, (i) mammary epithelial cells can be cultured with or without stromal components (26, 27), (ii) the direct effects of different hormones and growth factors on transformation can be studied, (iii) the molecular effects of carcinogens can be studied, (iv) the cellular origins of mammary cancers observed *in vivo* can be determined, and (v) the effect of hormones and growth factors on the metabolism to proximate carcinogens or on repair protein activity can be assayed (28–30).

Kittrell *et al.* (31) have used mouse MECs cultured in collagen gels for a short period of time and treated with the chemical carcinogen 7,12-dimethylbenz(*a*)anthracene followed by transplantation to the mammary fat pad to develop immortalized MEC lines that have a wide spectrum of neoplastic potential and different morphologic patterns of outgrowths. These lines have proven utility in analyzing the sequential events evolved in mammary carcinogenesis (32). Additionally the lines have been useful in testing the oncogenic capability of novel genes found in mammary cancers (22).

It would be of great interest to study the effect of null mutations of specific steroid receptors (33, 34) on the role of hormones and growth factors on the types of neoplasia produced in this culture system. The large variety of transgenic mice with varied patterns of growth and neoplastic potential now available also provide systems that might yield new insights into carcinogenesis when analyzed in this culture system (35).

Laduca and Sinha (36) have treated monolayers of rat MECs with MNU and then embedded the cells in collagen gels. They reported that microtumors, identified by histological analysis, formed in the gels. No further characterization has been forthcoming following this intriguing observation.

Great progress has been made in culturing rat MECs using reconstituted basement membrane (37). In this culture system, insulin, prolactin, progesterone, and EGF are required for optimal proliferation. With the optimal additives, MECs form distinct patterns of ductal branching or alveolar morphogenesis and undergo differentiation with synthesis of milk proteins and lipids. The optimization of culture conditions for rat MECs should enhance the feasibility of developing an *in vitro* transformation system. Transformed rat MECs could be assayed for by transplantation to the mammary fat pads (38) or subscapular fat pads of syngeneic hosts (39) or by xenografts to the mammary fat pads of nude mice (40).

Transformation of human breast epithelial cells with chemical carcinogens has been an extremely rare event (41). A major problem has been the lack of culture conditions for the successful propagation of human cells with a true luminal phenotype. Recent progress in developing selective media for the propagation of normal luminal epithelial cells and breast cancer cells and for the cultivation of selective lineages has greatly improved these model systems (42, 43).

The xenograft transplantation of human breast cancer cells to nude mice has been greatly improved by the co-injection of reconstituted basement membrane (44) or collagen gel (45). The success rate of transplantation of human breast cancers is greatly increased and tumor growth and metastasis enhanced when transplanted with basement membrane. The transplantation in collagen gels of human breast epithelial cells from reduction mammoplasties, presumed to be normal, always results in short tubular structures with a normal histomorphology. Transplantation of breast epithelial cells from breast cancer specimens results in outgrowths with an invasive pattern infiltrating the collagen as well as invasion into vascular spaces, nerves, and muscles. This pattern of malignancy is observed before the cancer reaches a palpable stage. Such assays should greatly aid studies involving the characterization of human luminal breast epithelial cells exposed to chemical carcinogens in culture.

ACKNOWLEDGMENTS. We thank Carol Slatten and Judith Yee for administrative assistance and Yu Chien Chou and Jerry Kapler for aid in the preparation of figures. We gratefully acknowledge Rebecca Osborn-Coolidge for the many contributions to the transformation project. This research was supported by NCI grants CA05388 and CA63369.

REFERENCES

1. W. Imagawa *et al.* (1994). Control of mammary gland development. In E. Knobil and J. D. Neill (eds.), *The Physiology of Reproduction*, vol. 2, 2nd ed., Raven Press, New York, pp. 1033–1065.
2. S. Nandi, R. C. Guzman, and J. Yang (1995). Hormones and mammary carcinogenesis in mice, rats, and humans: A unifying hypothesis. *Proc. Natl. Acad. Sci. USA* **92**:3650–3657.
3. I. H. Russo and J. Russo (1996). Mammary gland neoplasia in long-term rodent studies. *Environ. Health Persp.* **104**:938–967.
4. W. Imagawa, J. Yang, R. Guzman, and S. Nandi (2000). Collagen gel method for the primary culture of mouse mammary epithelium. Chapter 11 this volume.
5. W. Imagawa, G. K. Bandyopadhyay, and S. Nandi (1990). Regulation of mammary epithelial cell growth in mice and rats. *Endocrine Rev.* **11**:494–523.
6. B. K. Levay-Young, G. K. Bandyopadhyay, and S. Nandi (1987). Linoleic acid, but not cortisol, stimulates accumulation of casein by mouse mammary epithelial cells in serum-free collagen gel culture. *Proc. Natl. Acad. Sci. USA* **84**:8448–8452.
7. S. Miyamoto *et al.* (1988). Neoplastic transformation of mouse mammary epithelial cells by *in vitro* exposure to *N*-methyl-*N*-nitrosourea. *Proc. Natl. Acad. Sci. USA* **85**:477–481.
8. J. T. Emerman and D. R. Pitelka (1977). Maintenance and induction of morphological differentiation in dissociated mammary epithelium on floating collagen membranes. *In Vitro* **13**:316–328.
9. J. T. Emerman *et al.* (1977). Hormonal effects on intracellular and secreted casein in cultures of mouse mammary epithelial cells on floating collagen membranes. *Proc. Natl. Acad. Sci. USA* **74**:4466–4470.
10. J. Yang *et al.* (1979). Sustained growth and three-dimensional organization of primary mammary tumor epithelial cells embedded in collagen gels. *Proc. Natl. Acad. Sci. USA* **76**:3401–3405.
11. J. Yang *et al.* (1980). Sustained growth in primary culture of normal mammary epithelial cells embedded in collagen gels. *Proc. Natl. Acad. Sci. USA* **77**:2088–2092.
12. R. C. Guzman *et al.* (1982). Transplantation of mouse mammary epithelial cells grown in primary collagen gel cultures. *Cancer Res.* **42**:2376–2383.
13. R. C. Guzman *et al.* (1987). *In vitro* transformation of mouse mammary epithelial grown serum-free inside collagen gels. *Cancer Res.* **47**:275–280.
14. D. Medina (1973). Preneoplastic lesions in mouse mammary tumorigenesis. In H. Busch (ed.), *Methods in Cancer Research*, Academic Press, New York, pp. 3–53.
15. D. Medina (1996). The mammary gland: A unique organ for the study of development and tumorigenesis. *J. Mammary Gland Biol. Neoplasia* **1**:5–20.
16. K. B. DeOme *et al.* (1978). Detection of inapparent nodule-transformed cells in the mammary gland of virgin female BALB/cfC3H mice. *Cancer Res.* **38**:2101–2111.
17. K. B. DeOme *et al.* (1980). A survey of mouse mammary tissues from eight strains and two hybrid for the presence of nodule-transformed cells. In C. McGrath, M. J. Brennan, and M. A. Rich (eds.), *Cell Biology of Breast Cancer*, Academic Press, New York, pp. 79–91.
18. R. C. Guzman, R. C. Osborn, and K. B. DeOme (1981). Recovery of transformed nodule and ductal mammary cells from carcinogen treated C57BL mice. *Cancer Res.* **41**:1808–1811.
19. D. Medina, F. Shepherd, and T. Gropp (1978). Enhancement of the tumorigenicity of preneoplastic mammary lines by enzymatic dissociation. *J. Natl. Cancer Inst.* **60**:1121–1126.
20. S. Nandi, R. C. Guzman, and S. Miyamoto (1992). Hormones, cell proliferation, and mammary carcinogenesis. In J. Li, S. Nandi, and S. Li (eds.), *Hormonal Carcinogenesis*, Springer, New York, pp. 73–77.
21. S. Miyamoto *et al.* (1990). Transforming *c*-K-*ras* mutation is an early event in mouse mammary carcinogenesis induced *in vitro* by *N*-methyl-*N*-nitrosourea. *Mol. Cell Biol.* **10**:1593–1599.
22. T. K. Bera *et al.* (1994). Identification of a mammary transforming gene (MAT1) associated with mouse mammary carcinogenesis. *Proc. Natl. Acad. Sci. USA* **91**:9789–9793.
23. L. J. T. Young (2000). The cleared mammary fat pad and the transplantation of mammary gland morphological structures and cells. Chapter 6 this volume.

24. S. B. Rasmussen, L. J. T. Young, and G. H. Smith (2000). Preparing mammary gland whole mounts from mice. Chapter 7 this volume.

25. D. Shibata, W. J. Martin, and N. Arnheim (1988). Analysis of DNA sequences in forty year old paraffin embedded thin tissue sections: a bridge between molecular biology and classical histology. *Cancer Res.* **48:**4564–4566.

26. T. L. Woodward, J. W. Xie, and S. Z. Haslam (1998). The role of mammary stroma in modulating the proliferative response to ovarian hormones in the normal mammary gland. *J. Mammary Gland Biol. Neoplasia* **3:**117–132.

27. J. Xie and S. Z. Haslam (1997). Extracellular matrix regulates ovarian hormone dependent proliferation of mouse mammary epithelial cells. *Endocrinology* **138:**2466–2473.

28. R. C. Guzman *et al.* (1988). Metabolism of 7,12-dimethylbenz(a)anthracene by mouse mammary epithelial cells cultured serum free inside collagen gels. *Cancer Lett.* **40:**123–132.

29. T. A. Dutta-Choudhury, B. H. Bak, and R. C. Guzman (1991). Cellular levels of O^6-methylguanine-DNA-methyltransferase in mammary epithelial cells and liver from virgin, pregnant, and pituitary grafted mice. *Carcinogenesis* **12:**1795–1800.

30. M. A. M. S. Hamdan *et al.* (1992). Depletion of O^6-alkylguanine-DNA-alkyltransferase by O^6-benzylguanine in three-dimensional collagen cultures of normal human breast epithelial cells. *Carcinogenesis* **13:** 1743–1749.

31. F. S. Kittrell, C. J. Oborn, and D. Medina (1992). Development of mammary preneoplasias *in vivo* from mouse mammary cell lines *in vitro*. *Cancer Res.* **52:**1924–1932.

32. D. Medina (1996). Preneoplasia in mammary tumorigenesis. In R. Dickson and M. Lippman (eds.), *Mammary Tumor Cell Cycle, Differentiation, and Metastasis*, Kluwer Academic, Boston, pp. 37–69.

33. W. P. Bocchinfuso and K. S. Korach (1997). Mammary gland development and tumorigenesis in estrogen receptor knockout mice. *J. Mammary Gland Biol. Neoplasia* **2:**323–334.

34. J. P. Lydon *et al.* (1996). Reproductive phenotypes of the progesterone receptor null mutant mouse. *J. Steroid Biochem. Molec. Biol.* **56:**67–77.

35. R. D. Cardiff (1996). The biology of mammary transgenes: Five rules. *J. Mammary Gland Biol. Neoplasia* **1:**61–74.

36. J. R. Laduca and D. K. Sinha (1993). *In vitro* carcinogenesis of mammary epithelial cells by *N*-nitroso-*N*-methylurea using a collagen gel matrix culture. *In Vitro Cell. Develop. Biol.* **29A**(10)**:**789–794.

37. M. M. Ip and K. M. Darcy (1996). Three-dimensional primary culture model systems. *J. Mammary Gland Biol. Neoplasia* **1:**91–110.

38. L. J. Beuving (1968). Mammary tumor formation within outgrowths of transplanted hyperplastic nodules from carcinogen treated rats. *J. Natl. Cancer Inst.* **40:**1287–1291.

39. M. N. Gould, F. Biel, and K. H. Clifton (1977). Morphological and quantitative studies of gland formation from inocula of monodispersed rat mammary cells. *Exp. Cell. Res.* **107:**405–416.

40. S. Hwang *et al.* (1996). Hormone dependent and independent mammary tumor development from *N*-methyl-*N*-nitrosourea treated rat mammary epithelial cell xenografts in nude mouse: multiple pathways and H-ras activation. *Cancer Lett.* **101:**123–134.

41. M. R. Stampfer and P. Yaswen (1992). Factors influencing growth and differentiation normal and transformed human mammary epithelial cells in culture. In G. E. Milo, B. C. Casto, and C. F. Shuler (eds.), *Transformation of Human Epithelial Cells: Molecular and Oncogenetic Mechanisms*. CRC Press, Boca Raton, FL, pp. 117–140.

42. S. P. Ethier (1996). Human breast cancer lines as models of growth regulation and disease progression. *J. Mammary Gland Biol. Neoplasia* **1:**111–122.

43. J. Stingl *et al.* (1998). Phenotypic and functional characterization *in vitro* of a multipotent epithelial cell present in the normal adult human breast. *Differentiation* **63:**201–213.

44. R. R. Mehta *et al.* (1993). Growth and metastasis of human breast carcinomas with matrigel in athymic mice. *Breast Cancer Res. Treat.* **25:**65–71.

45. J. Yang *et al.* (1994). *Cancer Lett.* **81:**117–127.

Chapter 13

Establishment of Mouse Mammary Cell Lines

Daniel Medina and Frances Kittrell

Abstract.   The intent of this chapter is to briefly present a successful protocol for establishing mouse mammary epithelial cell lines in a reproducible manner. The chapter describes the establishment and characterization of cell lines *in vitro*, the requirements for *in vivo* transplantability, and tissue and cell banking. Unique reagents are also described. This method is applicable to normal as well as transformed mammary cell populations and could readily be exploited to establish mammary cell lines from transgenic and knockout mice as well as conventional mice.

Abbreviations.   extracellular matrix (ECM); adult bovine serum (ABS).

INTRODUCTION

Modern carcinogenesis studies rely heavily on *in vitro* systems to examine signaling pathways and agents that disturb such pathways and to understand the significant events in the regulation and development of tumor growth and function. Ideally, the results are translated into *in vivo* systems to validate the *in vitro* generated hypothesis. The strengths of the mouse mammary gland system have been well-defined *in vivo* stages of tumorigenesis and the ability to manipulate tumorigenesis *in vivo*. The ability to transplant mammary cell populations into their orthotopic site provides a powerful tool for testing the growth and functional properties of nontumorigenic as well as tumorigenic mammary cell populations maintained as *in vitro* cell lines. The realization of this ability was initially hampered by the lack of appropriate culture conditions and essential growth factors for growing and establishing mouse mammary epithelial cells, both normal and tumorous, *in vitro*. This deficiency was eliminated by the pioneering studies summarized in several papers (1–4).

The intent of this chapter is not to summarize the *in vitro* biology of mouse mammary cell lines. Several cell lines, characterized to various degrees, have been utilized for studies on mammary cell function. These include the COMMA-D cell line and its clonal derivatives: HC11, C1D9, SCp2 (4–6), NmuMG (7), C57NMG (8), CLS1 (9), IM2 (10), TM and FSK (11), EF (12), and others (13). These lines have proven useful as recipients in transfection experiments (13, 14) and for examining hormonal responsiveness and signaling pathways (6, 7). Most of these cell lines were established serendipitously, and the *in vivo* growth characteristics of many of these cell lines either have not been adequately tested or they fail to

Daniel Medina and Frances Kittrell   Department of Molecular and Cell Biology, Baylor College of Medicine, Houston, Texas 77030.

Methods in Mammary Gland Biology and Breast Cancer Research, edited by Ip and Asch. Kluwer Academic/Plenum Publishers, New York, 2000.

proliferate in the mammary fat pad. This chapter presents our experience in reproducibly establishing mouse mammary cell lines and testing their *in vivo* growth properties. The culture of mammary epithelial cells has been reported by several groups (3), and each group has its own preferences for the various steps. In several areas, cell culture is still subjective and an art, but the end result is reproducibility.

MATERIALS

Collagen Protocols

COLLAGEN PREPARATION

- Collect necessary supplies.
    Rat tails (may be stored wrapped in foil at −20°C).
    70% EtOH.
    100-mm petri dishes (weighed).
    Instruments (scalpel, scissors, pliers, forceps).
- Pull collagen fibers from skinned rat tails, using pliers.
- Wash by dipping collagen fibers in 70% EtOH.
- Roll washed fibers into bundles and place in preweighed 100-mm petri dishes.
- Dry open dishes in hood in front of UV light (overnight).
- Turn bundles over and expose to UV for about 1 h.
- Put lid on dishes (which will now be sterile inside).
- Weigh dishes with fibers.
- Transfer fibers to sterile 50-ml tubes and add acetic acid. Add fibers to sterile acetic acid solution (1 ml glacial acetic acid to 999 ml distilled H_2O) at a concentration of 6 mg collagen (tail fibers) per milliliter of acetic acid solution.
- Shake and place in refrigerator (shake two or three times a day for a week). The solution is very viscous.
- After one wash, centrifuge at 4400 rpm for 1 h.
- Immediately after centrifuge stops, pipette off supernatant and discard fibers. The supernatant is the collagen solution and is now approximately 2 mg/ml. The solution can be immediately used or stored at 4°C for 4–6 months.

COLLAGEN USAGE

1. To coat dishes with a thin collagen layer:
    - Dilute 1 ml of collagen solution (2 mg/ml) with 39 ml of 0.02 N acetic acid (1 ml of glacial acetic acid in 870 ml distilled H_2O).
    - Pipette diluted collagen solution (50 µg/ml) onto dishes to be coated. Use at least 5 µg/cm^2; therefore, a 60-mm dish requires 3 ml, and a 100-mm dish requires 8 ml.
    - Incubate at room temperature for 1 h.
    - Aspirate off liquid.
    - Rinse dishes with Solution A or PBS.
    - Use immediately or air-dry and store at 4°C for up to 1 week.
2. To plate cells in a layer of collagen:
    - Prepare the following: a mixture of 10× standard medium and 0.34 N NaOH at a ratio of 1.65 ml of 10× medium to 1 ml of 0.34 N NaOH.
    - Combine 1.5 ml of the above mixture with 8 ml of collagen and immediately pour into 100-mm petri dish (adjust total volume as needed for different size dishes).

- Let collagen layer harden in incubator for at least 5 min but no more than 2 h.
- Repeat step 2, adding cells in a small volume of medium to the mixture just before pouring on top of first layer.

Reagents

DIGESTION MEDIUM

DMEM:F12 buffered with HEPES (pH 7.6).
  100 units/ml pen–strep
  100 µg/ml gentamicin
  60 units/ml nystatin
  2 mg/ml collagenase
  100 units/ml hyaluronidase

GROWTH MEDIUM

DMEM:F12 buffered with HEPES (pH 7.6).
  10 µg/ml Insulin
  5 ng/ml epidermal growth factor
  1 mg/ml bovine serum albumin
  5 µg/ml linoleic acid complex (see next recipe)
  50 µg/ml gentamicin
  20 units/ml nystatin

LINOLEIC ACID—BSA

1. Fatty-acid-free BSA
   a. Mix 50 g of fatty-acid-free BSA in 250 ml of standard medium.
   b. Stir slowly (to avoid foaming) for 30 min at room temperature.
   c. Filter.
   d. Aliquot in 40-ml portions and store at −20°C.
2. Linoleic acid (LA)
   a. Dissolve 500 mg of LA in 25 ml sterile 0.1 M Na_2CO_3.
   b. Refrigerate overnight.
   c. Mix 25 ml of LA solution with 135 ml of Puck's Saline A and 40 ml of fatty-acid-free BSA (concentration is now 2.5 mg LA/ml).
   d. Gas with nitrogen in screw-capped glass tube.
   e. Heat in H_2O bath at 50°C for 1 h.
   f. Filter.
   g. Aliquot in 2-ml portions and store at −20°C. Protect from light.

SOLUTION A (20)

Glucose	1.80 g/L
NaCl	7.60 g/L
KCl	0.22 g/L
Na_2HPO_4	0.14 g/L
HEPES	7.15 g/L
Phenol Red	1.24 mg/L

Adjust pH to 7.6 with NaOH

DISPASE SOLUTION. Dispase 9.6 mg/ml dissolved in Solution A. Aliquot and store this 4× stock solution at −20°C. Thaw and dilute to 1× (2.4 mg/ml) with Puck's Saline A for use. Magnesium in Puck's Saline A helps the activity of dispase.

PUCK'S SALINE A

NaCl	8.0 g/L
KCl	0.4 g/L
Glucose	1.0 g/L
$MgCl_2 \cdot 6H_2O$	0.15 g/L
$NaHCO_3$	0.35 g/L
Phenol Red	5 mg/L

Adjust pH to 7.4

PRODUCTS AND CATALOG NUMBERS

DMEM:F12	Sigma	D-8900
EGF	Sigma	E-4127
Insulin	Sigma	I-5500
Linoleic acid	Sigma	L-1012
BSA (for LA)	Armour Biochemical	2295-02-3
BSA Fraction V	Sigma	A-9418
Nystatin	Sigma	N-1638
Gentamycin	Sigma	G-1272
Pen–Strep	Sigma	P-0906
Dispase (Grade II)	Boehringer–Mannheim	165–859
Collagenase A	Boehringer–Mannheim	1088–785
Hyaluronidase	Sigma	H-3884
ECMGel	Sigma	E-1270
10× Dulbecco's modified Eagle's medium	Sigma	D-2429

ESTABLISHMENT OF CELL LINES

A successful protocol for routinely establishing mammary cell lines from normal or neoplastic cell populations is based on the incorporation of three uncommon steps to the routine procedure (11). These steps are the use of low serum (2% adult bovine serum, ABS) in the growth medium, the initial seeding of the cells into collagen gels, and the use of the enzyme dispase rather than trypsin to serially passage the cells. The initial seeding in collagen gel and low serum concentration favor growth of epithelial cells over fibroblasts. The enzyme dispase causes less damage to the plasma membrane than does trypsin. The procedure outlined here has allowed us to routinely establish mammary epithelial cell cultures from normal virgin or pregnant gland in genetically normal (e.g., BALB/c) or genetically altered (e.g., p53 null) mice. In the original publication of this method, the success rate was virtually 100%. The protocol for digesting or making primary cultures of mouse mammary tissues is the same for normal (virgin or pregnant gland), preneoplastic, or tumor tissues. The time needed to digest each tissue may vary slightly from the 3 h noted here. Dissociated cells can be immediately plated *in* or *on* collagen or Matrigel for primary culture or frozen as a pellet for RNA extraction. All steps are performed under sterile or aseptic conditions. Media formulations and other recipes and protocols may be found at the end of this chapter. The basic elements of the culture procedure are as follows.

1. Remove the mammary glands from the host mouse aseptically and place in DMEM:F12 with antibiotics (same antibiotics as digestion media) to keep moist until mincing. The glands most frequently used are the thoracic (no. 2 and no. 3) glands and the inguinal (no. 4) glands. Lymph nodes should be discarded. Using sterile technique, mince tissue into very small pieces (<1 mm) with a scalpel or razor blade. Place minced tissue (1 g tissue/10 ml medium) in digestion medium (DMEM:F12 + antibiotics + collagenase + hyaluronidase) and shake at 37°C for approximately 3 h. The shaker should be set between 110 and 125 rpm. Shaking should be gentle but thorough. Small volumes (up to 15 ml) can be dissociated in a 50-ml conical tube placed at a 45° angle. Larger volumes can be put in an Erlenmeyer flask. The round shape of the Erlenmeyer flask facilitates proper shaking.

2. When tissue is thoroughly digested, so it visually appears as a cloudy homogeneous solution, centrifuge mixture at 1000 rpm (about $200 \times g$) for 5 min. Remove the supernatant and resuspend the cell pellet in 6–10 ml sterile phosphate buffered saline containing 5% adult bovine serum (PBS/ABS). Centrifuge, save pellet, resuspend, and repeat for a total of five washes with the PBS/ABS solution. Following the fifth wash, resuspend the cell pellet in the desired volume of growth medium and plate cells (2×10^6 cells/100 mm dish) or quickly freeze the cell pellet, using dry ice or liquid nitrogen for future RNA extraction. The majority of the cells will be single cells or tiny aggregates of 2–10 cells. Cells can be easily counted with a standard hemocytometer under 10× magnification. Number of cells recovered is highly dependent on tissue type used. Virgin mammary gland yields approximately 10^6 cells/100 mg. Pregnant or preneoplastic tissues yield approximately 5×10^6 cells/100 mg. Tumor cell yields vary drastically but are even higher than preneoplastic by three to five times.

3. Cells grown *in* collagen (see collagen protocol) or extracellular matrix gel (ECMGel) should not require serum added to the growth medium. Cells grown *on* collagen or ECMGel may require 1–2% serum. For establishment of stable cell lines, cells should be grown *in*, rather than *on*, collagen or ECMGel.

4. When cells have reached the desired density in collagen or ECMGel (2 to 4 weeks), they may be passaged and replated on a growth substrate or directly on plastic. The "desired" density is a subjective judgment, but the density of cells is more than sufficient if the gel starts to contract in the dish. To dissolve the collagen, use growth medium with 2 mg/ml collagenase added. Gently trace around the edge of the gel with a pipette to leave the gel floating in the collagenase solution. The gel should be allowed to dissolve completely (i.e., no clumps) (about 1 h at 37°C, unshaken) before the culture solution is centrifuged and washed in PBS with 5% ABS as in the dissociation step. As before, wash for a total of five times. Cells will now be single cells or small aggregates. Cells can be recovered from ECMGel by using dispase. Cells may now be plated directly on plastic or *on* a very thin layer of collagen or ECMGel. Cells can be grown in medium with 1–2% ABS. Cells grown *on* a collagen gel can be also recovered by using dispase (2.4 mg/ml).

5. Cell lines may be established from these monolayer cultures by using dispase to selectively remove spindle-shaped cells from the culture dishes. Epithelial islands usually will not be disturbed by a short treatment (5 min) with dispase, but the spindle-shaped cells will be easily removed. This differential dispase treatment can be used as needed in the early passages to purify the cuboidal epithelial population. Generally, epithelial cells require 10 to 30 min treatment with dispase. When these cells pass their crisis stage at about passages 3 to

5, they will begin to proliferate readily. Though tedious, the differential dispase treatment should yield purified epithelial populations that will immortalize to stable cell lines.

6. The key ingredient for success of this method is patience. Cells in passages 3 to 5 will undergo crisis and expand very slowly. Cells may stay at a given passage for 3 to 4 weeks before reaching a density that will allow passage. The culture media (5 ml for a T-25 flask or 14 ml for a T-75 flask) should continue to be changed twice a week. Replating of early cultures should always be at very low split ratios (1:2, 1:3); i.e., split the cells of one flask into two or three flasks, respectively. Once a cell line grows readily in culture so it can be subcultured weekly, then the split ratio can be modified to 1:5, then 1:10.

CHARACTERIZATION OF CELL LINES *IN VITRO*

Primary cultures of normal mammary epithelial cells will contain predominantly epithelial cells (≥90%), with the remaining 10% cells being myoepithelial cells and fibroblasts. The purity of the cultures over the first five passages (pre- and pericrisis) will depend on the growth medium used, the efficacy of the dispase treatment, and the vicissitudes of Nature. For most experimental aims, the cells should be characterized postcrisis when the cell line is relatively stable. Once established, the cell lines are reproductively stable for decades. Cells maintained in culture have been identified as epithelium according to several criteria, namely keratin-positive cells by immunocytochemical staining using antibodies that recognize keratins 8, 18, 19 (15); a cuboidal to polygonal morphology, in contrast to elongated bipolar cells characteristic of fibroblasts; hormone responsiveness in the synthesis of mammary-specific proteins such as casein (16); and *in vivo* growth after transplantation as mammary ducts, alveoli, or tumors (11). The cells will also exhibit membrane-localized cadherin staining, but staining for the estrogen receptor is not maintained (Medina, unpublished data). Myoepithelial cells express keratins 5 and 14, although occasional expression of keratin 14 by mammary epithelial hyperplastic outgrowth cells *in vivo* has been reported (17). Mammary epithelial cells established as cell lines retain expression of keratin proteins organized as filaments but may also express vimentin protein as filaments.

IN VIVO TRANSPLANTABILITY

The transplantation protocol, including fat pad clearing, is illustrated in several previous publications (18, 19) and in Chapter 6 in this volume. The successful transplantability into syngeneic mice of *in vitro* cultures is strikingly dependent on passage number and cell number inoculum. There is a close correlation between cell number and successful takes for inoculums between 1.0×10^5 to 7.5×10^5 cells/site. At the higher cell inoculum, there were no differences between cells grown on plastic prior to injection or injected as a cell suspension directly from collagen gels, and the success rate was greater than 95%. The injected cells gave rise to normal duct or to alveolar outgrowths. As long as the cell injections are performed under aseptic conditions, an immune response at the injection site is infrequent. An exception to this observation would be highly immunogenic tumors.

The frequency of successful normal growth *in vivo* depends on passage number. Successful normal growth is defined as the ability to produce duct or alveolar cells and to fill at least 25% of the fat pad by 8 weeks after transplantation. The success rates of cells in passages 1 and 2 are greater than 95%. However, once cells are maintained at longer passages, the *in vivo* transplantation success rate decreases markedly. Most of our cell lines lose *in vivo* normal growth capability between passages 4 and 6. However, COMMA-D retains *in vivo* growth potential up to passage 14, FSK4 up to passage 8, and TM12 up to passage 20.

The basis for the loss of *in vivo* growth has not been ascertained. Growth for successive passages *on* collagen gels or *in* collagen gels did not maintain *in vivo* growth capability. This loss of *in vivo* growth capability is also true for cell lines established from ductal or alveolar outgrowths. However, cell lines established from tumors maintain their ability to grow *in vivo* apparently indefinitely, since some of our cell lines, such as MOD, have been maintained in culture for over 14 years and still produce mammary tumors upon transplantation into syngeneic hosts.

The frequency of establishing a serially transplantable outgrowth line is remarkably high. The majority of the outgrowths were no longer serially transplantable after three successive transplant generations. Approximately 14% (9/65) of the cell populations injected into mammary fat pads gave rise to outgrowths that could be serially transplanted *in vivo* for greater than five successive transplant generations. Of the nine outgrowths that fulfilled the definition of serial transplantation, four showed ductal outgrowth and five, alveolar outgrowths. Seven of the nine outgrowth lines have been maintained in the fat pads by serial transplantation for up to 10 years and have retained their original morphology.

TISSUE AND CELL BANKING

Freezing down and rethawing of *in vitro* cell lines or *in vivo* outgrowths is frequently required in laboratories. We have had success with the following methods for freezing and reusing these two cell populations.

Cell lines are frozen down according to the following protocol.

- Remove cells from flask by using dispase. Commonly, we collect cells that have just reached confluency. One T25/T75 flask will equate to one aliquot.
- Dilute with an equal volume of standard growth medium (DMEM/F12) containing 2% serum to deactivate dispase. Centrifuge (*200 × g*, 5 min), remove supernatant, save pellet.
- Resuspend pellet in medium containing 7% DMSO and 2% ABS in DMEM/F12. Use a 2-ml cryogenic tube.
- Slowly freeze aliquots, lowering temperature at the rate of about 1°C/min by using an isopropanol-based freezing unit (Nalgene Cryo 1°C freezing container). Alternatively, you can freeze first at −20°C for ≤12 h before transferring the frozen cells to −80°C.
- Store short term at −80°C or long term in liquid nitrogen.

Frozen cell lines are recovered according to the following protocol.

- Quickly melt frozen aliquots by submersing vial in a 37°C water bath.
- Dilute with growth medium up to six times the volume of the frozen stock.
- Centrifuge (*200 × g*, 5 min), remove supernatant, resuspend pellet, and plate in growth medium (one aliquot per 100-mm dish or T25/T75 flask).

Tissue outgrowths are frozen down according to the following protocol.

- Excise tissue to be frozen taking care to remove any lymph nodes or excess fat pad not containing outgrowth or tumor.

- Mince tissue into ~1-mm-sized pieces.
- Place tissue in medium containing 7% DMSO and 2% ABS.
- Slowly freeze aliquots, lowering temperature at the rate of 1°C/min. Generally, the minced tissue from one inguinal fat pad will yield two aliquots.
- Store short term at −80°C or long term in liquid nitrogen.

Frozen tissue fragments are recovered with the following protocol.

- Quickly melt frozen aliquots by submersing in a 37°C water bath.
- Add extra medium to dilute concentration of DMSO. Note that fragments of mammary tissue will not usually pellet by centrifugation because of the high fat content; therefore, fragments of tissue outgrowths and tumors may be collected with forceps.
- For outgrowths, implant tissue in cleared mammary fat pads of syngeneic hosts. Tumor fragments ($\leq 1\ mm^2$) may be implanted with fine forceps or a trocar in the mammary fat pad or subcutaneously, respectively.

SUMMARY

These procedures demonstrate that mammary cells from a normal mammary gland can be established as *in vitro* cell lines reproducibly and retain *in vivo* growth capacity for at least four to six passages. A few of the *in vitro* cell lines retain *in vivo* growth capacity for normal or preneoplastic growth for 14–20 passages. A significant number of the *in vivo* outgrowths can be serially transplanted *in vivo* and then can be reestablished as stable *in vitro* cell lines at will. However, maintaining cell lines for prolonged passage *in vitro* results in loss of *in vivo* growth capability for the majority, but not all, of the cell lines. An understanding of the cellular and molecular basis for this loss of *in vivo* growth and successful resolution of this problem would greatly facilitate the use of normal and preneoplastic mammary cell lines to examine the mechanistic basis for tumor development. Currently, the majority of normal mammary cell lines represents populations derived from virgin mammary gland. It would be of interest to develop cell lines from putative stem cell populations (i.e., terminal end buds) and pregnant mammary gland. The latter is of particular interest, because the cell line that has been the most productive for experimental purposes and has produced normal morphogenesis *in vivo* for extended passages is the COMMA-1D line, which was generated from pregnant mammary gland. Finally, it is likely that cell lines from various transgenic or knockout mammary glands could easily be established by utilizing the methods discussed in this chapter. One major pitfall to this methodology remains and is the bane of all cell culturists, namely the problem of contamination by microorganisms. Therefore, it cannot be stressed frequently enough that it is critical to freeze down early passages (passages 3–10) and multiple aliquots.

ACKNOWLEDGMENT. We are grateful to Dr. Cynthia Zahnow for reviewing this protocol and discussing areas that were vague or confusing.

REFERENCES

1. J. T. Emerman, S. J. Burwen, and D. R. Pitelka (1979). Substrate properties influencing ultrastructural differentiation of mammary epithelial cells in culture. *Tissue and Cell* **11**:109–119.

2. J. Richards, D. Pasco, J. Yang, R. Guzman, and S. Nandi (1983). Comparison of the growth of normal and neoplastic mouse mammary cells on plastic, on collagen gels and in collagen gels. *Exp. Cell Res.* **146**:1–14.

3. B. K. Levay-Young, W. Imagawa, J. Yang, J. E. Richards, R. C. Guzman, and S. Nandi (1987). Primary culture systems for mammary biology studies. In D. Medina, W. Kidwell, G. Heppner, and E. Anderson (eds.), *Cellular and Molecular Biology of Mammary Cancer*, Plenum Press, New York, pp. 181–204.

4. K. G. Danielson, C. J. Oborn, E. M. Durban, J. S. Butel, and D. Medina (1984). Epithelial mouse mammary cell line exhibiting normal morphogenesis *in vivo* and functional differentiation *in vitro*. *Proc. Natl. Acad. Sci. U.S.A.* **81**:3756–3760.

5. C. Schmidhauser, M. J. Bissell, C. A. Myers, and G. F. Casperson (1990). Extracellular matrix and hormones transcriptionally regulate bovine beta-casein 5′ sequences in stably transfected mouse mammary cells. *Proc. Natl. Acad. Sci. U.S.A.* **887**:9118–9122.

6. A. Srebrow, Y. Friedmann, A. Ravanpay, C. W. Daniel, and M. J. Bissell (1998). Expression of *Hoxa-1* and *Hoxb-7* is regulated by extracellular matrix-dependent signals in mammary epithelial cells. *J. Cell Biochem.* **69**:377–391.

7. A. Bandyopadhyay, M. L. Cibull, and L. Z. Sun (1998). Isolation and characterization of a spontaneously transformed malignant mouse mammary epithelial cell line in culture. *Carcinogenesis* **19**:1907–1911.

8. A. B. Vaidya, E. Y. Lasfargues, J. B. Sheffield, and W. G. Coutinho (1978). Murine mammary tumor virus infection of an epithelial cell line established from C57BL/6 mouse mammary glands. *Virology* **90**:12–22.

9. L. W. Anderson, K. G. Danielson, and H. L. Hosick (1979). Epithelial cell line and subline established from premalignant mouse mammary tissue. *In Vitro* **15**:841–843.

10. E. Reichmann, R. Ball, B. Groner, and R. R. Friis (1989). New mammary epithelial and fibroblastic cell clones in coculture form structures competent to differentiate functionally. *J. Cell Biol.* **108**:1127–1138.

11. F. S. Kittrell, C. J. Oborn, and D. Medina (1992). Development of mammary preneoplasias *in vivo* from mouse mammary epithelial cells *in vitro*. *Cancer Res.* **52**:1924–1932.

12. L. M. Adams, S. P. Ethier, and R. L. Ullrich (1987). Enhanced *in vitro* proliferation and *in vivo* tumorigenic potential of mammary epithelium from BALB/c mice exposed to γ-radiation and/or 7,12-dimethylbenz(α)anthracene. *Cancer Res.* **47**:4425–4431.

13. F. Ciardello, R. Dono, N. Kim, M. G. Persico, and D. S. Salomon (1991). Expression of *cripto*, a novel gene of the epidermal growth factor gene family, leads to *in vivo* transformation of a "normal" mouse mammary epithelial cell line. *Cancer Res.* **51**:1051–1054.

14. T. K. Bera, R. C. Guzman, S. Mujamoto, D. K. Panda, M. Sasaki, K. Hanyu, J. Enami, and S. Nandi (1994). Identification of a mammary transforming gene (MAT1) associated with mouse mammary tumorigenesis. *Proc. Natl. Acad. Sci. U.S.A.* **91**:9789–9793.

15. B. B. Asch and H. L. Asch (1987). Structural components as markers of differentiation and neoplastic progression in mammary epithelial cells. In D. Medina, W. Kidwell, G. Heppner, and E. Anderson (eds.), *Cellular and Molecular Biology of Mammary Cancer*, Plenum Press, New York, pp. 29–46.

16. E. M. Durban, D. Medina, and J. S. Butel. (1985). Comparative analysis of casein synthesis during mammary cell differentiation in collagen and mammary gland development *in vivo*. *Dev. Biol.* **109**:288–298.

17. G. H. Smith, T. Mehrel, and D. R. Roop (1990). Differential keratin gene expression in developing differentiating preneoplastic and neoplastic mouse mammary epithelium. *Cell Growth Diff.* **1**:161–170.

18. D. Medina (1973). Preneoplastic lesions in mouse mammary tumorigenesis. *Meth. Cancer Res.* **7**:353–414.

19. D. Medina (1996). The mammary gland: A unique organ for the study of development and tumorigenesis. *J. Mam. Gland Biol. Neoplasia* **1**:5–19.

20. G. D. Shipley and R. G. Ham (1981). Improved medium and culture conditions for clonal growth with minimal serum protein and enhanced serum-free survival of Swiss 3T3 cells. *In Vitro* **17**:656–670.

Chapter 14

Whole Organ Culture of the Mouse Mammary Gland

Erika Ginsburg and Barbara K. Vonderhaar

Abstract. Whole mammary glands from pubescent mice, primed for 9 days with estrogen and progesterone, cultured in the presence of the lactogenic hormone mix of insulin, aldosterone, hydrocortisone, and prolactin develop pregnancy-like lobuloalveolar structures and synthesize milk protein. Withdrawal of prolactin from the medium (with or without the steroids) results in involution of the gland in a manner comparable to that which occurs *in vivo*. Reincubation with the four-hormone mix plus epidermal growth factor results in a second round of development. Thus, whole organ culture provides an excellent model system to study systematically the hormonal and growth factor requirements that regulate the biochemical events that occur during these processes.

Abbreviations. insulin (I); estradiol (E); progesterone (P); hydrocortisone (H); aldosterone (A); prolactin (PRL); epidermal growth factor (EGF); phosphate buffered saline (PBS).

INTRODUCTION

The mouse mammary gland serves as a model for studies of the regulation of growth and differentiation of epithelial cells as well as epithelial–stromal interactions. Extensive studies have been performed *in vivo* to understand the hormonal regulation of mammary gland differentiation; however, Ichinose and Nandi (1, 2) developed a model in which hormonal pretreatment of pubescent mice permitted normal lobuloalveolar development to a pregnancy-like state *in vitro*. Survival of the cultured glands in chemically defined, serum-free medium depended on insulin (I), but full differentiation occurred in the presence of the steroid hormones estradiol (E), progesterone (P), hydrocortisone (H), aldosterone (A), and prolactin (PRL). BALB/c mice required daily injections of E and P for 9 days prior to culture. When thoracic (no. 2) mammary glands were maintained in an atmosphere of 5% CO_2 : 95% O_2, full lobuloalveolar development and milk protein synthesis (3) occurred after 5–6 days.

Instead of 9 daily injections of E and P, slow-release cholesterol-based pellets containing the same ratio of E and P as the injections were used by Vonderhaar (4, 5). Glands from these primed mice developed lobuloalveolar structures within 6 days when cultured in the presence of the lactogenic mix of four hormones (IAH and PRL) even in the presence of 5%

Erika Ginsburg and Barbara K. Vonderhaar   Laboratory of Tumor Immunology and Biology, National Cancer Institute, National Institutes of Health, Bethesda, Maryland 20892.

Methods in Mammary Gland Biology and Breast Cancer Research, edited by Ip and Asch. Kluwer Academic/Plenum Publishers, New York, 2000.

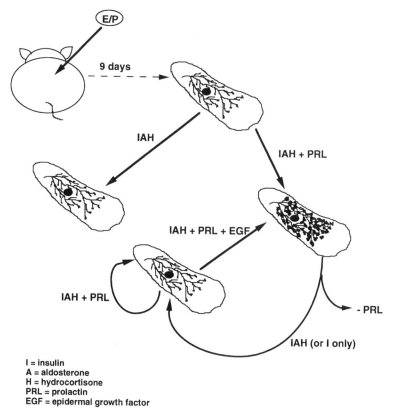

Figure 14-1. Schematic representation of developmental cycles of mouse mammary gland *in vitro*.

CO_2 in air. If epidermal growth factor (EGF) was also added to the media during the first round of development, the length of priming time could be decreased from 9 to 6 days with a concomitant increase in development (4). An additional significant improvement in overall development of the mammary gland occurs when 50% O_2 with 5% CO_2 in air is used as the incubator atmosphere during the 6 days in culture (5).

Other studies have shown that complete regression of the gland, following development in culture, takes place when PRL is withdrawn from the media for 9 to 15 days (6, 7). Media containing I alone or I, A, and H result in structures that resemble the involuted gland of the postlactational mother. Molecular events occurring during involution *in vitro* parallel those observed *in vivo* (8). Following PRL withdrawal and morphological involution in whole organ culture, a second cycle of development can be achieved by the addition of physiologic concentrations of EGF (7) in addition to IAH and PRL (Figure 14-1).

Thus, the whole organ culture method provides an excellent model for the systematic investigation of hormones necessary for growth, differentiation, and regression of the mammary gland and is a relatively simple technique that parallels events *in vivo*. Herein we describe the conditions successfully used in our laboratory for whole organ culture of the BALB/c mouse mammary gland.

MATERIALS AND INSTRUMENTATION

Sources

- Avertin (2,2,2-tribromoethanol): Aldrich Chemical Co., Milwaukee, WI
- Estradiol-17β, HEPES, insulin, aldosterone, hydrocortisone, progesterone, and cholesterol: Sigma, St. Louis, MO
- Hormone pellets: Innovative Research of America, Sarasota, FL, or prepared in-house as described in the following
- Whatman #105 lens paper: Schleicher and Schuell, Keene, NH
- Prosil-28: PCR Inc., Gainesville, FL
- Waymouth's 152/1, penicillin, streptomycin, gentamycin sulfate: Life Technologies, Inc., Gaithersburg, MD
- PRL: Hormone Distribution Program of the NIH (administered by Dr. Parlow; information on ordering is found in the January issue of Endocrine Society journals)
- EGF: Collaborative Research Products, Bedford, MA
- Pellet maker with punch and die; Parr Instrument Co., Moline, IL

Anesthesia

Animals are lightly anesthetized by use of Avertin or according to local IACUC (Institute Animal Care and Use Committee) regulations. Avertin is prepared freshly at 25 mg/ml in distilled water and is dissolved by mixing end-over-end. Animals are injected intraperitoneally with 0.04 ml/g body weight.

Pellets

A mixture of E, P, and cholesterol at a ratio of $1:1000:2002$ is dissolved in 100% ethanol and then dried down under a nitrogen gas stream. Individual E–P pellets are then made from 10 mg powder using a pellet maker fitted with a 0.2-cm punch and die. Pellets may also be purchased from Innovative Research of America.

Siliconizing Lens Paper

Prior to siliconizing, sheets of loose-weave lens paper (we recommend Whatman #105) are placed in a shallow dish and covered with ethyl ether for 20–30 min at room temperature; the ether is then removed by aspiration. Subsequently this same procedure is performed three times with 95% ethanol for 20–30 min and four times with distilled water for 15 min. The sheets are then dried overnight at 37°C. The dried sheets are then soaked in the siliconizing agent (Prosil-28 diluted with distilled water at $1:100$) for 30 min at room temperature. After aspiration of the excess siliconizing agent, the sheets are washed, as before, four times with distilled water for 15 min. Again the papers are dried at 37°C. The dried lens paper is cut into pieces large enough to hold one entire no. 4 gland (about 1.5×1.5 cm). The pieces are placed in a glass petri dish and autoclaved. Once the papers undergo the initial washes they should only be handled with forceps or gloved hands; after sterilization, only with sterile forceps. Siliconizing the lens paper is essential to make it float.

Media

Basal developmental medium consists of Waymouth's 152/1 supplemented with penicillin (100 U/ml), streptomycin (100 μg/ml), gentamycin sulfate (50 μg/ml), 20 mM HEPES, I (5 μg/ml), A (100 ng/ml), H (100 ng/ml), and PRL (1 μg/ml). Stock solutions of I, A, H, and PRL can be prepared ahead of time at these recommended concentrations: I at 2 mg/ml in 5 mM HCl, A and H at 5 mg/ml in 100% ethanol, and PRL at 2 mg/ml in 0.01 M sodium bicarbonate, pH 8.7. A and H can be stored in the refrigerator for months as long as evaporation is prevented, but I and PRL should be made fresh after 7–10 days if refrigerated. Both peptide hormones in solution can be stored frozen for up to 6 months. EGF is prepared at 100 μg/ml in sterile PBS and stored in the refrigerator for up to 4 weeks.

Incubator

For best results a tri-gas incubator capable of sustaining a gas mix of 50% O_2 and 5% CO_2 in air is required (see Comment 1). Actual gas concentrations in the incubator chamber should be tested with a Fyrite test kit rather than relying on the indicators of the incubator. It is also possible to use a conventional dual-gas incubator to deliver 5% CO_2 in air; the development of the gland is less striking and takes several days longer. Gastight incubation boxes flushed with a known quantity of O_2 may also be used, but the results, due to a less-controlled gas environment, are variable.

METHODS

Priming

Two methods of priming have proven successful (see Comment 2). The initial work from several laboratories (2, 3, 6, 7) utilized daily subcutaneous injections of E (1 μg) and P (1 mg) in a distilled water or 0.9% saline suspension. This method suffers from daily spikes of hormone concentration in the serum and is labor intensive. We have adapted the technique of slow-release pellets, which is labor saving and less traumatic to the mice. After an initial rapid rise in E and P concentrations in the serum, the level of these hormones decreases and then remains constant at two to four times the basal level after 24 h (9). Thus, female BALB/c mice (see Comment 3), 24–28 days of age, are primed with a 10-mg cholesterol-based pellet of E and P. Mice are lightly anesthestized with Avertin or according to local IACUC regulations and pellets are inserted subcutaneously into the intrascapular region by using a trocar or fine forceps through a small incision; the wound is then secured with a surgical clip.

Culture

After 9 days of priming with E and P, the abdominal no. 4 glands (see Comment 4) are removed aseptically, stretched individually on dry, sterile siliconized lens paper (see Comment 5), and placed into 35-mm sterile petri dishes to which 2 ml Waymouth's 152/1 serum-free media containing the requisite hormones and growth factors for testing is added (see Comment 6). The glands from no more than three animals at a time are removed and temporarily placed in a sterile dish with a small amount of sterile medium without hormones in order to keep the glands moist until they are stretched on the lens paper. If the glands are to be used for biochemical or molecular analysis, the lymph node should be removed before culturing. Frequently, 0.1% BSA is included in the media to prevent adsorption of the hormones and growth factors to the plastic, but it is not essential. Glands are maintained in a tri-gas incubator in an atmosphere of 50% O_2 and 5% CO_2 in air.

The media must be replaced initially after 24 h, then every second day for a total of 5–7 days to obtain complete lobuloalveolar development. Involution is achieved by withdrawing PRL (with or without A and H) from the media. To assess involution, glands are removed from culture at various times up to 15 days after removal of PRL. A second round of full lobuloalveolar development is achieved when glands thus involuted for 9 to 15 days (see Comment 7) are reincubated in the presence of IAH + PRL + EGF (60 ng/ml) (Figure 14-2).

At any time during culture, glands may be removed and whole-mounted and stained with carmine alum or hematoxylin–eosin (see Chapter 7 by Rasmussen *et al.* in this volume) for morphological analysis, fixed and sectioned for histological analyses, or quick-frozen at −80°C for subsequent protein, DNA, or RNA extraction. To ensure that whole-mounted glands retain their shape following whole organ culture, it is best to stretch them on glass slides and allow them to air-dry for approximately 10 min before submerging them in the fixative.

Assessing Morphogenesis

The morphological results of whole organ culture can be assessed by assigning a relative developmental score based on separate readings of coded samples by independent observers (2, 5, 10). At best, this method is semiquantitative. A more quantitative morphometric analysis is based on the technique developed by Michna *et al.* (11) and adapted by Plaut *et al.* (12) The gland, starting at the lymph node, is photographed using a light microscope at a 25-fold magnification. The resulting 3-inch × 5-inch photograph is marked with a circle, which covers an area of 24 cm^2. Where appropriate, multiple areas from the same gland may be counted by using a smaller circle. Replicates of multiple glands in the same hormone conditions must be assessed. The number of end buds, alveolar buds, or lobuloalveoli (see Figure 14-2 for examples) encompassed by the circle are counted as individual units based on the following characteristics: end buds are defined as large bulbous structures at the ends of ducts, alveolar buds are defined as round to slightly lobular structures composed of no more than 5 alveoli, and lobuloalveoli are defined as groups of greater than 5 alveoli organized into discrete lobules located along or at the end of a duct. An upper limit of 30 structures per designated area can be assessed.

COMMENTS

1. Many of the original studies of whole organ culture suggested a gas mix of 95% O_2 : 5% CO_2. Not only is this mix not achievable in modern incubators but it presents the danger of explosion. We carefully tested various O_2 levels and found that 50% O_2 with 5% CO_2 in air gives optimal results (5).

2. Priming prior to removal of the glands is necessary for lobuloalveolar development *in vitro*. In 1964, Ichinose and Nandi (1) suggested that this requirement "is tentative, since appropriate alteration of the culture system might permit such differentiation of untreated tissues entirely *in vitro*." To date, such conditions have not been discovered despite attempts using a variety of combinations of peptide and steroid hormones and growth factors *in vitro* (9). However, recent studies (13) have shown that priming with P alone in ovariectomized mice allowed glands to develop lobuloalveolar structures in culture, although not as extensively as E–P primed glands.

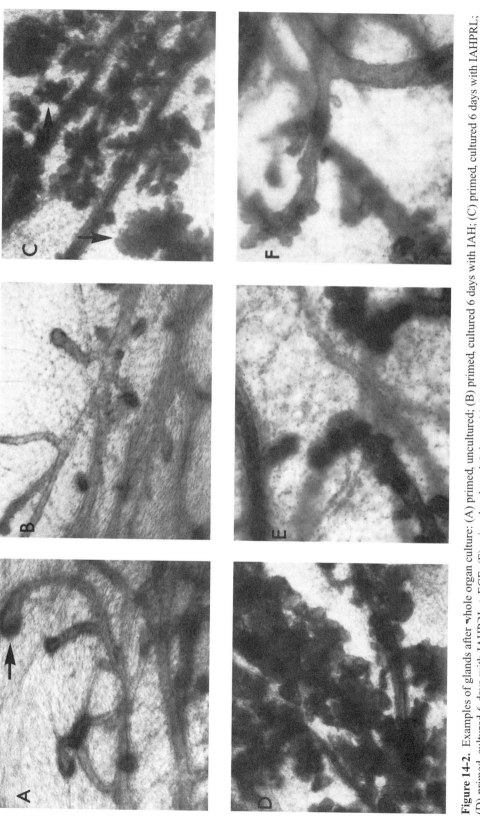

Figure 14-2. Examples of glands after whole organ culture: (A) primed, uncultured; (B) primed, cultured 6 days with IAH; (C) primed, cultured 6 days with IAHPRL; (D) primed, cultured 6 days with IAHPRL + EGF; (E) primed, cultured 6 days with IAHPRL + EGF and then 9 days with I alone; (F) primed, cultured 6 days with IAHPRL + EGF and then 15 days with IAH alone. Horizontal arrow in panel A indicates a teminal end bud; horizontal arrow in panel C indicates an alveolar bud; vertical arrow in panel C indicates a lobuloalveolus. Magnification 40×.

3. In this chapter we outlined the optimal conditions for culture of whole mammary glands from BALB/c mice. Other strains of mice as well as rats can be used. Rats do not need priming and have a reduced requirement for steroids in the culture medium (14). For some strains of mice the time of priming is altered. For instance, RIII mice require only 5 days of priming, whereas C57BL and A/Crgl mice require 15 days. The optimal hormonal requirement of each strain of mouse for full lobuloalveolar development *in vitro* also varies (15).

4. Using the original conditions of priming and culture, Banerjee *et al.* (16) found that the no. 2 thoracic gland gave the maximal development in 5 days compared to the no. 4 abdominal (next best) and no. 3 thoracic (least developed) glands. Under our conditions we found development of the nos. 2 and 4 glands to be comparable. Hence, we routinely use only the no. 4 glands for culture because of the ease and accuracy of clean dissection from the mice. The thoracic glands can then be used for biochemical and morphological analysis of the uncultured gland, or they can be cultured in order to maximize the use of tissue from a single mouse. Glands from mice older than 5–6 weeks at the onset of whole organ culture cannot be used because of poor diffusion of nutrients and hormones into the larger, thicker tissue.

5. Instead of siliconized lens paper, others have used sterile Dacron polyester rafts on a stainless steel grid (2, 6) to maintain the gland in or on the medium. In our experience it is necessary to stretch the gland out on lens paper or a Dacron raft to maintain its shape. Without stretching the gland out on some device, the gland balls up and does not develop. We prefer the siliconized lens paper because it is easy to manipulate, allows the gland to float on the medium, and facilitates medium changes. In our experience, whether the glands are submerged or floated on the medium makes no difference in the ultimate developmental outcome of the cultures.

6. Initial studies by Ichinose and Nandi (1, 2) used I, A, E, P, PRL, and growth hormone (GH) in the developmental culture medium. Of the hormones listed, both P and GH appeared to make a minimal contribution. An effect of thyroxine was also reported, which depended on the concentration of PRL in the medium (17). Subsequent studies (6) found that the most effective hormonal combination for morphogenesis and milk protein synthesis in cultures of BALB/c mammary glands was I, A, H, and PRL. EGF will also enhance morphogenesis in glands from BALB/c mice even when used in the first round of development (5). Barlow *et al.* (12) found that physiological concentrations of estrogen were critical for lobuloalveolar development of the BALB/c mammary glands in whole organ culture in phenol red–free medium.

7. Removal of all hormones except I results in the most rapid and extensive involution, which is complete at 9 days; retaining I, A, and H in the media results in complete involution at 15 days. If involution is allowed to proceed beyond 15 days in the presence of IAH, the second round of development cannot be achieved. We have successfully taken glands through three rounds of development, although the extent of the final development was diminished.

CONCLUSIONS

Whole organ culture offers advantages over other culture systems, chief among which is the presence of all cell types in their proper orientation to one another. The basic conditions for effective culture of the glands from BALB/c mice are presented here to serve as a starting point for use of the technique in different strains of mice. To use this technique effectively, the optimal conditions of hormone priming and time in culture with appropriate mixes and concentrations of hormones and growth factors should be worked out for each strain. When this is done, the whole organ culture method is a powerful tool for studying hormones and growth factors involved in lobuloalveolar development of the mammary gland and the consequent induction of milk synthesis as well as involution.

REFERENCES

1. R. R. Ichinose and S. Nandi (1964). Lobuloalveolar differentiation in mouse mammary tissues *in vitro*. *Science* **145**:496–497.
2. R. R. Ichinose and S. Nandi (1966). Influence of hormones on lobulo-alveolar differentiation of mouse mammary glands *in vitro*. *J. Endocrin.* **35**:331–340.
3. P. M. Terry, M. R. Banerjee, and R. M. Lui (1977). Hormone-inducible casein messenger RNA in a serum-free organ culture of whole mammary gland. *Proc. Natl. Acad. Sci. USA* **74**:2441–2445.
4. B. K. Vonderhaar, Hormones and growth factors in mammary gland development. In C. M. Veneziale (ed.), *Control of Cell Growth and Proliferation*, 1984, Van Nostrand, Reinhold, New York, pp. 11–33.
5. K. Plaut, M. Ikeda, and B. K. Vonderhaar (1993). Role of growth hormone and insulin-like growth factor I in mammary development. *Endocrinology.* **133**:1843–1848.
6. B. G. Wood, L. L. Washburn, A. S. Mukherjee, and M. R. Banerjee (1975). Hormonal regulation of lobulo-alveolar growth, functional differentiation and regression of whole mouse mammary gland in organ culture. *J. Endocrinol.* **65**:1–6.
7. Q. J. Tonelli and S. Sorof (1980). Epidermal growth factor requirement for development of cultured mammary gland. *Nature* **285**:250–252.
8. C. S. Atwood, M. Ikeda, and B. K. Vonderhaar (1995). Involution of mouse mammary glands in whole organ culture: a model for studying programmed cell death. *Biochem. Biophys. Res. Commun.* **207**:860–867.
9. C. S. Atwood, R. C. Hovey, J. P. Glover, G. Chepko, E. Ginsburg, E. Robinson, Jr., and B. K. Vonderhaar (2000). Progesterone induces ductal side branching in the mammary glands of pubertal mice. *J. Endocrinol.* (in press)
10. R. A. Knazek, S. C. Liu, J. S. Bodwin, and B. K. Vonderhaar (1980). Essential fatty acids are required in the diet for development of the mouse mammary gland. *J. Natl. Cancer Inst.* **64**:377–382.
11. H. Michna, Y. Nishino, M. R. Schneider, T. Louton, and M. F. elEtreby (1991). A bioassay for the evaluation of antiproliferative potencies of progesterone antagonists. *J. Steroid Biochem. Mol. Biol.* **38**:359–365.
12. J. Barlow, T. Casey, J. F. Chiu, and K. Plaut (1997). Estrogen affects development of alveolar structures in whole-organ culture of mouse mammary glands. *Biochem. Biophys. Res. Commun.* **232**:340–344.
13. K. Plaut, R. Maple, E. Ginsburg, and B. Vonderhaar (1999). Progesterone stimulates DNA synthesis and lobulo-alveolar development in mammary glands in ovariectomized mice. *J. Cell. Physiol.* **180**:298–304.
14. W. G. Dilley and S. Nandi (1968). Rat mammary gland differentiation *in vitro* in the absence of steroids. *Science* **161**:59–60.
15. D. V. Singh, K. B. DeOme, and H. A. Bern (1970). Strain differences in response of the mouse mammary gland to hormones *in vitro*. *J. Natl. Cancer Inst.* **45**:657 675.
16. M. R. Banerjee, B. G. Wood, and D. L. Kinder (1973). Whole mammary gland organ culture: selection of appropriate gland. *In Vitro* **9**:129–133.
17. D. V. Singh and H. A. Bern (1969). Interaction between prolactin and thyroxine in mouse mammary gland lobulo-alveolar development *in vitro*. *J. Endocrinol.* **45**:579–583.

Chapter 15

Working with the Mouse Mammary End Bud

Charles W. Daniel and Gary B. Silberstein

Abstract. Terminal end buds (TEB) are bulbous, rapidly growing structures responsible for formation of mammary ducts during puberty. Regulation of TEB branching, turning, and extent of growth creates the characteristic pattern of the mammary tree. In this chapter we describe two methods of isolating the TEB, one by simple dissection and the other by enzymatic digestion. A procedure is proposed for the isolation of cap cells, the basal layer of the TEB that differentiates into myoepithelium and which may contribute to other mammary stem cell populations.

Abbreviation. terminal end bud (TEB); minimal essential medium (MEM).

INTRODUCTION

At the beginning of puberty, around 3–4 weeks of age in the mouse, the mammary gland undergoes a spurt of extremely rapid growth, creating the mammary ductal tree that will later serve as scaffolding for secretory lobules. This period of ductal elongation and branching is allometric, indicating that the growth rate of mammary ductal epithelium during puberty is disproportionately more rapid than that of other organs in the body. By 6–7 weeks of age the mammary ducts have approached the available limits of the fat pad and ductal elongation ceases. This growth cessation is due to tissue-level inhibitory influences (1) and occurs even though mammogenic hormones required for growth remain present. In the postpubertal adult, additional growth may occur in the form of side branching in response to the hormones of the estrous cycle; the complexity of this later development depends on whether the strain of mouse in question displays a pronounced luteal phase during the ovarian cycle.

Mammary ducts are composed of two layers of cells: the lumenal epithelium forming the inner layer, surrounded and entirely enclosed by the thin monolayer of longitudinally arranged myoepithelial cells, which synthesize the basal lamina and may mediate interactions between the periductal stroma and lumenal cells. Both of these tissue types are growth quiescent, displaying only the level of DNA synthesis and mitosis required for cell replacement due to the sporadic loss of cells (2). In addition to these differentiated cell types, experimental and morphological evidence demonstrates the presence of scattered stem cells. These may be of more than one type, one presumably responsible for the growth of secretory epithelium

Charles W. Daniel and Gary B. Silberstein   **Department of Biology, University of California, Santa Cruz, California 95065.**

Methods in Mammary Gland Biology and Breast Cancer Research, edited by Ip and Asch. Kluwer Academic/Plenum Publishers, New York, 2000.

during pregnancy, and another for additional ductal elongation, as illustrated by regeneration and growth of ductal cells transplanted into gland-free fat pads of suitable hosts (3, 4).

End buds create the mammary gland. The highly mitotic TEBs supply differentiating myoepithelium and lumenal epithelium for the formation of mature ducts and, presumably, provide the stem cell population as well. They represent the focal point of action of regulatory hormones, growth factors, and cytokines, and are a nexus for stroma–epithelium interactions. Their rate of growth, direction of turning, and bifurcation—with occasional trifurcation—determines mammary patterning and the final extent of development of the ductal tree.

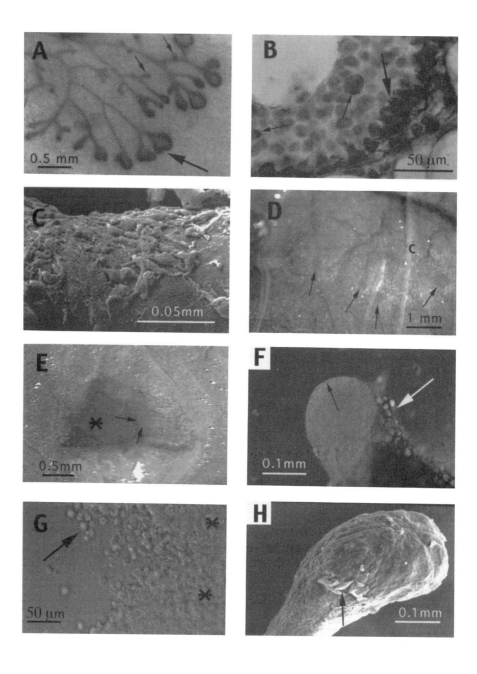

End buds are illustrated in Figure 15-1A. The first and most intensively studied type of end bud is the terminal end bud (TEB). Terminal end buds are responsible for ductal elongation and the formation of the major branches of the ductal tree. A second bud type, the lateral bud (LB), forms along the sides of differentiated ducts and increases pattern complexity by adding branches. Typically these laterals are short, for the LBs can travel only a small distance before approaching another mammary duct, resulting in growth cessation and regression of the LB to form a nonmitotic terminal structure. During pregnancy, additional orders of fine side branching appear, along with alveolar buds that give rise to functionally differentiated tissue.

Mitotic activity and DNA synthesis in the TEB have been described (2, 5). In active TEBs most cells are traversing the mitotic cycle, resulting in a remarkable rate of ductal elongation of about 0.5 mm/day in a large bud. The TEB, like the differentiated duct, consists of two readily distinguished layers. The lumenal epithelium is multilayered, accounting for the large size of these structures in comparison to mature ducts, in which the lumenal epithelium consists of one or a very few layers. In the TEB there are no differentiated myoepithelial cells. In their place are the basal cap cells, a monolayer of cuboidal undifferentiated cells that is, in a formal topological sense, continuous with the basal layer of the skin. Cap cells display characteristics of undifferentiated cells in having few cell–cell adhesions with each other or with the underlying cell mass; rounded nuclei with diffuse chromatin, and undistinguished cytoplasm containing no remarkable accumulations of organelles, complete this picture (6).

Cap cells are the undifferentiated progenitor population for myoepithelium. This is convincingly shown by morphology, in which the progressive accumulation of myofilaments can be traced with electron microscopy (6) and by various molecular markers (7, 8). Cap cells also contribute to the lumenal epithelial population, a well-documented observation that has received little attention in the literature. Williams and Daniel (6) showed by differential staining that small clusters of cap cells appear to break away from their basal location and sink into the multilayered lumenal cell mass of the TEB.

Figure 15-1. Micrographs showing several aspects of mouse mammary end bud. (A) Portion of a whole mount hematoxylin-stained preparation of a no. 4 mammary gland from a 5-week animal in puberty. The rapidly growing TEBs (large arrow) often form a semicircular array, which may aid in their identification *in situ.* The indentation in the indicated TEB probably indicates that this bud will bifurcate to form a major branch point. Small arrows indicate lateral buds (LB) that arise at widely spaced intervals. (B) Histological section of a TEB showing immunostaining of laminin, which is found in cap cells (large arrow) and in certain lumenal cells (small arrows). These laminin-containing lumenal cells can easily be distinguished by color differences, but even here the presence of laminin in the cytoplasm makes these cells stand out from other lumenal cells in which the density is due mainly to nuclear stain. (C) Flank region of a TEB showing connective tissue cells attached to the basal lamina. Cap cells and differentiating myoepithelial cells are beneath the basal lamina and are not visible. (D) TEBs viewed *in situ* in the no. 3 fat pad. Arrows point to the tips of several TEBs, and the subtending ducts in some cases can be seen to extend upwards. C: Collagen strands. (E) A dissection showing a partially revealed TEB. The asterisk indicates a region of the no. 3 fat pad that has been torn away to reveal the exposed tip of a TEB (arrows). In this preparation, the TEB is seen as a smooth-surfaced hemisphere protruding slightly into the torn area of the fat pad. (F) Phase-contrast image of a TEB dissected as described. The monolayer of cap cells can be seen (black arrow), and adherent adipocytes with other ECM material are indicated by the white arrow. (G) Cap cells that have been released as a result of treatment with testicular hyaluronidase. Asterisks indicate the multilayered lumenal epithelium, which has retained its structural integrity. (H) TEB after collagenase digestion. Note that the basal lamina is intact. A small number of presumed fibrocytes are attached to the lamina in the flank region (arrow). Size bars are in some cases approximations and are intended to give a relative idea of comparative size relationships.

More recently, similar observations have been made through the use of immunohisto-chemical staining for P-cadherin, an adhesion molecule specific for cap and myoepithelial cells, and laminin, a component of the basal lamina made in the epithelium only by basal cells (Figure 15-1B). In all cases observed, as the cap cells entered the lumenal layers the molecular markers persisted for a short time but were gradually lost as the cap cells appeared to take on a lumenal identity. It could be argued that these results do indicate not cell migration but merely that occasional groups of lumenal cells express unusual markers. This appears unlikely in view of direct observational evidence using phase-contrast time-lapse microcinematography of freshly isolated, living TEBs. In these studies the migration of cap cells into deeper lumenal layers was directly and unequivocally observed (6).

These observations raise the intriguing possibility that cap cells, in addition to representing myoepithelial stem cells may, by migration and subsequent cell changes, seed the end bud with undifferentiated stem cells that then become scattered throughout the subtending ducts. These cells could be the source of one or more of the putative stem cell classes identified by Chepko and Smith (3). An alternative and more prosaic possibility is that, following migration, they differentiate into ordinary lumenal cells with limited developmental potential, or perhaps disappear altogether through apoptosis.

That cap cells may represent a pluripotent mammary stem cell population is a testable hypothesis. If a population of isolated cap cells, injected into cleared fat pads, proved capable of regenerating complete mammary glands containing all the expected cell types, with potential for normal ductal development and full functional differentiation, this would constitute formal proof of a stem cell population. Because of the central importance of the stem cell question, we first describe how cap cells can be isolated. At this point they could be implanted directly and, equally interesting, cultured to increase their numbers and to investigate their ability to differentiate *in vitro* under controlled conditions. Although this experiment, to our knowledge, has not been attempted and could hardly be described as trivial, the individual steps have been worked out and it does appear feasible to the determined investigator.

MATERIALS AND INSTRUMENTATION

- Stereo dissecting microscope with zoom or stepwise variable magnification. It is useful, though not essential, to use a dual-head model or an instrument equipped with a phototube and a color CCD video pickup, attached to a good-quality monitor; consultation with colleagues is often useful in these technique-sensitive procedures.
- Light source for illumination of mammary glands in anesthetized mice during surgery. Units with dual flexible fiber optic cables are the most useful, since the angle and intensity of illumination must be frequently adjusted to visualize end buds *in situ*, and small differences in the angle at which light strikes the tissue can determine whether an end bud is visible.
- Standard surgical instruments used in mouse surgery. Very sharp, good-quality jeweler's forceps are particularly important, and at least two pair are recommended.
- Female mice approximately 5 weeks of age. Strains with pigmented hair are preferred because the coloration frequently helps to identify the nipple and often increases contrast in the fat pad itself, making glandular elements more easily visible.
- Clinical centrifuge.

- Dulbecco's minimal essential medium (Sigma D-5530) or other chemically defined tissue culture medium.
- Collagenase (Worthington Biochemical 4206 or Sigma type 3).
- Testicular hyaluronidase (Sigma Type I–S, cat. no. H3506).
- Penicillin–streptomycin (Gibco/BRL 15140-031) or other broad-spectrum tissue culture antibiotic.
- 35-mm culture dishes.

METHODS

Surgical Removal of the TEB and Cap Cell Isolation

BACKGROUND. TEBs can be partially isolated by dissection, avoiding the use of enzymes, though mammary ducts cannot. To understand this distinction it is useful to review the relationship between epithelial elements of the mammary ductal tree and the fibrous periductal stroma that surround them. As the rapidly growing end bud invades the adipose-rich stroma, its basal lamina is in direct contact with adipocytes, blood vessels, collagen fibers, and other elements of the mammary fat pad. The end bud tip is not invested in an organized fibrous tunic, as is the subtending duct. On the contrary, the advancing TEB displays an unusual basal lamina that is rich in hyaluronic acid (9), a specialization that provides a slippery, nonadhesive surface facilitating invasion of the TEB through the fat pad.

Distal to the TEB tip, in the "flank" region where the end bud narrows, fibrocytes and mesenchyme-like cells attach to the basal lamina (Figure 15-1C). It is not known whether these cells represent a distinct subpopulation of fibroblasts, but it is apparent that their morphology is different from those in the periductal stroma. This is most readily explained by shape changes associated with adhesion to the basal lamina substrate, which here becomes increasingly rich in sulfated proteoglycans (10). These stromal cells synthesize a tough fibrous extracellular matrix, presumably in response to unidentified paracrine interactions between the epithelium and its contiguous stroma. This periductal tunic consists in large part of Type I collagen, but also contains fibronectin and a myriad of other extracellular matrix molecular types. This dense fibrous envelope stabilizes the differentiated duct and partially inhibits further growth by discouraging promiscuous formation of lateral buds. This inhibitory role is accomplished by accumulation in the periductal matrix of TGFβ1, a powerful inhibitor of mammary ductal growth (10, 11).

PROCEDURE. Because the hyaluronate-rich TEB tip lacks adhesions to surrounding stroma, it can be readily pulled away from the fat pad by using simple instruments such as sharp jeweler's forceps or needles. The mouse is anesthetized, immobilized, and the ventral abdominal skin deflected to reveal the no. 3 thoracic mammary glands (these glands are thinner than no. 4 glands and it is more often possible to visualize glandular elements *in situ*). At this age the enlarged end buds are usually aligned in an arc and, with practice, can be identified as clear areas in the otherwise highly refractile adipose tissue (Figure 15-1D). Each end bud is about 0.25–0.5 mm, with a few as large as 1 mm. Grasp the region of the subtending duct with blunt serrated forceps; using the sharp point of jeweler's forceps, tear away the adipose tissue from the TEB tip. A TEB thus isolated is illustrated in Figure 15-1E–1F.

A region of the gland containing one or more partially exposed end buds may be removed with iris scissors and placed in a 35-mm petri dish containing MEM supplemented with 1 mg/ml testicular hyaluronidase. This enzyme (and probably others, such as Type IV collagenase) will dissolve the exposed basal lamina, revealing the underlying cap cells. Gentle pressure, such as the application of a fragment of coverslip, can stimulate release of the cap cells (Figure 15-1G), which can then be collected with a micropipette and transferred to another container for subsequent culturing or transplantation. The reason that cap cells are released in an almost pure form is that, being undifferentiated, their P-cadherin intercellular adhesions are quite weak compared to the tight E-cadherin junctions interconnecting lumenal cells. Removal of cap cells would probably be accelerated by use of calcium-free medium, but it is likely that this would loosen the lumenal tissue and make contamination with lumenal cells more likely.

Identification of the TEB *in situ* and its dissection is technically challenging and requires practice. This surgical isolation of the TEB has been filmed and will be incorporated into an instructional video. Further information can be obtained through the Biology of the Mammary Gland Homepage *http://mammary.nih.gov/index.html*, at which a link will become available to a site providing information on how to obtain the video.

To our knowledge, the isolation of cap cells (or any other mouse mammary stem cell) has never been attempted. Nevertheless, in the hands of a patient operator, our success in demonstrating the release of cap cells into the medium (Figure 15-1G) indicates that it is feasible. Certainly this is an experiment worth the effort. The isolation of stem cells from any tissue is something of a holy grail of embryology and cell biology. One has only to think of the dramatic consequences of the isolation and culture of embryonic stem cells and their genetic manipulation in culture, making possible the *in vitro* study of differentiation and the creation of gene-targeted animals. Successful isolation, characterization, and subsequent genetic manipulation of a mammary stem cell could have profound implications for future study of breast cancer and for elucidating the genetic regulation of mammary development.

Enzymatic Isolation of the TEB and Other Mammary Structures

BACKGROUND.   Using collagenase it is now a routine procedure to isolate mammary epithelial organoids for culture (12). A modification of these methods makes possible the isolation of entire branches of the mammary tree or, on occasion, the entire mammary tree, extending from the primary duct to the most distal TEBs. These isolates provide an alternative source for end buds, which can be easily cut away from their subtending ducts, and one that has the potential for the isolation of multiple TEBs. It is possible that sufficient TEB tissue could be obtained, for example, for use in microarray analysis of patterns of gene expression.

This procedure provides a different kind of preparation from the surgical isolates described previously. With enzymatic digestion the periductal stroma is removed, leaving bare the basal lamina of the end buds and ducts, except for occasional adherent fibrocytes and other cellular elements (Figure 15-1H).

PROCEDURE
1. Remove no. 4 or no. 3 mammary glands. Dissect out and discard lymph nodes from no. 4 glands. Do not mince the glands, as is done in procedures for isolation of mammary cells for culture. If only the TEBs are of interest, it may be desirable to use only the portion of the gland that contains them, though TEBs may be difficult to identify in the relatively thick no. 4 gland.
2. Incubate each pair of glands overnight for roughly 12 h at 37°C in about 25 ml Dulbecco's minimal essential medium (or equivalent) containing 1.0 mg/ml of collagenase and supplemented only with an antibiotic such as penicillin–streptomycin.

Conical 50-ml centrifuge tubes, capped and placed in an upright position, are convenient for this incubation.

3. Using fresh collagenase solution, place the glands in a petri dish, and under the microscope gently pull away stromal elements from the mammary epithelium. If this is unsuccessful, encourage digestion and dissociation by gentle agitation, such as a platform rocker or gyratory-type shaker; examine the preparations periodically and continue the manual dissection.

4. It may be useful to centrifuge the tissue at $100 \times g$ for 1–2 min to remove fat and adipocytes that have been released. This may be repeated if indicated. It may also be useful to examine the preparations with an inverted phase microscope.

5. When the epithelial tissues have been sufficiently released from stromal elements, they may be transferred to fresh medium lacking collagenase.

CRITICAL ISSUES

None of these procedures are "cookbook" issues, and different conditions, concentrations, and times may need to be used.

PITFALLS

In attempting to isolate cap cells an important pitfall is possible contamination with other cell types. Identification of cap cells with specific markers therefore becomes important, if not essential, and here, unfortunately, there are no specific procedures to follow. One surface marker for cap and myoepithelial cells is P-cadherin. This marker can certainly be used for immunostaining (13) and possibly adapted to cell sorting. Another specific marker that could be useful to distinguish cap from lumenal cells is laminin (unpublished observations; Figure 15-1B). Myofibrils are not useful as markers in these undifferentiated cells. In rats, *Thy-1* has been identified as a marker for cap cells (14) but has not been investigated in the mouse. Additional ideas might be obtained by consulting the contributions of Glukhova and colleagues (8) and Stingl and co-workers (15).

Assuming that isolation of cap cells is successful, the question arises as to what cultural conditions would be most favorable for maintaining their undifferentiated character. A definitive answer is, of course, not available, but one may speculate based on information available from animal studies. The chemical environment in culture should initially be simple, consisting of little more than chemically defined medium only cautiously supplemented with hormones (perhaps insulin), growth factors, or other bioactive materials. Differentiation factors, such as retinoic acid, transforming growth factor type β, and combinations of mammogenic hormones that stimulate functional differentiation, should logically be avoided in the first experiments. With respect to the physical environment, differentiation of cap cells *in situ* is accompanied by changes in the basal lamina, which becomes depleted in hyaluronate and richer in sulfated proteoglycans (9). By this reasoning, a substrate rich in hyaluronic acid might be useful in maintaining the undifferentiated character of these cells. Ultimately, of course, the test for the presence of the genuine stem cell is the ability of cloned populations to develop into identifiable mammary cell types *in vitro* or to regenerate mammary gland when injected into cleared fat pads *in vivo*, an enticing possibility indeed.

REFERENCES

1. C. W. Daniel, G. B. Silberstein, K. Van Horn, P. Strickland, and S. Robinson (1989). TGF-beta 1-induced inhibition of mouse mammary ductal growth: developmental specificity and characterization. *Dev. Biol.* **135**:20–30.
2. F. Bresciani (1968). Topography of DNA synthesis in the mammary gland of the C3H mouse and its control by ovarian hormones: an autoradiographic study. *Cell Tissue Kinetics* **1**:51–63.
3. G. Chepko and G. H. Smith (1997). Three division-competent, structurally-distinct cell populations contribute to murine mammary epithelial renewal. *Tissue Cell* **29**:239–253.
4. E. C. Kordon and G. H. Smith (1998). An entire functional mammary gland may comprise the progeny from a single cell. *Development* **125**:1921–1930.
5. C. W. Daniel and G. B. Silberstein (1987). Postnatal development of the rodent mammary gland. In M. C. Neville and C. W. Daniel (eds.), *The Mammary Gland: Development, Regulation, and Function*, Plenum Press, New York, pp. 3–36.
6. J. M. Williams and C. W. Daniel (1983). Mammary ductal elongation: Differentiation of myoepithelium during branching morphogenesis. *Dev. Biol.* **97**:274–290.
7. A. Sonnenberg, H. Daams, M. A. Van Der Valk, J. Hilkens, and J. Hilgers (1986). Development of mouse mammary gland: Identification of stages in differentiation of luminal and myoepithelial cells using monoclonal antibodies and polyvalent antiserum against keratin. *J. Histochem. Cytochem.* **34**(8):1037–1046.
8. M. Glukhova, V. Koteliansky, X. Sastre, and J. P. Thiery (1995). Adhesion systems in normal breast and in invasive breast carcinoma. *Am. J. Pathol.* **146**:706–716.
9. G. B. Silberstein and C. W. Daniel (1982). Glycosaminoglycans in the basal lamina and extracellular matrix of the developing mouse mammary duct. *Dev. Biol.* **90**:215–222.
10. G. B. Silberstein, P. Strickland, S. Coleman, and C. W. Daniel (1990). Epithelium-dependent extracellular matrix synthesis in transforming growth factor-beta 1-growth-inhibited mouse mammary gland. *J. Cell Biol.* **110**:2209–2219.
11. G. B. Silberstein and C. W. Daniel (1987). Reversible inhibition of mammary gland growth by transforming growth factor-beta. *Science* **237**:291–293.
12. G. H. Smith (1996). Experimental mammary epithelial morphogenesis in an *in vivo* model: Evidence for distinct cellular progenitors of the ductal and lobular phenotype. *Breast Cancer Res. Treatment* **39**:21–31.
13. C. W. Daniel, P. Strickland, and Y. Friedmann (1995). Expression and functional role of E- and P-cadherins in mouse mammary ductal morphogenesis and growth. *Dev. Biol.* **169**:511–519.
14. R. Dulbecco, M. Unger, B. Bowman, and P. Syka (1983). Epithelial cell types and their evolution in the rat mammary gland determined by immunological markers. *Proc. Natl. Acad. Sci. USA* **80**:1033–1037.
15. J. Stingl, C. J. Eaves, U. Kuusk, and J. T. Emerman (1998). Phenotypic and functional characterization *in vitro* of a multipotent epithelial cell present in the normal adult human breast. *Differentiation* **63**:201–213.

Chapter 16

Isolation and Culture of Normal Rat Mammary Epithelial Cells

Kathleen M. Darcy, Danilo Zangani, Ping-Ping H. Lee, and Margot M. Ip

Abstract. Primary culture models offer researchers the opportunity to study the factors that regulate physiologically relevant development of normal mammary epithelial cells under defined conditions. This chapter provides detailed methods for the isolation and culturing of normal mammary epithelial cells. Briefly, excised rat mammary glands are mechanically and enzymatically disaggregated, and organized clusters of mammary epithelial cells are isolated as mammary epithelial organoids. The recovered organoids, free of associated stromal fibroblasts and adipocytes, are then cultured within a complex reconstituted basement membrane rich in laminin, type IV collagen, and sulfated proteoglycans. In the presence of serum-free medium supplemented with insulin, prolactin, progesterone, hydrocortisone, and epidermal growth factor, functionally immature mammary epithelial cells from pubescent virgin rats undergo extensive proliferation, branching morphogenesis, and functional differentiation *in vitro*. Adaptations of these protocols allow mammary gland biologists and breast cancer researchers to isolate and culture various types of normal and malignant mammary cells.

Abbreviations. bovine serum albumin (BSA); double-distilled water (ddH$_2$O); dimethyl sulfoxide (DMSO); extracellular matrix (ECM); epidermal growth factor (EGF); Engelbreth–Holm–Swarm (EHS); fetal bovine serum (FBS); mammary epithelial organoids (MEO); phosphate buffered saline (PBS); reconstituted basement membrane (RBM).

INTRODUCTION

A major obstacle to progress in the fields of mammary gland biology and breast cancer research has been the difficulty of developing defined *in vitro* models that support physiologically relevant development of normal mammary epithelial cells. Presently, primary culture models are the best at providing the essential cell–cell and cell–extracellular matrix (ECM) interactions required for proper development of these cells *in vitro*. In general, organized clusters of mammary epithelial cells, termed mammary epithelial organoids (MEO), are isolated from intact mammary glands and then cultured on or within a substratum such as collagen, laminin, or a combination of ECM components, in the presence of serum-containing or serum-free medium supplemented with specific combinations of steroids and/or polypeptides

Kathleen M. Darcy   GOG Statistical and Data Office, Roswell Park Cancer Institute, Buffalo, New York 14263.   Danilo Zangani, Ping-Ping H. Lee, and Margot M. Ip   Department of Pharmacology and Therapeutics, Roswell Park Cancer Institute, Buffalo, New York 14263.

Methods in Mammary Gland Biology and Breast Cancer Research, edited by Ip and Asch. Kluwer Academic/Plenum Publishers, New York, 2000.

(1). The developmental potential and responsiveness of the primary mammary epithelial cells
are influenced not only by the culture conditions but also by the choice of the mammary gland
donor and the isolation method (1).

This chapter provides detailed methods for the isolation and culturing of mammary
epithelial cells from normal pubescent virgin rats. Figure 16-1 provides an overview of these
procedures, and Table 16-1 indicates the composition of the defined serum-free primary
culture medium. This isolation method can be used to isolate normal MEO from a variety of
mammary gland sources, including rats, mice, or humans at different developmental stages,
or that may vary in their ability to develop mammary tumors. Alternatively, this procedure
can be used to isolate mammary tumor organoids from primary or metastatic mammary
tumors. Furthermore, the serum-free primary culture conditions can be used to support the
in vitro development of various types of normal and tumor-derived MEO. Additionally, we
have found that growth of some mammary cell lines, including two rat mammary tumor lines
(NMU and RBA) and the HC11 mouse mammary epithelial cell line, can be supported by
this medium.

MEO ISOLATION   **RBM Preparation**

Gland Disaggregation	MEO Selection	Procedure
Mechanically mince glands into 1-2 mm³ pieces. Enzymatically digest with dispase and collagenase overnight with minimal agitation	Use density to remove adipocytes. Use size to remove large tissue fragments and single cells. Use adherence to remove stromal cells	Tumor Homogenization. Urea Extraction. Extensive Dialysis. Test for Sterility. Evaluate Biological Activity

PRIMARY CULTURE CONDITIONS

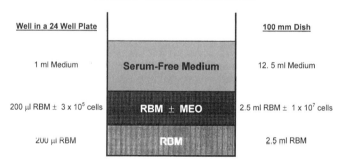

Figure 16-1. An overview of the isolation of mammary epithelial organoids (MEO), the preparation
of the reconstituted basement membrane (RBM), and the primary culture conditions. When isolating
MEO, the appropriate mammary glands are excised from the donor rat, mechanically and enzymatically disaggregated, and the various selection steps used to remove adipocytes, large tissue fragments,
single cells, and adherent stromal cells. The RBM is extracted from the EHS sarcoma, and the recovered matrix is rich in ECM components as well as growth factors (5, 12, 13). The use of dialysis tubing
with a cutoff of 12,000–14,000 kDa permits the removal of small proteins and growth factors. Primary
MEO can be cultured within the RBM on top of a layer of RBM in tissue culture wells or dishes in the
presence of defined serum-free medium.

Table 16-1. Details Regarding the Preparation and Composition of Optimal Primary Culture Medium

Component	Source	Solvent	Stock conc.	Final conc.
DMEM/F12 medium	Sigma (D-2906)	ddH$_2$O	1×	1×
Fatty-acid-free BSA	Sigma (A-6003)	DMEM/F12	10 mg/ml	1 mg/ml
Gentamicin	Gibco (15750-060)	Liquid reagent	50 mg/ml	50 μg/ml
Bovine insulin	Sigma (I-5500)	0.01 N HCl	10 mg/ml	10 μg/ml
Human apo-transferrin	Sigma (T-2252)	DMEM/F12	5 mg/ml	5 μg/ml
Ovine prolactin	NIDDK-NIH	0.01 N NH$_4$OH	1 mg/ml	1 μg/ml
Progesterone	Sigma (P-0130)	100% ethanol	1 mg/ml	1 μg/ml
Hydrocortisone	Sigma (H-4001)	100% ethanol	1 mg/ml	1 μg/ml
Ascorbic acid	Sigma (A-0278)	DMEM/F12	0.88 mg/ml	0.88 μg/ml
Mouse EGF	Collaborative (40001) or UBI (01-101)	DMEM/F12	10 μg/ml	10 ng/ml

MATERIALS AND INSTRUMENTATION

The equipment required for basic cell culture includes (1) a laminar airflow cabinet, (2) a 37°C humidified incubator with 4–5.5% CO$_2$, (3) an inverted tissue culture microscope with phase contrast optics and a mounted camera, (4) a biological microscope, (5) a refrigerated centrifuge for 15- and 50-ml tubes at speeds up to 4500 × g, (6) balances, (7) a pH meter, (8) a hemocytometer, and (9) a liquid nitrogen cryotank. The following materials are recommended for isolating and culturing primary mammary epithelial cells: (1) sterile Falcon tissue culture flasks (T75 and T175 flasks), 100-mm dishes, 24-well plates, tubes (50-ml polypropylene conical tubes and 15-ml polystyrene conical tubes), and pipettes; (2) Corning 500-ml filter units (0.22 μm and 0.45 μm); (3) Nalgene cryovials (2-ml size) and a slow-freeze cryochamber. High-quality deionized and distilled water or double-distilled water (ddH$_2$O) should be used for reagent and media preparation. An autoclave should be available to sterilize glassware, stir bars, and surgical equipment.

DETAILED METHODS

Isolation of Mammary Epithelial Organoids

MATERIALS. The materials required to excise abdominal and inguinal mammary glands from rats include dissecting scissors, surgical forceps with and without teeth, scalpel with appropriate surgical blades, dissecting board, pins or tape to hold down the legs of the animal, ice bucket with ice, and sterile 50-ml conical tubes. The materials required for isolating MEO from intact mammary glands include (1) fetal bovine serum (FBS), phenol red–free DMEM/F12 medium and trypan blue from Sigma (St. Louis, MO); (2) gentamicin from Gibco BRL Life Technologies, Inc. (Grand Island, NY); (3) grade II dispase (Cat. No. 165859) from Roche Molecular Biochemicals (Indianapolis, IN); (4) class 3 collagenase (Cat. No. 4183) from Worthington Biochemical (Freehold, NJ); (5) sheets of 530-μm (Cat. No. 3-530/50) and 60-μm (Cat. No. 3-60/45) Nitex filter from Tetko (Depew, NY); (6) sterile dissecting scissors, forceps with teeth, a 30-ml glass beaker, syringes, and 22- and 25-gauge needles.

PREPARATION OF STERILE 530-μm AND 60-μm NITEX FILTERS. Cut a 5-cm-square piece of 530-μm Nitex filter, a 15-cm-square piece of 60-μm Nitex filter, and 12-cm- and 34-cm-square pieces of heavy-duty aluminum foil. Fold each piece of foil in half twice, cut out a semicircle with a radius of 1.5 cm or 3.8 cm at the center of the folded edge of the small or large piece of foil, respectively. Unfold each piece of foil once, and with the circles superimposed, slip the piece of 530-μm or 60-μm Nitex filter between the small or large pieces of foil, respectively. Fold all four sides of the foil around the filter to secure it in place. For the 60-μm filter, repeatedly fold all four sides of the foil plus filter in small increments to pull the filter as tight as possible. The edge of the 60-μm filter can be secured to the foil with a strip of autoclave tape. Wrap the filters individually in foil, and autoclave. The final dimension of the 530-μm filter should be approximately 5 cm × 5 cm, whereas the 60-μm filter should be approximately 12 cm × 12 cm.

SOLUTIONS AND MEDIA

1. Saline with 1000 units/ml penicillin G: Supplement a 1-L bottle of sterile 0.9% NaCl with 10^6 Units penicillin G (Marsam Pharmaceuticals, Inc., Cherry Hill, NJ). Store at 4°C for up to 3 months.
2. Phenol red–free DMEM/F12 medium: Prepare medium in 1-L batches from powder as recommended by Sigma. Each liter of medium should be supplemented with 1.2 g of sodium bicarbonate and sterilized by passage through a 0.2-μm filter. Store medium in the dark for up to 1 month at 4°C.
3. Digestion solution: Prepare fresh DMEM/F12 medium with 5% (v/v) FBS, 50 μg/ml gentamicin, 0.2% (w/v) class 3 collagenase, and 0.2% (w/v) grade II dispase, and sterilize by passing the solution through a 0.45-μm filter.
4. Adherence medium: Prepare DMEM/F12 medium with 5% (v/v) FBS and 50 μg/ml gentamicin, and sterilize by passing the medium through a 0.2-μm filter.
5. Cryopreservation medium: Prepare DMEM/F12 medium with 50% (v/v) FBS, 10% (v/v) dimethyl sulfoxide (DMSO), and 50 μg/ml gentamicin, and sterilize by passing the medium through a 0.2-μm filter before adding the DMSO.
6. Citric acid solution: Prepare 0.1 M citric acid in ddH$_2$O. For long-term storage, sterilize the solution by passing it through a 0.2-μm filter and store at 4°C.
7. Nuclei preparation buffer: Prepare 20 mM Tris, pH 7.4 at 4°C, with 3 mM CaCl$_2$, 2 mM MgCl$_2$, and 0.3% (v/v) Nonidet-P 40. For long-term storage, sterilize by passing the buffer through a 0.2-μm filter before adding the detergent, and store at 4°C.
8. Trypan blue solution: Prepare 0.25% (w/v) trypan blue in ddH$_2$O. For long-term storage, pass the solution through a 0.2-μm filter and store at 4°C.

PROTOCOL FOR ISOLATING MAMMARY EPITHELIAL ORGANOIDS (MEO)

1. Euthanize rats by asphyxiation with CO_2, extend and secure the legs of each rat on a dissecting board as indicated in Figure 16-2A, and then wet down the fur with 70% alcohol. Using forceps and scissors, make a midline then four side incisions as indicated in Figure 16-2A, and note the location of the six pairs of bilateral mammary glands (Figure 16-2B).
2. Use a scalpel blade and forceps to pull back the skin from both sides of the abdomen and then to dissociate the bilateral abdominal (no. 4), cranial inguinal (no. 5), and caudal inguinal (no. 6) mammary glands. Remove nipples, skin, and muscle from the excised mammary glands. Transfer the glands to sterile 50-ml tubes containing ice-cold sterile saline with 1000 units/ml penicillin G.

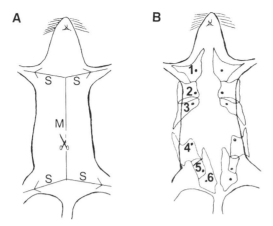

Figure 16-2. Schematic of a rat and the position of the six pairs of mammary glands. The six pairs of mammary glands in the rat are exposed by making a long ventral midline incision (M) and four short ventral incisions (S) from the ends of the midline incision across the arms and legs as indicated in (A). (B) Schematic of the bilateral cervical (no. 1), cranial thoracic (no. 2), caudal thoracic (no. 3), abdominal (no. 4), cranial inguinal (no. 5), and caudal inguinal (no. 6) mammary glands.

When possible, work in a laminar flow cabinet and exercise standard sterile culture techniques.

3. Weigh excised mammary glands in a preweighed sterile 100-mm tissue culture dish and then keep the glands ice-cold while preparing 10 ml of digestion solution per gram of mammary gland. Transfer small batches of mammary gland (~5 g) to a sterile 30-ml beaker with ~15 ml of digestion solution, and then use sterile scissors to mince glands into uniform 1–2 mm^3 pieces. The mincing job is often easier if the glands are first cut into four to five pieces.

4. Transfer the minced mammary gland fragments and the remaining digestion solution to a T175 flask, and incubate the flask horizontally in a 37°C humidified CO_2 incubator for 11–19 h. The digestion is complete when a majority of the floating fragments of mammary gland settle to the bottom of the flask as small lobular organoids (MEO). Light-microscopic examination should reveal that most of the MEO have a smooth surface and are devoid of loosely associated (fuzzy) connective tissue, fibroblasts, and/or adipocytes (Figure 16-3A).

5. Stand the flask in the vertical orientation, allow the free lipid to form a layer above the digestion medium, and carefully aspirate away the upper lipid layer. Split the digest into sterile 50-ml tubes and collect the cells by a 10 min 500 × g centrifugation at 4°C; during this centrifugation step prepare 100 ml of adherence medium and place an autoclaved 530-μm filter on top of a sterile 50-ml tube and an autoclaved 60-μm filter on top of a sterile 100-mm tissue culture dish for use in steps 6–8. After centrifugation of the cells, aspirate off the supernatant and the upper lipid layer, wipe down the sides of the tube with sterile cotton swabs to remove the fatty residue, carefully resuspend the pellets in each tube in DMEM/F12 medium using a 10-ml pipette, repeat the centrifugation step, and gently resuspend the pellets in each tube in a total of 40 ml with DMEM/F12 medium.

6. Pass the cell suspension through the 530-μm Nitex filter and collect the single cells and MEO filtrate in 50-ml tubes. Large tissue fragments, blood vessels, and nerve bundles should be retained on the filter.

7. Pass the 530-μm filtrate through the 60-μm Nitex filter to retain the MEO on the filter and to allow the single cells and small MEO to drop into the underlying 100-mm dish. Take care not to overload the filter with MEO, since clogged filters will trap single cells. Recover the MEO retained on the 60-μm filter by gently flipping the 60-μm filter on top of another sterile 100-mm dish and dropping 5–10 ml of adherence medium on the 60-μm filter to release the MEO into the underlying dish.

8. Pass the recovered MEO through a sterile 530-μm filter, and transfer the filtrate and the remaining adherence medium to a T75 flask with a small sterile stir bar. Transfer three 1-ml aliquots of well-mixed MEO suspension to 15-ml tubes for nuclei isolation and counting (see step 9). Incubate the remaining MEO in the T75 flask in the horizontal orientation in a 37°C humidified CO_2 incubator for 4 h, and gently swirl the flask every 30 min to allow fibroblasts, preadipocytes, and organoids with associated stromal cells to adhere selectively to the flask and be subsequently removed from the nonadherent MEO.

9. During the 4-h adherence incubation, evaluate cell density in the set-aside MEO suspension. Pass the aliquoted MEO suspension through a 1-ml syringe with a 22-gauge needle 10–15 times and incubate the cell suspension with 7 ml of 0.1 M citric acid solution for 90 min in a 37°C humidified CO_2 incubator. Collect the isolated nuclei and residual cells using a 10-min $2560 \times g$ centrifugation at 4°C, resuspend the pellet in 1–5 ml of ice-cold nuclei preparation buffer (depending on the size of the pellet), and pass the suspension through a 6-ml syringe with a 25-gauge needle 10–15 times to break up residual intact cells. Using a hemocytometer, count the nuclei in 10 μl of a mixture of 90 μl nuclei suspension and 10 μl of trypan blue solution and calculate cell number per milliliter as well as cell recovery per gram of starting mammary gland.

10. Nonadherent MEO recovered from the T75 flask after the 4-h incubation (Figure 16-3A) can be used to set up a primary culture study, as described in the subsequent "Primary Culture Conditions" section, or banked as follows. Transfer the nonadherent MEO from the T75 flask to sterile 50-ml tubes and pellet the MEO, using a 10-min $500 \times g$ centrifugation at 4°C. Aspirate off the supernatant and suspend the MEO in cryopreservation medium at a density of $2–5 \times 10^7$ cells/ml in Nalgene cryovials. Slowly freeze MEO for 2 to 24 h in a Nalgene cryocontainer at −80°C and store the vials of MEO in a cryotank.

Preparation of the Reconstituted Basement Membrane

MATERIALS. The Engelbreth–Holm–Swarm (EHS) sarcoma (Cat. No. CRL-2108) can be obtained from American Type Tissue Collection (ATTC) (Rockville, MD) and is carried in female CD2F1 mice. Dissecting scissors, forceps, 3-ml and 20-ml syringes, 18-gauge and 22-gauge needles, 50-ml polypropylene conical tubes, 250-ml glass beaker, 70% alcohol in a dispensing bottle, nonsterile gauze, magnetic stir plate, stir bars, 50-ml and 250-ml graduated cylinders, and liquid nitrogen are required to transplant and harvest the EHS sarcoma. A −80°C freezer is required for storage of excised tumors.

The reconstituted basement membrane (RBM) is prepared from the EHS sarcoma by a modification (2–4) of the procedure of Kleinman *et al.* (5). Alternatively, the RBM can be

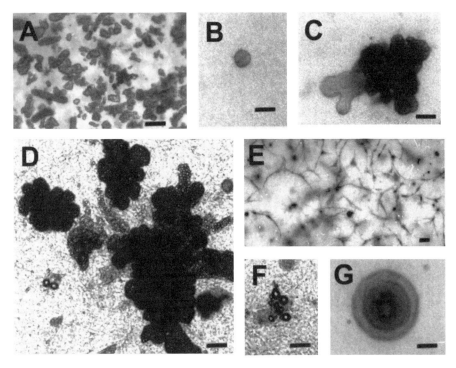

Figure 16-3. Light-microscopic appearance of normal rat MEO. (A) Morphological appearance of newly isolated MEO. With time in culture, a majority of the recovered organoids develop into lobular (B), multilobular (C, D), and lobuloductal (D) MEO. These MEO can also be classified as end bud (B), end bud–alveolar hybrid (C), or alveolar (D). Fibroblasts, stained with a tetrazolium dye to improve the contrast of these stromal cells, are shown in (E). A small cluster of adipocytes is shown in (F) and a lobular squamous colony is shown in (G). The magnification bars in (A)–(G) represent 100 µm.

purchased as the Matrigel reagent from Collaborative Research (Bedford, MA). The materials required to prepare the RBM include (1) a polytron homogenizer with a large probe (Kinematica, Steinhofhalde, Switzerland), (2) Sepcor 250-ml flat-bottomed centrifugation bottles, (3) Spectra/por molecular porous dialysis tubing with a molecular weight cutoff of 12,000 to 14,000 kDa and a diameter of 4.5 cm, and (4) a fixed-angle rotor that can handle flat-bottomed 250-ml bottles with the accompanying temperature-controlled centrifuge for speeds up to $25,000 \times g$. A magnetic stir plate, dialysis clamps, stir bars, beakers, graduated cylinders, dialysis chambers, sterile 50-ml polypropylene conical tubes, and sterile Falcon 24-well tissue culture plates are also required. Finally, N-ethylmaleimide and streptomycin can be obtained from Sigma, chloroform from Fisher Scientific (Fair Lawn, NJ), and phenol red–free RPMI 1640 medium (Cat. No. 3200-084) from Gibco BRL Life Technologies, Inc. (Grand Island, NY).

BUFFERS AND MEDIA

1. Phosphate-buffered saline (PBS): Prepare PBS (137 mM NaCl, 2.7 mM KCl, 4.3 mM Na_2HPO_4, and 1.4 mM KH_2PO_4, pH 7.5 in ddH_2O), pass through a 0.2-µm filter, and store at 4°C.
2. PBS with streptomycin: Supplement PBS with 2 mg/ml streptomycin sulfate and store at 4°C.

3. High-salt buffer: Prepare fresh ice-cold 50 mM Tris, pH 7.4 at 4°C with 3.4 M NaCl, 4 mM EDTA, and 2 mM *N*-ethylmaleimide, and store overnight at 4°C.
4. Urea buffer: Prepare fresh ice-cold 50 mM Tris, pH 7.4 at 4°C with 150 mM NaCl and 2 M urea, and store overnight at 4°C.
5. Tris-saline buffer: Prepare ice-cold 50 mM Tris, pH 7.4 at 4°C with 150 mM NaCl, and store at 4°C.
6. Tris-saline buffer with chloroform: Just before use, add chloroform, to a final concentration of 0.55% (v/v), to ice-cold Tris-saline buffer.
7. Phenol red–free RPMI 1640 medium: Prepare sterile medium from powder as recommended by Gibco, store at 4°C, and supplement with 50 μg/ml gentamicin just before use.

PROTOCOL FOR ESTABLISHING THE EHS SARCOMA
1. Rapidly thaw the EHS tumor suspension from ATTC in a 37°C water bath.
2. Transfer tumor suspension to a sterile 50-ml conical tube and dilute out the DMSO in the suspension at least 10-fold using PBS.
3. Centrifuge the tumor suspension at $500 \times g$ for ~1 min at 4°C, aspirate off the supernatant, and suspend the pellet in ~1 ml PBS with streptomycin. The volume may need to be adjusted to permit the tumor suspension to pass through a 22-gauge syringe.
4. Swab the hind limbs of two recipient mice with 70% ethanol; then use a 3-ml syringe with a 22-gauge needle to inject 0.5 ml of tumor suspension intramuscularly. Allow the tumor to grow out for ~5 weeks. Injection at two sites reduces the number of mice required for tumor passage. Moreover, mice with two tumors show no signs of morbidity and ambulation is not impaired.
5. Excise the EHS sarcoma from the hind limb of a mouse sacrificed by cervical dislocation and transplant each tumor into 10 mice. When the transplanted tumors consistently grow out in ~3 weeks, they can be used for standard transplanting, harvesting, and preparation of the RBM.

PROTOCOL FOR TRANSPLANTING AND HARVESTING THE EHS SARCOMA
1. Sacrifice donor mice by cervical dislocation and excise nonnecrotic EHS sarcoma from the hind limbs. Pool together small pieces of tumor from several donor mice to minimize transplant variability.
2. Generate a tumor suspension by passing 1 g of tumor in 20 ml PBS in a 50-ml tube through a 20-ml syringe without a needle and then through the same syringe with an 18-gauge needle. Fill the tube to 50 ml with PBS.
3. Centrifuge the tumor suspension at $500 \times g$ for ~1 min at 4°C, aspirate off the supernatant, wash the pellet in 50 ml PBS, and repeat the centrifugation step. Suspend the final pellet in a total of 110 ml PBS with streptomycin in a glass beaker with a stir bar, using a magnetic stir plate.
4. Swab the hind limbs of recipient mice with 70% ethanol, then use a 3-ml syringe with a 22-gauge needle to inject 0.5 ml of tumor suspension intramuscularly. Allow the tumor to grow out in the mice for ~3 weeks. The tumor can be injected into one or both legs of the animal.
5. Excise the EHS sarcoma from the hind limbs of mice sacrificed by cervical dislocation, freeze the tumor in liquid nitrogen, and store it at −80°C.

PROTOCOL FOR PREPARING THE RBM FROM THE EHS SARCOMA. *Throughout this procedure the tumor and extract should be kept in beakers in ice or at 4°C.*

1. Transfer a set quantity of EHS sarcoma from a −80°C freezer to a beaker and allow the tumor to thaw overnight at 4°C (100 g of tumor will give approximately 150 ml of RBM).

2. Homogenize the tumor in 2 ml of ice-cold high-salt buffer per gram of tumor, using one or two 30-s pulse[s] of a polytron set at 45% output. The tumor suspension should have a thick grainy consistency and a blood-red color. Centrifuge the tumor suspension in 250-ml Sepcor bottles at 4°C for 15 min at ~12,000 × g and discard the supernatant.

3. Repeat the homogenization and centrifugation steps twice; after the third centrifugation homogenize the tumor pellets in 1 ml of ice-cold urea buffer per gram of original tumor, using two 30-s pulses of a polytron set at 45% output. Extract the viscous tumor homogenate overnight at 4°C with gentle stirring.

4. Centrifuge the extract in Sepcor bottles at ~23,500 × g for 20 min at 4°C, transfer the supernatant to a storage bottle, and keep it at 4°C until the end of step 5. Homogenize the residual pellets in 0.5 ml of ice-cold urea buffer per gram of original tumor, using one 30-s pulse of a polytron set at 45% output, and reextract the homogenate for 1 h at 4°C with gentle stirring. In preparation for step 5, during the second extraction, clamp off one end of the dialysis tubing and preequilibrate the tubing for at least 1 h in Tris-saline buffer at 4°C.

5. Centrifuge the second extract in Sepcor bottles at 4°C for 20 min at ~23,500 × g. Working at 4°C, pool the recovered supernatants in a storage bottle and transfer the pooled supernatants into the dialysis tubing. Clamp off the other end of the dialysis tubing.

6. Dialyze the RBM against Tris-saline buffer containing 0.55% (v/v) chloroform, then two changes of Tris-saline buffer, and finally sterile phenol red–free RPMI 1640 medium with 50 μg/ml gentamicin. Each dialysis should be carried out at 4°C with at least 10 volumes of ice-cold buffer or media relative to the RBM and with gentle stirring for 6–18 h. For convenience, the dialysis buffers are generally changed at the beginning and end of the working day.

7. Working in a laminar airflow cabinet and using standard sterile technique, spray the dialysis bag with 70% alcohol, cut open the bag with sterile scissors, and pool the ice-cold RBM into a sterile 500-ml storage bottle or a sterile beaker in ice. The recovered RBM should have a smooth consistency and a pale beige to rose color.

8. Aliquot the RBM into sterile 50-ml tubes in ice, quickly freeze all but one aliquot of RBM in liquid nitrogen, and store the frozen RBM at −20°C or lower. An aliquot of each batch of RBM should be immediately checked for sterility (see step 9) and then a thawed aliquot can be evaluated at varying dilutions for the ability to support physiological development of primary MEO cultured in the presence of optimal primary culture medium. See the next section for the protocol to evaluate the biological activity of a new batch of RBM.

9. To evaluate RBM sterility, plate 200 μl of 100% RBM into wells in a 24-well tissue culture plate, using a repeater pipette with a 5-ml combitip, allow the RBM to solidify at 37°C for 1–2 h, add 1 ml of medium to each well, and periodically examine the RBM cultured for 2–3 weeks in a humidified 37°C incubator for contamination (usually seen in 2–3 days).

Primary Culture Conditions

MATERIALS.   In addition to the RBM, the following materials are required for culturing primary MEO: (1) progesterone, hydrocortisone, bovine insulin, ascorbic acid, fatty-acid-free fraction V bovine serum albumin (BSA), phenol red–free DMEM/F12 medium, and apo-transferrin from Sigma; (2) gentamicin from Gibco BRL Life Technologies, Inc.; (3) culture-grade mouse EGF from Collaborative Research (Bedford, MA) or Upstate Biotechnology, Inc. (Lake Placid, NY); (4) ovine prolactin from the National Hormone and Pituitary Program (National Institute of Diabetes and Digestive and Kidney Diseases, Bethesda, MD; see application request in *Endocrinology*); (5) sterile glass beakers and stir bars; (6) ice buckets with ice.

MEDIUM

Optimal Primary Culture Medium.   Prepare F12/DMEM medium as described in the section on isolation of mammary epithelial organoids and supplement the medium with 10 µg/ml insulin, 1 µg/ml prolactin, 10 ng/ml EGF, 1 µg/ml progesterone, 1 µg/ml hydrocortisone, 5 µg/ml apo-transferrin, 880 ng/ml ascorbic acid, 1 mg/ml fatty-acid-free BSA, and 50 µg/ml gentamicin as indicated in Table 16-1. The culture medium should be sterilized by passage through a 0.2-µm filter, and it can be stored in the dark at 4°C for up to 3 weeks. Fresh culture medium should be prepared at the beginning of each experiment.

PROTOCOL FOR EVALUATING THE BIOLOGICAL ACTIVITY OF A NEW BATCH OF RBM

1. Thaw an aliquot of RBM overnight at 4°C and dilute the RBM by 10% to 50%, using ice-cold DMEM/F12. Plate 200 µl of ice-cold undiluted RBM as well as each dilution of RBM into appropriate wells in a 24-well plate, and allow the RBM to solidify for 1 to 2 h at 37°C.
2. Quickly thaw banked MEO in a 37°C water bath, bring volume up to 50 ml with DMEM/F12 medium, collect cells by a 10-min $250 \times g$ centrifugation at 4°C, and gently suspend 1.5×10^6 cells in each milliliter of undiluted or diluted RBM. For each type of RBM, plate 200 µl of RBM with 3×10^5 cells into appropriate pre-coated wells in the 24-well plate. Allow the RBM to solidify at 37°C for 2–4 h, add 1 ml of optimal primary culture medium per well, and culture the cells for at least 21 days in a humidified CO_2 incubator at 37°C.
3. Change the medium every 3.5 days and periodically examine the individual cultures with an inverted light microscope with phase contrast optics for morphological changes in the primary MEO (Figure 16-3A–D) and for the outgrowth of fibroblasts (Figure 16-3E), adipocytes (Figure 16-3F), and/or squamous colonies (Figure 16-3G) (3, 4, 6). A suitable batch of RBM will not break up during media removal or addition and will permit 80–95% of the isolated MEO to develop into lobular, multilobular, and lobuloductal organoids (Figure 16-3B–D).

PROTOCOL FOR SETTING UP A STANDARD PRIMARY CULTURE STUDY

1. Calculate the total volume of RBM and quantity of MEC required for the primary culture study and scale up these values by 15%. MEO cultured within wells in a 24-well plate are ideal for quantification of cell number (2), ^{3}H-thymidine incorporation (2, 7), and casein accumulation (4, 6, 8), as well as for basic histological and electron microscopic analysis (2–4). Cultures set up in 100-mm dishes are better for evaluating gene expression, protein expression and localization, apopto-

sis, and signal transduction (9, 10, and unpublished data). Plating densities below 5×10^5 cells/ml RBM result in sporadic and inconsistent outgrowth patterns. In addition, densities higher than 1×10^8 cells/ml RBM are beyond the cellular capacity of the RBM.

2. Thaw the appropriate amount of RBM overnight at 4°C, pool the RBM in a sterile container in ice, and, if necessary, dilute the RBM with ice-cold DMEM/F12 medium. Add 200 µl or 2.5 ml of ice-cold diluted RBM to appropriate wells in 24-well tissue culture plates or to 100-mm dishes, respectively. Allow the RBM to solidify for 1–2 h at 37°C.

3. Set up the experimental cultures using newly isolated MEO or banked MEO (quickly thaw in a 37°C water bath and bring volume up to 50 ml with DMEM/F12 medium). Recover the MEO in sterile 50-ml tubes, using a 10-min $250 \times g$ centrifugation at 4°C. Gently suspend the MEO at a density of 1.5×10^6 cells/ml of ice-cold diluted RBM in a sterile beaker in ice with a sterile stir bar, and plate 200 µl of RBM alone or with 3×10^5 cells into appropriate wells in each 24-well plate. Alternatively, suspend the MEO at a density of 4×10^6 cells/ml of ice-cold diluted RBM in a sterile beaker in ice with a sterile stir bar, and plate 2.5 ml of RBM alone or with 1×10^7 MEC into each 100-mm dish.

4. Allow the RBM to solidify at 37°C for 2–4 h, add 1 ml per well or 12.5 ml per dish of primary culture medium, and culture the cells for up to 21 days in a humidified CO_2 incubator at 37°C. Change the medium every 3.5 days or as necessary for the experimental protocol.

COMMENTS AND PITFALLS

In planning primary culture studies, 2–3 g of abdominal and inguinal mammary glands can be removed from each female (50–60-day-old) Sprague-Dawley rat, and $1–3 \times 10^7$ mammary epithelial cells can be recovered per gram of mammary gland. When first starting this procedure in the laboratory and occasionally thereafter, we recommend that an aliquot of the recovered MEO be fixed in 10% (v/v) phosphate buffered formalin, paraffin-embedded, sectioned, and stained with hematoxylin and eosin. Histological evaluation of the recovered MEO should reveal that these organoids are primarily composed of functionally immature mammary epithelial cells and are devoid of morphologically distinct fibroblasts, adipocytes, and connective tissue. Paraffin blocks should also be prepared from the cells cultured within the RBM to evaluate the types of cells that are developing *in vitro*. The presence of skeletal muscle, fibroblasts, adipocytes, or immune cells in the primary culture can arise from technical problems associated with excising mammary glands or in isolating the MEO.

Several lots of collagenase can be evaluated from companies such as Worthington Biochemical to select a batch that effectively dissociates minced mammary gland fragments into large numbers of MEO devoid of loosely associated stromal tissue. A majority of the recovered MEO should not only remain viable when cultured within the RBM in the presence of optimal primary culture medium, but should also develop into classical mammary end bud as well as alveolar organoids composed primarily of luminal epithelial cells. A convenient digestion time should be a secondary consideration in evaluating new batches of collagenase, since the digestion solution can always be prepared on the basis of collagenase activity per milliliter of solution. For reference, a batch of class 3 collagenase from Worthington Biochemical with an activity of 154 Units/g typically digests minced mammary glands from virgin rats into a high proportion of relatively pure MEO in 13.5–14 h. When needed, the digest in the T175 flask can be swirled during the incubation to speed up the digestion, but special care should be taken since MEO exposed to collagenase and dispase for prolonged periods are very fragile.

It should be emphasized that the isolation procedure results in the recovery of an enriched, not pure, population of mammary epithelial cells. The recovered MEO are primarily composed of functionally immature mammary epithelial cells, and these organized cell clusters are held together by junctional complexes. The primary culture conditions just described not only stimulate functionally immature MEO to undergo extensive proliferation but also induce mammary-specific branching morphogenesis and functional differentiation reminiscent of that observed in rat mammary glands during late pregnancy and lactation. Conditions have also been identified that induce the cultured MEO to undergo apoptosis (9, 10). This model is ideal for studying the full spectrum of developmental events in normal mammary epithelial cells. Like the *in vivo* situation, mammary epithelial development *in vitro* is asynchronous. The asynchronous nature of normal mammary epithelial cells make mechanistic studies challenging to undertake and interpret.

Although the RBM plays an essential role in inducing and maintaining physiologically relevant development of primary MEO *in vitro*, several drawbacks are associated with using this complex ECM. The consistency and biological activity of the RBM varies between preparations, requiring that pilot studies be carried out on each batch of RBM to identify batches and dilutions that support selective survival and induce the maximal outgrowth of normal mammary epithelial cells. Most batches of RBM can be used at a 70% concentration, but some batches break up even when used undiluted. Although the type and magnitude of biological responses observed between experiments that use the same batch of RBM are very consistent, there can be variability in the magnitude of responses observed for different batches of RBM. This type of variability makes it difficult to combine data from primary culture studies using different batches of RBM.

Because the RBM interferes with many biological assays, control samples of RBM alone should be evaluated with samples of MEO cultured within the RBM to determine the contribution of the RBM. When needed, the RBM can be mechanically and/or enzymatically removed from the cultured MEO prior to sample preparation or processing. For enzymatic digestion, a 1:1 mixture of culture medium and 2% (w/v) dispase in PBS is added to the well, the contents of the well are transferred to a 50-ml tube, and digestion is allowed to proceed at 37°C in a gyroshaker at 250 rpm. Unfortunately, these procedures are often time-consuming for multiple samples, disrupt cell–ECM interactions, and/or may damage the cells, thus complicating the evaluation of short-term effects on gene or protein expression, or changes in signal transduction.

As indicated in the introduction, researchers can elect to isolate MEO from mammary glands excised from pregnant or lactating rats, using our standard isolation protocol, but the digestion should be reduced to 4–5 h; moreover, because of the greater epithelial content of these mammary glands the cell recovery per animal is increased by ~15-fold (7). It is important to realize that MEO recovered from pregnant or lactating rats will be primarily composed of functionally differentiated mammary epithelial cells, and these cells are restricted in their developmental potential. To isolate mammary tumor organoids, the standard protocol can be used, but the digestion should only take 9–12 h (Varela and Ip, submitted).

When necessary, the primary culture conditions can be scaled down to perform experiments in 96-well plates. These adjustments make this model more feasible for studies employing scarce reagents or human breast tissue. Also note that modifications of the primary culture model (11, 14) and/or have made it possible to study stromal–epithelial interactions in normal or malignant mammary epithelial cells cultured in transwell inserts with mammary fibroblasts, adipocytes, epithelial cells, and/or tumor cells in the lower culture well. Finally, the combination and concentrations of steroids and polypeptides can be varied to mimic a specific developmental stage or to evaluate the biological effects of a wide variety of natural and synthetic compounds.

ACKNOWLEDGMENTS. We would like to recognize Dr. Hillary Hahm for her work in developing the MEO isolation and primary culture model, and we want to thank the various members of the Ip laboratory who have modified and improved these procedures over the years. We are grateful to Drs. Hynda Kleinman and George Martin for providing us with the EHS tumor and their procedures for transplanting the sarcoma and preparing the RBM. This work was supported by NIH CA33240 and CA64870, DAMD17-94-J-4159, and NIH Cancer Center grant CA16056.

REFERENCES

1. M. M. Ip and K. M. Darcy (1996). Three-dimensional mammary primary culture model systems. *J. Mammary Gland Biol. Neoplasia* **1**:91–110.
2. H. A. Hahm and M. M. Ip (1990). Primary culture of normal rat mammary epithelial cells within a basement membrane matrix. I: Regulation of proliferation by hormones and growth factors. *In Vitro Cell. Dev. Biol.* **26**:791–802.
3. K. M. Darcy, J. D. Black, H. A. Hahm, and M. M. Ip (1991). Mammary organoids from immature virgin rats undergo ductal and alveolar morphogenesis when grown within a reconstituted basement membrane. *Exp. Cell Res.* **196**:49–65.
4. K. M. Darcy, S. F. Shoemaker, P.-P. H. Lee, M. M. Vaughan, J. D. Black, and M. M. Ip (1995). Prolactin and epidermal growth factor regulation of the proliferation, morphogenesis, and functional differentiation of normal rat mammary epithelial cells in three dimensional primary culture. *J. Cell. Physiol.* **163**:346–364.
5. H. K. Kleinman, M. L. McGarvey, J. R. Hassell, V. L. Star, F. B. Cannon, G. W. Laurie, and G. R. Martin (1986). Basement membrane complexes with biological activity. *Biochemistry* **25**:312–318.
6. M. M. Ip, S. F. Shoemaker, and K. M. Darcy (1992). Regulation of rat mammary epithelial cell proliferation and differentiation by tumor necrosis factor alpha. *Endocrinology* **130**:2833–2844.
7. L. M. Varela and M. M. Ip (1996). Tumor necrosis factor-α: A multifunctional regulator of mammary gland development. *Endocrinology* **137**:4915–4924.
8. H. A. Hahm, M. M. Ip, K. Darcy, J. D. Black, W. K. Shea, S. Forczek, M. Yoshimura, and T. Oka (1990). Primary culture of normal rat mammary epithelial cells within a basement membrane matrix. II: Functional differentiation under serum-free conditions. *In Vitro Cell. Dev. Biol.* **26**:803–814.
9. K. M. Darcy, A. L. Wohlhueter, D. Zangani, M. Vaughan, J. A. Russell, S. F. Shoemaker, E. Horn, R. Huang, L. M. Varela, and M. M. Ip (1999). Selective changes in EGF receptor expression and function during the proliferation, differentiation and apoptosis of mammary epithelial cells. *Eur. J. Cell Biol.* **78**:511–523.
10. M. M. Ip, P. A. Masso-Welch, S. F. Shoemaker, W. K. Shea-Eaton, and C. Ip (1999). Conjugated linoleic acid inhibits proliferation and induces apoptosis of normal rat mammary epithelial cells in primary culture. *Exp. Cell Res.* **250**:22–34.
11. D. Zangani, K. M. Darcy, S. Shoemaker, and M. M. Ip (1999). Adipocyte-epithelial interactions regulate the *in vitro* development of normal mammary epithelial cells. *Exp. Cell Res.* **247**:399–409.
12. S. Inoue and C. P. Leblond (1985). The basement-membrane-like matrix of the mouse EHS tumor. I: Ultrastructure. *Am. J. Anat.* **174**:373–386.
13. S. Vukicevic, H. K. Kleinman, F. P. Luyten, A. B. Roberts, N. S. Roche, and A. H. Reddi (1992). Identification of multiple active growth factors in basement membrane matrigel suggests caution in interpretation of cellular activity related to extracellular matrix components. *Exp. Cell Res.* **202**:1–8.
14. K. M. Darcy, D. Zangani, W. K. Shea-Eaton, S. F. Shoemaker, P.-P. H. Lee, L. H. Mead, A. Mudipalli, R. Megan, and M. M. Ip (2000). Mammary fibroblasts simulate growth, alveolar morphogenesis and functional differentiation of normal rat mammary epithelial cells. *In Vitro Cell. Dev. Biol.* In press.

Chapter 17

Characterization of Normal Human Breast Epithelial Cell Subpopulations Isolated by Fluorescence-Activated Cell Sorting and Their Clonogenic Growth *In Vitro*

John Stingl, Connie J. Eaves, and Joanne T. Emerman

Abstract. Luminal-cell-restricted, myoepithelial-cell-restricted, and mixed progenitors of the human mammary epithelium can be isolated by fluorescence-activated cell sorting of cells harvested from 3-day primary cultures of normal mammary tissue. Useful markers that allow these populations to be distinguished are MUC1, CALLA, $\alpha6$ integrin, and epithelial-specific antigen. The progenitor content of the sorted cell subpopulations is detected in a 9- to 12-day colony assay in which the cells are cultured in a serum-free medium with NIH 3T3 feeders to optimize the growth of luminal and myoepithelial progenitors plated at low densities. Efficiencies of colony formation of 1–20% and colony sizes of >100 cells are routinely observed in such cultures. The different types of colonies can be readily identified by their gross morphology and their expression of a variety of luminal- and myoepithelial-cell-specific proteins.

Abbreviations. fluorescence-activated cell sorting (FACS); human breast epithelial cells (HBEC); Ham's F12/Dulbecco's modified Eagle's medium/Hepes (F12/DME/H); penicillin (P); streptomycin (S); bovine serum albumin (BSA); insulin (INS); hydrocortisone (HC); cholera toxin (CT); tris hydroxymethyl amino methane hydrochloride (TRIS); fetal bovine serum (FBS); Hank's balanced salt solution supplemented with sodium azide and FBS (HFN); propidium iodide (PI); mammary gland mucin (MUC1); common acute lymphoblastic leukemia antigen (CALLA); fluorescein isothiocyanate (FITC); R-phycoerythrin (PE); epithelial-specific antigen (ESA); epithelial cell adhesion molecule (Ep-CAM); $\alpha6$ integrin ($\alpha6$); immunoglobulin (IgG); epidermal growth factor (EGF); serum-free medium (SF medium); human mammary fibroblasts (HMF); red blood cell (rbc); alkaline phosphatase anti-alkaline phosphatase (APAAP).

INTRODUCTION

The human mammary epithelium is composed of different cell types. Luminal epithelial cells line the lumen of the ducts and alveoli of the mammary tree, and underlying these are the

John Stingl and Joanne T. Emerman   Department of Anatomy, University of British Columbia, Vancouver, British Columbia, V6T 1Z3 Canada.   Connie J. Eaves   Department of Medical Genetics, University of British Columbia, Terry Fox Laboratory, British Columbia Cancer Agency, Vancouver, British Columbia Canada.

Methods in Mammary Gland Biology and Breast Cancer Research, edited by Ip and Asch. Kluwer Academic/Plenum Publishers, New York, 2000.

Normal human mammary tissue

Enzymatic dissociation

Three day culture

Cell harvesting and labelling for FACS

Seeding of immunophenotypically distinct cells
in an in vitro HBEC colony forming assay

9-12 days

Analysis of colonies

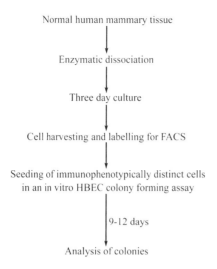

Figure 17-1. General protocol for studying the clonal growth of immunophenotypically distinct HBEC isolated from primary cultures of HBEC.

smooth muscle-like myoepithelial cells. As well, a population of cells having a phenotype intermediate between luminal and myoepithelial cells has been described and postulated to represent the mammary epithelial stem compartment (1, 2). Recently, we have identified a similar intermediate cell type present in short-term cultures of freshly isolated human mammary tissue (3). This work has come from a major commitment of our laboratory to understand the stem cell biology of the resting human adult mammary gland. The specific approach we have taken has revolved around the identification of culture conditions that support the growth of luminal and myoepithelial cell lineages from single isolated precursors. This methodology has then been combined with fluorescence-activated cell sorting (FACS) of the original precursor-containing cell suspensions to enable the growth and differentiation of immunophenotypically distinct human breast epithelial cell (HBEC) subpopulations to be examined (Figure 17-1). This chapter describes the methods for generating initial primary human breast epithelial cell cultures from normal adult human mammary tissue, the cell markers used to identify different HBEC populations and their use in isolating discrete subpopulations of HBEC, the culture conditions used to optimize the yield of different types of colonies from single HBEC, and the different types of colonies thus obtained.

MATERIALS AND INSTRUMENTATION

Items required for each key procedure

1. *Mammary Tissue Dissociation and Initiation of Primary Cultures*: cooler with ice; 220-ml (8 oz) specimen containers; forceps; scalpels; glass petri dish; 250-ml Bellco ridged dissociation flasks (Bellco Glass, Inc., Vineland, NJ); aluminum foil; parafilm; rotary shaker in a 37°C incubator; 50-ml centrifuge tubes; culture vessels
2. *Cell Labeling and Cell Sorting*: cooler with ice; 15-ml centrifuge tubes; 20-μm mesh (BioDesign Inc., New York); 25-mm Swinnex filter holders (Millipore Corporation, Bedford, MA); 20-ml syringes; 12 × 75 mm polystyrene tubes; fluorescence-activated cell sorter (FACStar[PLUS], Becton Dickinson, San Jose, CA); 1.5-ml microfuge tubes

3. **HUMAN BREAST EPITHELIAL CELL COLONY-FORMING ASSAY**: 60-mm tissue culture dishes; dissecting microscope

METHODS

Reagents and Reagent Preparation

MAMMARY TISSUE DISSOCIATION AND INITIATION OF PRIMARY CULTURES

1. Transport medium: Ham's F12/Dulbecco's modified Eagle's medium [F12/DME mixed 1:1 (v:v)] (StemCell Technologies, Vancouver, B.C., Canada) supplemented with 10 mM Hepes (H) (Sigma Chemical Co., St. Louis, MO) and 5% calf serum (Gibco Laboratories, Grand Island, NY)
2. Dissocation medium: F12/DME/H supplemented with 100 U/ml penicillin (P) (StemCell), 100 µg/ml streptomycin (S) (StemCell), 20 mg/ml bovine serum albumin (BSA, Fraction V) (Gibco), 5 µg/ml insulin (INS) (Sigma), 0.5 µg/ml hydrocortisone (HC) (stock solution is dissolved in ethanol) (Sigma), 10 ng/ml cholera toxin (CT) (Sigma), 100 U/ml hyaluronidase (Sigma), and 300 U/ml collagenase (Sigma) (collagenase is a low-trypsin crude preparation at 300 U/mg) (Cat. No. C9891, Sigma). For preparation of the 10× collagenase and hyaluronidase stock, dissolve collagenase at 3×10^3 U/ml and hyaluronidase at 10^3 U/ml together in F12/DME/H and store at −70°C.
3. Red blood cell lysis solutions: 0.155 M NH$_4$Cl (8.3 g NH$_4$Cl + 1 L H$_2$O) and 0.170 M tris(hydroxymethyl amino methane hydrochloride) (TRIS) pH 7.65 (2.06 g TRIS + 0.1 L H$_2$O).
4. Primary culture growth medium: F12/DME/H supplemented with 100 U/ml P, 100 µg/ml S, 1 mg/ml BSA, 1 µg/ml INS, 0.5 µg/ml HC, and 10 ng/ml CT. Five percent fetal bovine serum (FBS) (Gibco) is included in the primary culture medium for the first 24 h.

HARVESTING PRIMARY CULTURES AND CELL SORTING

1. Trypsinization solution: 0.05% trypsin (Gibco) and 0.025% EDTA (Sigma) in saline
2. Staining buffer and miscellaneous reagents: Hank's balanced salt solution (StemCell) suppplemented with 0.02% sodium azide (w/v) (Sigma) and 2% FBS (HFN)
3. 1 mg/ml DNAse I (Sigma) in HFN
4. Dispase (50 caseinolytic units/ml in Hank's balanced salt solution) (Collaborative Biomedical Products, Bedford, MD)
5. Human serum (Red Cross)
6. 1 mg/ml propidium iodide (PI) (Sigma) dissolved in phosphate buffered saline

ANTIBODIES RECOGNIZING THE FOLLOWING EPITOPES

1. Mammary gland mucin MUC1 (also commonly known as polymorphic epithelial mucin, epithelial membrane antigen, episialin, and eight other names; see Ref. 4 for structure and biology of this mucin), IgG1 clone HMFG-2 (gift from Dr. J. Taylor-Papadimitriou, Imperial Cancer Research Fund, U.K.; also commercially available from Novocastra Laboratories, Newcastle upon Tyne, U.K.) used as an undiluted supernatant, and IgG1 clone 214D4 (gift from Dr. J. Hilkens, The Netherlands Cancer Institute) used at 1:100 dilution of the supernatant.

2. Common acute lymphoblastic leukemia antigen (CALLA/CD10), IgG1 clone SS2/36 (DAKO, Mississauga, Ont., Canada) conjugated directly either to fluorescein isothiocyanate (FITC) or R-phycoerythrin (PE). Both used at 1:10 dilution.

3. Epithelial specific antigen/epithelial cell adhesion molecule (ESA/Ep-CAM), IgG1 clone VU-1D9 (Novocastra) used at 1:100 dilution (0.4 μg/ml), and IgG1clone Ber-EP4 conjugated directly to FITC (DAKO) used at 1:10 dilution.

4. IgG1 control antibodies directly conjugated to FITC or PE (DAKO) used at a 1:10 dilution are used as negative controls for the CALLA and ESA primary antibodies that are directly conjugated to FITC or PE.

5. α6 integrin (CD49f), IgG2 clone GoH3 (PharMingen Canada, Mississauga, Ont., Canada) used at 1:100 dilution (5 μg/ml). HFN supplemented with normal rat serum to a final concentration of 10% is used as a negative control for α6 integrin binding.

6. Goat anti-mouse IgG (H + L) directly conjugated to PE (Jackson Immuno-Research Laboratories, Inc., West Grove, PA) used at 1:125 dilution.

7. Goat anti-rat IgG (H + L) directly conjugated to FITC (Jackson) used at 1:100 dilution.

8. Keratin 14, IgG3 clone LL002 (Novocastra) diluted 1:20 (5 μg/ml).

9. Keratin 8/18, IgG1 clone 5D3 (Novocastra) diluted 1:40 (2 μg/ml).

10. Keratin 19, IgG1 clone RCK 108 (DAKO) diluted 1:80 (0.5 μg/ml).

11. An IgG1 mouse monoclonal recognizing dextran (a gift from Dr. Peter Lansdorp, Terry Fox Laboratory, Vancouver, B.C., Canada) diluted to 5 μg/ml was used as a negative control for the HMFG-2, 214D4, K14, K8/18, and K19 staining experiments presented herein.

HBEC COLONY-FORMING ASSAY

1. Serum-free growth medium (adapted from Refs. 5, 6, and 7): Primary culture medium supplemented with 10 ng/ml epidermal growth factor (EGF) [Collaborative; medium here referred to as serum-free (SF) medium].

2. Feeder layer: NIH 3T3 mouse fibroblasts (American Type Culture Collection, Rockville, MD) irradiated at 5×10^3 cgy and seeded at 4×10^3 cells/cm^2 in 60-mm culture dishes in F12/DME/H + 5% FBS + 5 μg/ml insulin.

3. Fixative: acetone:methanol (1:1) at −20°C.

4. Staining solution: Wright's Giemsa (Fisher Scientific, Vancouver, B.C., Canada).

Detailed Procedures

INITIATION OF PRIMARY HBEC CULTURES.   Prior to the reduction mammoplasty surgery, two 220-ml specimen containers filled with 100 ml of F12/DME/H supplemented with 5% calf serum are delivered to the operating room on ice in a cooler (the size of the specimen container depends on how much surgical tissue the surgeon will provide). Following the surgery, the specimens are returned immediately to the laboratory and transferred aseptically to a glass petri dish with forceps. The patient's age and specimen characteristics (e.g., size, consistency, appearance, etc.) are then recorded. With a pair of scalpels, the sample is minced until the pieces of tissue are approximately 3 mm^3, and the specimen is transferred to a Bellco dissociation flask. Dissociation medium is then added such that the total volume of the mixture is no higher than the widest point of the dissociation flask and the minced tissue is well suspended within the medium and is easily swirled about (e.g., there should be more

dissociation medium than minced tissue). If the surgical samples are large, several dissociation flasks are needed. The flask is then covered with sterile aluminum foil and placed onto
a rotary shaker inside a 37°C incubator for 16–24 h. Should the incubator not be equilibrated
at 5% CO_2, the flask must also be wrapped with parafilm to prevent the dissociation mixture
from becoming too alkaline. Digestion is complete when all large tissue pieces have been
digested and the suspension is made up of single cells and organoids (e.g., the suspension
can be drawn into a 10-ml pipette). It is not uncommon to have occasional undigested pieces
of tissue following 16–24 h of digestion, especially if the starting material is tough and fibrous.
Usually these few pieces are discarded, but if they are numerous they can be collected by
allowing the suspension to settle. The supernatant containing the organoids can then be
decanted, fresh dissociation media added to the tissue pieces, and the suspension dissociated
until completion. The epithelial-cell-rich pellet in the supernatant is collected by centrifuging the cell suspension in 50-ml centrifuge tubes at 80 g for 4 min. The supernatant from this
first centrifugation can be saved as a crude source of human mammary fibroblasts (HMF).
To obtain these, the cells are centrifuged at 100 g for 10 min and then resuspended and cultured in standard tissue culture flasks in F12/DME/H supplemented with 5% FBS and 5 µg/ml
insulin (a more detailed procedure to separate stromal fibroblasts, pericytes, and blood vessels
from one another is described in Ref. 8).

Typically, a large red blood cell (rbc) pellet cosediments with the epithelial pellet of the
first centrifugation. Unless the pellet is to be frozen in liquid nitrogen (in which the rbc do
not survive), the rbc are selectively lysed by an ammonium chloride treatment. To perform
this, the pellet is resuspended in 2 ml of primary culture growth medium to which 9 ml of
0.155 M NH_4Cl and 1 ml of 0.170 M TRIS are added. The suspension is then incubated for
15 min in a 37°C water bath. The suspension is then centrifuged at 100 g for 5 min and the
supernatant discarded. The epithelial pellet is resuspended in primary culture growth medium
supplemented with FBS to a final concentration of 5% and aliquoted into 25- or 75-cm^2 tissue
culture flasks at a subconfluent density (approximately 25%). After 24 h, the media is changed
to the serum-free primary culture growth medium, and the culture is maintained for a further
2 days *in vitro* before harvesting the cells for analysis or sorting using the FACS. When freshly
isolated single HBEC are required, a 15–30 min treatment with a phosphated buffered saline
solution containing 0.05% trypsin, 0.02% EDTA, and 0.4 mg/ml DNAse treatment of the
HBEC organoids followed by cell filtration can be used (9).

The initial 3-day culture period allows nonadherent blood cells and debris to be washed
away, while allowing the organoids to flatten out onto the tissue culture plastic and to become
easier to harvest into a single cell suspension. Exposure to a minimal growth medium (no
EGF or serum, serum is present only in the first 24 h to promote cell attachment) during this
period reduces proliferation and HBEC lineage selection while maintaining cell viability.
Although serum has been reported to promote luminal cell survival (10, 11), it also promotes
stromal cell growth (6) and is thus better avoided for the latter 48-h culture period in order
to select in favor of HBEC. However, to date, we have not examined specifically the effects
of inclusion of EGF and serum in the presort culture medium on the subsequent phenotypes
of HBEC obtained.

CELL STAINING AND FACS.   Three-day primary cultures are incubated with prewarmed
trypsin solution and gently agitated until all cells are released from the plastic substratum.
An equal volume of cold HFN is added to the trypsin solution, and the cell suspension is centrifuged at 100 g for 5 min. After disposal of the supernatant, 1 ml of HFN, 100 µl of dispase,
and 50 µl of DNAse I are added to the epithelial pellet, and the suspension is warmed to 37°C

in a water bath for 5 min to promote disaggregation of any cell clumps. The suspension is then diluted with 10 ml of cold HFN and filtered through a 20-μm mesh. Cell clumps adhering to the mesh can be washed off and recultured. The filtrate is centrifuged at $100g$ for 5 min, the resulting pellet is diluted with 1 ml of cold HFN supplemented with 10% human serum, and the suspension incubated for 30 min on ice to reduce nonspecific antibody binding. For all preblocking and antibody incubation steps, the cell concentration should not exceed 10^7 cells/ml. The cell suspension is then aliquoted into (typically) four 12×75 polystyrene tubes (polypropylene tubes are not used because they do not make a good vacuum seal with the flow cytometer). The first tube is stained with control antibodies, the second and third with single-label antibodies (conjugated directly or indirectly to PE or FITC), and the fourth is double labeled (for selection of sort markers, see subsection "Cell Markers That Distinguish Subpopulations of HBEC"). The single-label cells are used for setting single color parameter compensation. Thirty-minute incubations on ice are used for all antibodies followed by two 3-ml washes with cold HFN. On the last wash, the cells are diluted with 1 μg/ml of PI in 10 ml of cold HFN, and the suspension filtered a second time through a 20-μm mesh. Propidium iodide is added to the last wash to allow identification and exclusion of PI⁺ (dead) cells from subsequent analysis or sorting procedures. The filtrate is then centrifuged, and the resultant pellet resuspended with 300–600 μl of cold HFN supplemented with 0.1 mg/ml DNAse I. Viable (PI⁻) cells are sorted into 1.5-ml microfuge tubes containing cold SF medium supplemented with 10% FBS. During all staining, incubation, and sorting procedures, the cells are kept in the dark and maintained on ice.

An important consideration for separating cells by flow cytometry is achievement of a single-cell suspension, since the cells must pass through a small orifice (70 μm on the FAC-STAR^{PLUS}) when being sucked into the flow cytometer. The purity of the sort is limited by the ability to disaggregate dissimilar cells as well. The protocols described here rely on a short presort culture period, treatment with a variety of enzymes (trypsin, dispase, and DNAse), inclusion of the metabolic inhibitor sodium azide, two filtration steps through a 20-μm mesh (one at the beginning of cell labeling and one immediately prior to cell sorting), and maintenance of the cells on ice in an attempt to generate single-cell suspensions.

HBEC COLONY-FORMING ASSAY. We have observed that successful primary cultures can be routinely initiated from >80% of breast reduction samples isolated from premenopausal women. The probability of obtaining successful HBEC cultures appears to be related to the developmental stage of the tissue (12). It has been known for a long time that HBEC grow poorly at low densities unless feeder layers are provided (13). More recently we confirmed that NIH 3T3 mouse embryonic fibroblasts, when irradiated at 5×10^3 cgy and seeded at 4×10^3 cells/cm² (subconfluent), promoted the growth of HBEC colonies. To obtain HBEC colonies, HBEC (sorted or unsorted) are simply seeded at 2×10^3 cells per 60-mm culture dish (approximately 100 cells/cm²) in SF medium supplemented with 5% FBS. After 48 h, the medium is switched to SF medium and the cultures are maintained for a further 7 to 10 days with no further medium changes. To score colonies, the plates are fixed in acetone : methanol (1 : 1), air-dried, rinsed with H_2O, and stained with Wright's Giemsa. The colony number and phenotype (see the following) are then best scored under a dissecting microscope. Alternatively, the cells can be stained immunohistochemically to detect specific epitopes. In this case, it may be necessary to grow the cells on collagen-coated glass coverslips, depending on the fixatives and microscope to be used. With this procedure, HBEC colony-forming efficiencies of 1–20% and colony sizes of 2 to >100 cells are routinely observed.

The importance of feeders in promoting colony growth by HBEC is illustrated in Figure 17-2, which demonstrates the proliferation of HBEC subcultured from a 3-day primary culture

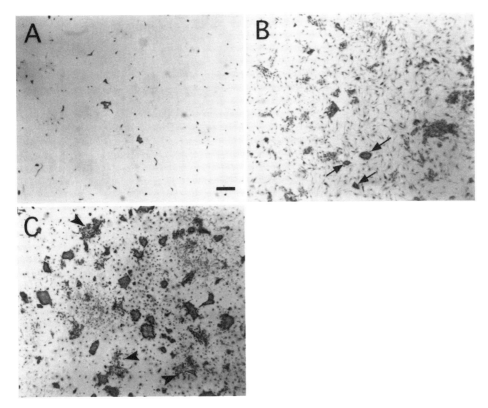

Figure 17-2. Effect of HMF and NIH 3T3 feeders on HBEC colony formation. Unsorted HBEC isolated from a 3-day primary culture were seeded at 500 cells/cm^2 in the absence of any feeder (A), in the presence of an irradiated HMF feeder (B), or in the presence of irradiated NIH 3T3 feeders (C), maintained for 11 days in SF medium, and then stained with Wright's Giemsa. Note that the majority of the colonies in the presence of the HMF feeder have a myoepithelial cell phenotype and that only a few colonies exhibiting a luminal cell phenotype are observed (arrows). In the presence of the NIH 3T3 feeders, abundant luminal cell colonies are observed in addition to the myoepithelial cell colonies (arrowheads). Bar = 10^3 μm.

initiated from mammary tissue from a 29-year-old woman and seeded at 500 cells/cm^2 in the absence of any feeder cells (Figure 17-2A), in the presence of irradiated (at 5×10^3 cgy) passaged HMF (Figure 17-2B), and in the presence of irradiated murine embryonic fibroblasts (NIH 3T3 cells) (Figure 17-2C). Although Figure 17-2 is at low magnification, myoepithelial cells can be identified by their dispersed cell arrangement (arrowheads in Figure 17-2C), whereas the luminal cells can be identified by their close cell arrangement with one another (arrows in Figure 17-2B; the morphology of myoepithelial and luminal HBEC are described in more detail in the "Phenotype of HBEC Colonies" section). Although both HMF and NIH 3T3 cells support clonogenic growth of luminal and myoepithelial cells in a serum-free medium, we have consistently observed threefold more and larger colonies of cells exhibiting a luminal morphology in cultures containing NIH 3T3 feeders compared to HMF feeders (unpublished observations).

PHENOTYPE OF HBEC COLONIES.   When HBEC are seeded at low densities and then cultured for another 9 to 12 days, a spectrum of colony phenotypes is observed (Figures

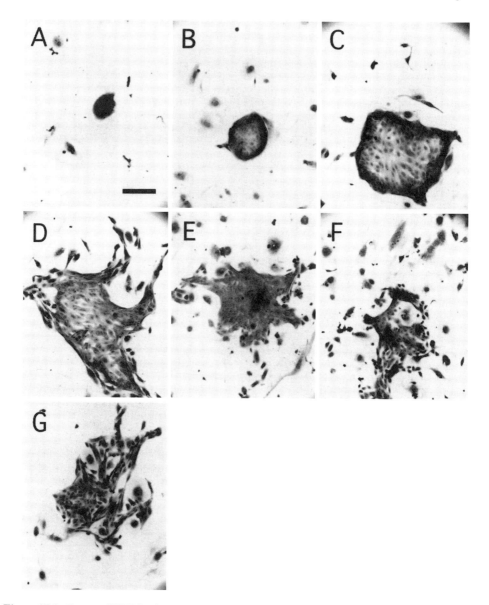

Figure 17-3. Range of HBEC colony morphologies observed after 11 days in culture. All colonies were generated from the same original primary HBEC culture. Colony phenotypes include pure luminal colonies (A–C), mixed phenotypes (D–F), and pure myoepithelial cell colonies (G). Bar = 250 μm.

17-3A–G). Colonies range from being composed entirely of cells exhibiting luminal characteristics (Figures 17-3A–C) to colonies composed exclusively of cells exhibiting myoepithelial characteristics (Figure 17-3G), with others containing a mixture of these cell types (Figures 17-3D–F). Pure luminal cell colonies are typically composed of tightly arranged cells with indistinct cell borders. In the larger colonies in which only luminal cells are seen, the cells located at the periphery of the colony are more closely arranged than the more centrally located cells, which suggests the formation of a central lumen (Figures 17-3B, C). This effect, particularly evident when the cells are cultured in the presence of NIH 3T3 cells, could be due to the fact that HMF (14) and NIH 3T3 cells (15) are a source of hepatocyte growth factor, a cytokine involved in HBEC epithelial cell polarization (reviewed in Ref. 16). The cells produced in the colonies derived from luminal-cell-restricted progenitors express the typical luminal epitopes keratin 8/18 (Figure 17-4A), keratin 19 (Figure 17-4B), MUC1 (Figure 17-4C), and ESA/Ep-CAM (data not shown) (3), and show low levels of expression of keratin 14 (colony indicated by arrow in Figure 17-4D) similar to the distribution of keratins within the mammary epithelium *in vivo* (as described in Ref. 17). We have previously speculated that the progenitors that generate these luminal-cell-restricted colonies may be alveolar progenitors since they generate alveolar-like structures with cuboidal epithelial cells arranged around a central lumen when cultured in a three-dimensional collagen gel matrix (3).

Pure colonies of myoepithelial cells are composed of highly refractile dispersed teardrop-shaped cells that express keratin 14 (lower colony in Figure 17-4D) and CALLA (18) but do not express keratin 19 (Figure 17-5A). Karsten and collegues reported expression of MUC1 by a minor population of cells expressing a myoepithelial-like phenotype (18), but we have not observed MUC1 staining by the myoepithelial cells seen in pure colonies of these

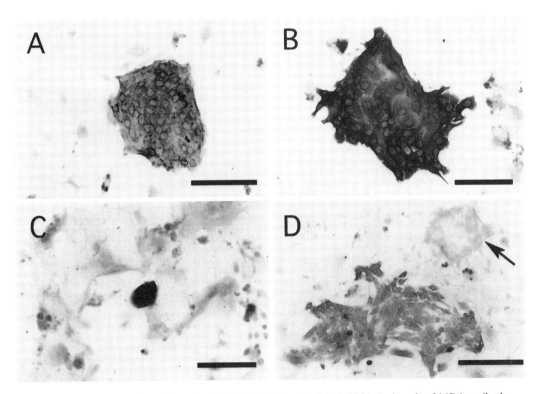

Figure 17-4. Expression of keratin 8/18 (A), keratin 19 (B), MUC1 (using the 214D4 antibody, C), and keratin 14 (arrow in D) in pure luminal cell colonies. HBEC were seeded at low density on collagen-coated glass coverslips in the presence of NIH 3T3 feeders and were then cultured in SF medium. After 10 days, the coverslips were fixed in −20°C acetone. The expression of the various epitopes was visualized by using the alkaline phosphatase anti-alkaline phosphatase (APAAP) technique, and the cells were counterstained with Wright's Giemsa. Background staining with a negative control antibody is shown in Figure 17-6F. Bar in (A) and (D) = 250 μm. Bar in (B) and (C) = 100 μm.

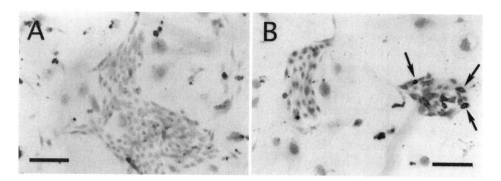

Figure 17-5. Expression of keratin 19 (A) and keratin 8/18 (B) in pure myoepithelial cell colonies. Note the heterogeneous expression of keratin 8/18 (arrows) in the colony on the right in (B). These cells were prepared like those in Figure 17-4. Background staining with a negative control antibody is shown in Figure 17-6F. Bar = 250 µm.

cells. Although the term *myoepithelial* is used to describe these keratin 14⁺–keratin 19⁻ cells herein, these cells are not differentiated myoepithelial cells since they do not express smooth muscle actin, which is a more accurate marker for the myoepithelial lineage (19). The lack of smooth muscle actin expression in these cells is related to the culture conditions in which the cells are maintained, since smooth muscle expression is inversely correlated with the proliferative status of these cells (20). The cells of these pure myoepithelial colonies correspond to the type II or "basal" cells described by others (18, 21), which have been reported to express histo–blood group antigen H type 2 (18) and are deficient in gap junctional intercellular communication (22). Interestingly, we have observed a heterogeneous expression of keratin 8/18 in myoepithelial cell colonies (keratin 8/18⁺ myoepithelial cells in a myoepithelial colony are indicated by the arrows in Figure 17-5B), and a similar finding has been noted by others (17, 18, 23).

The mixed colonies typically contain a central core of cells that may be piled up on one another or flattened, but generally have poorly defined cell borders. The cells express the typical luminal epitopes keratin 8/18 (Figure 17-6A), keratin 19 (Figure 17-6B), MUC1 (Figure 17-6C), and ESA (data not shown) (3), but are negative for the myoepithelial-specific keratin 14 (arrows in Figure 17-6E). The centrally located cells are different from those in the pure luminal colonies in that the more distal cells usually do not pile up on one another as if trying to form a lumen. Instead, keratin 14–expressing cells emerge at the periphery of the centrally located keratin 14⁻ cells (Figure 17-6E). These primitive myoepithelial cells also express keratins 8/18 (arrowheads in Figure 17-6A), whereas myoepithelial cells maintained *in vitro* for extended periods of time down-regulate expression of this protein (3, 24). We have previously proposed that the progenitors that generate these mixed (luminal–myoepithelial) colonies may in fact be ductal progenitors rather than alveolar progenitors, since we have found that these cells generate branching ductal-like structures when cultured in a three-dimensional collagen gel matrix (3).

CELL MARKERS THAT DISTINGUISH SUBPOPULATIONS OF HBEC

MUC1 and CALLA.   MUC1 and CALLA were originally described as markers of HBEC by O'Hare and colleagues (24). These authors reported that fluorescently labeled antibodies that

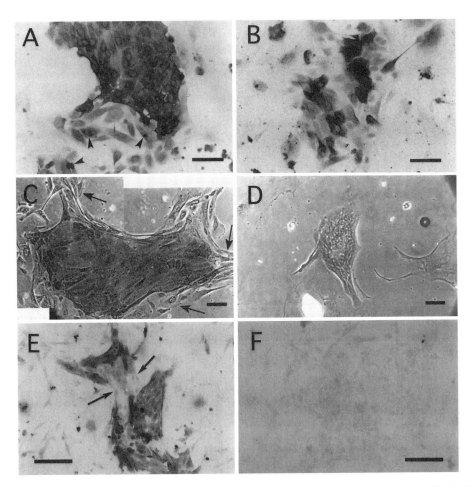

Figure 17-6. Expression of keratin 8/18 (A), keratin 19 (B), MUC1 (using the 214D4 antibody, C), and keratin 14 (E) in mixed colonies. Note in (A) the keratin-expressing teardrop-shaped cells (arrowheads) emerging from the periphery of the closely arranged centrally located cells. Note in (C) the MUC1⁻ cells (arrows) surrounding the MUC1⁺ cells. Note in (E) the centrally located keratin 14–negative cells (arrows). The cells in all panels, except for those in (C) and (D), were prepared like those in Figures 17-4 and 17-5. Cells in (C) and (D) were grown on tissue culture plastic in the presence of NIH 3T3 feeders in SF medium for 12 days. The culture was fixed in −20°C acetone:methanol, and expression of MUC1 was visualized by using the APAAP technique. (D) Control background staining for (C); (F) Background control staining for (A), (B), and (E). Cells in (A), (B), and (E) were counterstained with Wright's Giemsa. Bar in (A)–(D) = 100 μm. Bar in (E) and (F) = 250 μm.

recognize MUC1 identify luminal cells, whereas those specific for CALLA identify myoepithelial cells in freshly dissociated as well as cultured HBEC. Our experience generally confirms these observations (3), although we have also encountered some variability in the type of progenitors selected, depending on the clone of anti-MUC1 antibody utilized (see also Refs. 25 and 26). For example, the dot plots in Figures 17-7A and 17-B demonstrate the differences observed when two different anti-MUC1 antibodies [HMFG-2 (27) and 214D4] are used in conjunction with CALLA to stain cells from a 3-day culture of dissociated normal human mammary tissue. In this example, only 10% of the total cell population is stained with

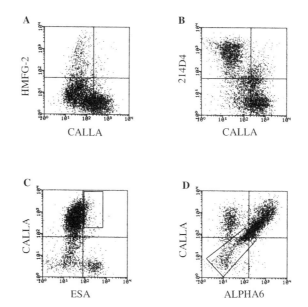

Figure 17-7. Dot plots generated from analysis of cells in 3-day primary HBEC cultures. Cells were stained with HMFG-2/goat anti-mouse-PE and CALLA-FITC (A), 214D4/goat anti-mouse-PE and CALLA-FITC (B), CALLA-PE and ESA-FITC (C), or with CALLA-PE and α6/goat anti-rat-FITC (D). The crossed lines are adjusted such that cells stained with isotype control antibodies are all situated within the lower left quadrant. Box in (C) represents the ESA$^+$CALLA$^+$ fraction, which is enriched for bipotent progenitors, whereas the box in (D) represents the fraction enriched for luminal-cell-restricted progenitors. Dot plots (A) and (B) are generated from a single primary culture, whereas dot plots (C) and (D) are from separate cultures.

HMFG-2, whereas 42% of the cells stain positively with 214D4. Conversely, we have found HMFG-2 to be more reliable than 214D4 for identifying progenitors of pure luminal colonies (manuscript in preparation).

We have also observed that the CALLA$^+$ subpopulation isolated from primary short-term cultures of dissociated normal mammary tissue contains progenitors of mixed and pure myoepithelial cell colonies as well as fibroblasts that invariably contaminate primary and early-passage HBEC cultures (3). Expression of CALLA by human (28) and rat (29) mammary fibroblasts has also been reported by others. Since these stromal cells can constitute a significant portion of our short-term (3-day) primary cultures, CALLA, at least in combination with MUC1, is not a useful discriminating marker for isolating HBEC subpopulations. However, the proportion of contaminating fibroblasts harvested from the primary HBEC cultures can be reduced by performing a partial trypsinization to remove these cells (along with some of the loosely adherent myoepithelial cells) prior to cell harvesting or by seeding the freshly dissociated HBEC pellet in a culture vessel in the presence of 5% FBS for 2–4 h to allow the initial preferential attachment of fibroblasts and then transfer of the less rapidly adherent HBEC organoids to new culture vessels (21).

ESA. ESA, also known as epithelial cell adhesion molecule [Ep-CAM, (30)] and EGP-40 (31), is a homophilic Ca^{2+}-independent cell adhesion molecule specific for most epithelial cells (32). When normal resting adult mammary tissue is stained to detect ESA, expression is localized primarily to the basal and lateral cell membranes of luminal epithelial cells and more weakly on basal cells (32). When normal mammary tissue is maintained *in vitro*, only cells that are closely arranged and have indistinct cell borders stain as ESA positive (3). Thus, all the cells generated from luminal-cell-restricted progenitors as well as the centrally located closely arranged cells of mixed luminal–myoepithelial cell colonies express ESA. Teardrop-shaped myoepithelial cells express no-to-low levels of this protein, and stromal cells also do not express this protein. The ESA^+ cells of the luminal cell compartment can be further divided into those that are destined to differentiate into luminal/alveolar cells and those that will form mixed or pure myoepithelial colonies by expression of CALLA (Figure 17-7C) (3). The ESA^+CALLA^- subpopulation is enriched for luminal-restricted progenitors, whereas the ESA^+CALLA^+ subpopulation (box in Figure 17-7C) is enriched for progenitors of mixed and pure myoepithelial colonies. The ESA^-CALLA^+ subpopulation is composed of a mixture of HMF, myoepithelial cells, and intermediate progenitors that no longer express ESA.

Alpha-6 Integrin (α6) and CALLA.   Alpha-6 integrin has previously been localized on myoepithelial cells in sectioned human breast tissue (33). Figure 17-7D shows an example of a FACS dot plot showing the results of staining cells from a 3-day culture of HBEC with anti-α6 and anti-CALLA. The upper-left-hand quadrant represents mammary fibroblasts ($α6^-CALLA^+$), whereas the HBEC population is distributed as a diagonal grouping of events extending from the lower left quadrant ($α6^-CALLA^-$) to the upper right quadrant ($α6^+CALLA^+$). We have found that the $α6^{-to\pm}CALLA^{-to\pm}$ subpopulation (box in Figure 17-7D) ($-$ to $\pm$ = negative to intermediate expression) is enriched for luminal-cell-restricted progenitors, as wells as $CALLA^-$ stroma cells, whereas the $α6^+CALLA^+$ subpopulation in the upper-right-hand quadrant is enriched for progenitors that generate mixed/intermediate colonies and myoepithelial-restricted colonies (unpublished observations).

For routine selection of bipotent progenitors and myoepithelial-restricted progenitors, we have found the $α6^+CALLA^+$ and ESA^+CALLA^+ subpopulations to be suitable. However, the α6/CALLA combination has the advantage that the stromal, luminal, and bipotent plus myoepithelial subpopulations can be separately isolated in a single separation step by using a combination of two antibodies. Populations of myoepithelial-restricted progenitor cells can be obtained by enriching for the ESA^- fraction of passaged HBEC. We have found that up to 90–100% enrichment of certain types of clonogenic HBEC progenitors can be isolated by using the markers described here.

COMMENTS AND CRITICAL ISSUES

All of the procedures and data presented are based on analysis of HBEC progenitors isolated from 3-day primary cultures initiated with normal mammary tissue. To date, we have not examined the distribution of markers expressed on freshly isolated HBEC, and thus it is difficult to comment on changes in phenotype that may be induced in their initial 3-day period in culture.

The wide spectrum of breast epithelial colony morphologies and sizes that can be obtained *in vitro* as described here and elsewhere (3, 29, 34) demonstrates that it is not accurate to rigidly categorize an individual HBEC as luminal or myoepithelial. It seems clear that the classically defined "luminal cell" compartment is biologically heterogeneous as indicated by the heterogeneous staining of some "typical" luminal Type I cells with the myoepithelial markers keratin 14 (3, 17, 18, 24) and CALLA (18). Similarly, the staining of Type II myoep-ithelial cells with the luminal markers keratin 18 (3, 18) and MUC1 (18) invites reconsider-ation of how this compartment is viewed. Obviously, intermediates exist since both MUC1 and keratin 14 have been demonstrated to be expressed within a single cell (35).

The majority of mammary tumors express keratin 19, MUC1, and ESA/Ep-CAM (32, 36, 37). Human breast epithelial cell selection strategies that utilize luminal-cell-specific markers might give the best enrichment of malignant HBEC, although the data reviewed here show that nonmalignant luminal cells and their progenitors would be copurified in such an approach. Epithelial-specific antigen/Ep-CAM would likely be the most suitable marker for this since this epitope is specific for most epithelial cells, is not expressed by neural, mus-cular, or connective tissue (32), and appears to distinguish adenocarcinoma cells in serous effusions (38, 39). Alternatively, a variety of antibodies have been developed that recognize novel epitopes present on MUC1 that are unmasked via aberrant glycosylation during tumor progression (40–43). As a result, these antibodies show preferential binding to malignant HBEC over normal HBEC. However, malignant HBEC are also notoriously difficult to grow and to distinguish from contaminating nonmalignant HBEC *in vitro* (reviewed in Ref. 44), although several novel systems have been reported to promote the selective growth of malig-nant HBEC. These include the use of a reconstituted basement membrane (45, 46), culture conditions that simulate the microenvironment of breast tumors (47), and optimization of other culture parameters (48).

ADVANTAGES AND PITFALLS OF FACS ISOLATION METHODOLOGIES

The main advantage of separating HBEC by FACS rather than by immunomagnetic methods (9, 28) is that subtle but discrete differences in epitope expression can be better exploited to separate different subpopulations, with the resultant populations isolated >99% pure with respect to the parameters chosen. FACS also affords the opportunity to combine multiple parameters, including cell size (forward light scatter), cell granularity (orthogonal light scatter), cell viability (exclusion of viability dyes), and other phenotypes as well as analy-sis of the expression of different antigens, which greatly increases the resolution of subpop-ulations. The characterization of HBEC by flow cytometry can also be extended to include an analysis of intracellular epitopes such as keratins and steroid hormone receptors (49), DNA content, and other parameters that change during cell cycle progression, as well as others that do not. (However, a more detailed review of these general features of flow cytometry are beyond the scope of this Chapter, and the reader is directed to Ref. 50).

The main disadvantage of using the FACS to obtain subpopulations of HBEC is the capital cost of the equipment, the expertise required for operating it, and the limited number of cells that can be isolated in comparison to other immunologic methods. For example, the number of MUC1$^+$ and CALLA$^+$ cells that could be isolated from cultured (28) and freshly isolated (9) HBEC suspensions by using positive selection with antibodies specific for MUC1 and CALLA conjugated to superparamagnetic beads (28) or Dynabeads (9) was 10-fold higher than the numbers routinely obtainable by sorting. Thus, for obtaining bulk populations or as a preliminary step to flow cytometry, immunomagnetic separation techniques provide an important alternative. However, where the number of cells ultimately required is small, as for the analysis of progenitor populations in the studies reviewed here, the low yield of cells may not be a limiting consideration, and the purity and resolution afforded by the FACS out-weigh this disadvantage.

ACKNOWLEDGMENTS. The authors thank Darcy Wilkinson and Dianne Reid for excellent technical assistance and Gayle Thornbury for operating the flow cytometer. We also thank Drs. Patty Clugston, Jane Sproul, and Richard Warren for supplying the surgical specimens. Grants from the British Columbia Health Research Foundation, the Canadian Breast Cancer Research Initiative of the National Cancer Institute of Canada, and funds from Novartis supported this work. C. J. Eaves is a Terry Fox Cancer Research Scientist of the National Cancer Institute of Canada.

REFERENCES

1. P. S. Rudland (1991). Histochemical organization and cellular composition of ductal buds in developing human breast: Evidence of cytochemical intermediates between epithelial and myoepithelial cells. *J. Histochem. Cytochem.* **39:**1471–1484.
2. P. S. Rudland, R. Barraclough, D. G. Fernig, and J. A. Smith (1997). Mammary stem cells in normal development and cancer. In C. Potten (ed.), *Stem Cells*, Academic Press, San Diego, CA, pp. 147–232.
3. J. Stingl, C. J. Eaves, U. Kuusk, and J. T. Emerman (1998). Phenotypic and functional characterization *in vitro* of a multipotent epithelial cell present in the normal adult human breast. *Differentiation* **63:**201–213.
4. S. Patton, S. J. Gendler, and A. P. Spicer (1995). The epithelial mucin, MUC1, of milk, mammary gland and other tissues. *Biochim. Biophys. Acta* **1241:**407–423.
5. J. Yang, A. Balakrishnan, S. Hamamoto, C. W. Beattie, T. K. Gupta, S. R. Wellings, and S. Nandi (1986). Different mitogenic and phenotypic responses of human breast epithelial cells grown in two versus three dimensions. *Exp. Cell Res.* **167:**563–569.
6. J. T. Emerman and D. A. Wilkinson (1990). Routine culturing of normal, dysplastic and malignant human mammary epithelial cells from small tissue samples. *In Vitro Cell. Dev. Biol.* **26:**1186–1194.
7. B. M. Gabelman and J. T. Emerman (1992). Effects of estrogen, epidermal growth factor, and transforming growth factor-β on the growth of human breast epithelial cells in primary culture. *Exp. Cell Res.* **201:**113–118.
8. L. Ronnov-Jessen, B. van Deurs, J. E. Celis, and O. W. Petersen (1990). Smooth muscle differentiation in cultured human breast gland stromal cells. *Lab Invest.* **63:**532–543.
9. J. J. Gomm, P. J. Browne, R. C. Coope, Q. Y. Liu, L. Buluwela, and R. C. Coombes (1995). Isolation of pure populations of epithelial and myoepithelial cells from the normal human mammary gland using immunomagnetic separation with Dynabeads. *Anal. Biochem.* **226:**91–99.
10. S. P. Ethier, M. L. Mahacek, W. J. Gullick, T. J. Frank, and B. L. Weber (1993). Differential isolation of normal luminal mammary epithelial cells and breast cancer cells from primary and metastatic sites using selective media. *Cancer Res.* **53:**627–635.
11. J. J. Gomm, R. C. Coope, P. J. Browne, and R. C. Coombes (1997). Separated human breast epithelial and myoepithelial cells have different growth factor requirements *in vitro* but can reconstitute normal breast lobuloavleolar structure. *J. Cell Physiol.* **171:**11–19.
12. J. Russo, M. J. Mills, M. J. Moussalli, and I. H. Russo (1989). Influence of human breast development on the growth properties of primary cultures. *In Vitro Cell. Dev. Biol.* **25:**643–649.
13. H. S. Smith, S. Lan, R. Ceriani, A. J. Hackett, and M. R. Stampfer (1981). Clonal proliferation of cultured nonmalignant and malignant human breast epithelia. *Cancer Res.* **41:**4637–4643.
14. B. Niranjan, L. Buluwela, J. Yant, N. Perusinghe, A. Atherton, D. Phippard, T. Dale, B. Gusterson, and T. Kalamati (1995). HGF/SF: a potent cytokine for mammary growth, morphogenesis and development. *Development* **121:**2897–2908.
15. J. V. Soriano, M. S. Pepper, T. Nakamura, L. Orci, and R. Montesano (1995). Hepatocyte growth factor stimulates extensive development of branching duct-like structures by cloned mammary gland epithelial cells. *J. Cell Sci.* **108:**413–430.
16. J. V. Soriano, M. S. Pepper, L. Orci, and R. Montesano (1998). Roles of hepatocyte growth factor/scatter factor and transforming growth factor-β1 in mammary gland ductal morphogenesis. *J. Mammary Gland Biol.* **3:**133–150.
17. J. Taylor-Papadimitriou, M. Stampfer, J. Bartek, A. Lewis, M. Boshell, E. B. Lane, and I. M. Leigh (1989). Keratin expression in human mammary epithelial cells cultured from normal and malignant tissue: Relation to *in vivo* phenotypes and influence of medium. *J. Cell Sci.* **94:**403–413.

18. U. Karsten, G. Papsdorf, A. Pauly, B. Vojtesek, R. Moll, E. B. Lane, H. Clausen, P. Stosiek, and M. Kasper (1993). Subtypes of non-transformed human mammary epithelial cells cultured *in vitro*: histo-blood group antigen H type 2 defines basal cell-derived cells. *Differentiation* **54**:55–66.

19. W. Bocker, B. Bier, G. Freytag, B. Brommelkamp, E.-D. Jarasch, G. Edel, B. Dockhorn-Dworniczak, and K. W. Schmid (1992). An immunohistochemical study of the breast using antibodies to basal and luminal keratins, alpha-smooth muscle actin, vimentin, collagen IV and laminin. *Virchows Arch [A]* **421**:315–322.

20. O. W. Petersen and B. van Deurs (1988). Growth factor control of myoepithelial cell differentiation in cultures of human mammary gland. *Differentiation* **39**:197–215.

21. C.-Y. Kao, C. S. Oakley, C. W. Welsch, and C.-C. Chang (1997). Growth requirements and neoplastic transformation of two types of normal human breast epithelial cells derived from reduction mammoplasty. *In Vitro Cell. Dev. Biol.—Animal* **33**:282–288.

22. C.-Y. Kao, K. Nomata, C. S. Oakley, C. W. Welsch, and C.-C. Chang (1995). Two types of normal human breast epithelial cells derived from reduction mammoplasty: phenotypic characterization and response to SV40 transfection. *Carcinogenesis* **16**:531–538.

23. S. Dairkee and H. W. Heid (1993). Cytokeratin profiles of immunomagnetically separated epithelial subsets of the human mammary gland. *In Vitro Cell. Dev. Biol.* **29A**:427–432.

24. M. J. O'Hare, M. G. Ormerod, P. Monoghan, E. B. Lane, and B. A. Gusterson (1991). Characterization *in vitro* of luminal and myoepithelial cells isolated from the human mammary gland by cell sorting. *Differentiation* **46**:209–221.

25. C. S. Foster, P. A. W. Edwards, E. A. Dinsdale, and A. M. Neville (1982). Monoclonal antibodies to the human mammary gland. *Virchows Arch. [A]* **394**:279–293.

26. P. A. W. Edwards and I. M. Brooks (1984). Antigenic subsets of human breast epithelial cells distinguished by monoclonal antibodies. *J. Histochem. Cytochem.* **32**:531–537.

27. J. Burchell, H. Durbin, and J. Taylor-Papadimitriou (1983). Complexity of expression of antigenic determinants recognized by monoclonal antibodies HMFG-1 and HMFG-2, in normal and malignant human mammary epithelial cells. *J. Immunol.* **131**:508–513.

28. C. Clarke, J. Titley, S. Davies, and M. J. O'Hare (1994). An immunomagnetic separation method using superparamagentic (MACS) beads for large-scale purification of human mammary luminal and myoepithelial cells. *Epith. Cell Biol.* **3**:38–46.

29. S. R. Dundas, M. G. Ormerod, B. A. Gusterson, and M. J. O'Hare (1991). Characterization of luminal and basal cells flow-sorted from the adult rat mammary parenchyma. *J. Cell Sci.* **100**:459–471.

30. S. V. Litvinov, M. P. Velders, H. A. M. Bakker, G. J. Fleuren, and S. O. Warnaar (1994). Ep-CAM: a human epithelial antigen is a homophilic cell-cell adhesion molecule. *J. Cell Biol.* **125**:437–446.

31. B. Simon, D. K. Podolsky, G. Moldenhauer, K. J. Isselbacher, S. Gattoni-Celli, and S. J. Brand (1990). Epithelial glycoprotein is a member of a family of epithelial cell surface antigens homologous to nidogen, a matrix adhesion protein. *Proc. Natl. Acad. Sci. U.S.A.* **87**:2755–2759.

32. U. Latza, G. Niedobitek, R. Schwarting, H. Nekarda, and H. Stein (1990). Ber-EP4: new monoclonal antibody which distinguishes epithelia from mesothelia. *J. Clin. Pathol.* **43**:213–219.

33. G. K. Koukoulis, I. Virtanen, M. Korhonen, L. Laitinen, V. Quaranta, and V. E. Gould (1991). Immunohistochemical localization of integrins in the normal, hyperplastic, and neoplastic breast. *Am. J. Pathol.* **139**:787–799.

34. M. J. Smalley, J. Titley, and M. J. O'Hare (1998). Clonal characterization of mouse mammary luminal epithelial and myoepithelial cells separated by fluorescence-activated cell sorting. *In Vitro Cell. Dev. Biol.—Animal* **34**:711–721.

35. S. H. Dairkee, C. M. Blayney-Moore, H. S. Smith, and A. J. Hackett (1986). Concurrent expression of basal and luminal markers in cultures of normal human breast analyzed using monoclonal antibodies. *Differentiation* **32**:93–100.

36. J. Sloane and M. G. Ormerod (1981). Distribution of epithelial membrane antigen in normal and neoplastic tissues and its value in diagnostic tumor pathology. *Cancer* **47**:1786–1795.

37. J. Bartek, J. Taylor-Papadimitriou, N. Miller, and R. Millis (1985). Patterns of expression of keratin 19 as detected with monoclonal antibodies in human breast tissues and tumors. *Int. J. Cancer* **36**:299–306.

38. M. E. Bailey, R. W. Brown, D. R. Mody, P. Cagle, and I. Ramzy (1996). Ber-EP4 for differentiating adenocarcinoma from reactive and neoplastic mesothelial cells in serous effusions. Comparison to carcinoembryonic antigen, B72.3 and Leu-M1. *Acta Cytol.* **40**:1212–1216.

39. M. Delahaye, F. van der Ham, and T. H. van der Kwast (1997). Complementary value of five carcinoma markers for the diagnosis of malignant mesothelioma, adenocarcinoma metastasis, and reactive mesothelioma in serous effusions. *Diag. Cytopath.* **17**:115–120.

40. J. Burchell, S. Gendler, J. Taylor-Papadimitriou, A. Girling, A. Lewis, R. Mullis, and D. Lamport (1987). Development and characterization of breast cancer reactive monoclonal antibodies directed to the core protein of the human milk mucin. *Cancer Res.* **47**:5476–5482.

41. P. X. Xing, J. Prenzoska, K. Quelch, and I. F. C. McKenzie (1992). Second generation anti-MUC1 peptide monoclonal antibodies. *Cancer Res.* **52**:2310–2317.

42. M. V. Croce, A. G. Colussi, M. R. Price, and A. Segal-Eiras (1997). Expression of tumor associated antigens in normal, benign and malignant human epithelial tissue: a comparative immunohistochemical study. *Anticancer Res.* **17**:4287–4292.

43. S. Fiorentini, E. Matczak, R. C. Gallo, M. S. Reitz, I. Keydar, and B. A. Watkins (1997). Humanization of an antibody recognizing a breast cancer specific epitope by CDR-grafting. *Immunotechnology* **3**:45–59.

44. S. P. Ethier (1996). Human breast cancer cell lines as models of growth regulation and disease progression. *J. Mammary Gland Biol.* **1**:111–121.

45. O. W. Petersen, L. Ronnov-Jessen, A. R. Howlett, and M. J. Bissell (1992). Interaction with basement membrane serves to rapidly distinguish growth and differentiation pattern of normal and malignant human breast epithelial cells. *Proc. Natl. Acad. Sci. U.S.A.* **89**:9064–9068.

46. L. M. Bergstraesser and S. A. Weitzman (1993). Culture of normal and malignant primary human mammary epithelial cells in a physiological manner simulates *in vivo* growth patterns and allows discrimination of cell type. *Cancer Res.* **53**:2644–2654.

47. S. Dairkee, G. Deng, M. R. Stampfer, F. M. Waldman, and H. S. Smith (1995). Selective cell culture of primary breast carcinoma. *Cancer Res.* **55**:2516–2519.

48. N. Pandis, S. Heim, G. Bardi, J. Limon, N. Mandahl, and F. Mitelman (1992). Improved technique for short-term culture and cytogenetic analysis of human breast cancer. *Genes Chrom. Cancer* **5**:14–20.

49. I. Brotherick, T. W. J. Lennard, S. Cook, R. Johnstone, B. Angus, M. P. Winthereik, and B. K. Shenton (1995). Use of the biotinylated antibody DAKO-ER 1D5 to measure oestrogen receptor on cytokeratin positive cells obtained from primary breast cancer cells. *Cytometry* **20**:74–80.

50. H. M. Shapiro (1994). *Practical Flow Cytometry.* Alan R. Liss, Inc., New York.

Chapter 18

Isolation and Culture of Human Breast Cancer Cells from Primary Tumors and Metastases

Stephen P. Ethier, Cheryl A. Ammerman, and Michele L. Dziubinski

Abstract.   Over the years, a number of groups have developed culture media and conditions that support the growth of normal human mammary epithelial cells from a variety of lineages, and these cell systems have increased our understanding of human mammary gland biology. In contrast, it remains difficult to isolate and culture human breast cancer cells from primary tumors and metastatic specimens. Our laboratory has now developed 13 human breast cancer cell lines. Some of these cell lines originated from primary tumor specimens, others were derived from chest wall recurrences in patients who had prior surgery, and some of the cell lines were derived from pleural effusion metastases. The cell lines that we have obtained exhibit an array of genetic alterations representative of the genomic diversity of uncultured human breast cancers. In addition, these cells are cultured under well-defined conditions (most cell lines are grown in serum-free media) that allow detained cellular studies to be carried out that complement the genetic analyses of these cell lines. This chapter outlines the culture methods and approaches that we have used to develop this panel of cell lines. Our methods emphasize certain key features that we feel are essential for the isolation and culture of breast cancer cells. These features are all focused on developing culture conditions that allow for the slow emergence of cancer cells in the relative absence of normal cells, which proliferate rapidly under highly-growth-factor-enriched conditions. Thus, selective growth media and methods for enriching cell populations for cancer cells while minimizing the presence of normal epithelial and stromal elements are important for the expansion of breast cancer cells in vitro. It is still not possible to develop cell lines from every breast cancer specimen obtained in the laboratory. Thus, whereas the cell lines we have developed have resulted in improvements in our understanding of breast cancer cell biology, much work remains to be done to understand why some breast cancer cells fail to grow *in vitro* while growing robustly in the patient. Improving our knowledge of the factors that influence breast cancer cell viability and proliferation will be important for development of novel therapeutic strategies for breast cancer.

Abbreviations.   balanced salt solution (BSS); common acute lymphoblastic antigen (CALLA); cyclin D1 (CCND1); comparative genomic hybridization (CGH); cholera toxin (CT); chest wall nodule (CWN); dimethyl sulfoxide (DMSO); estradiol (E2); epidermal growth factor (EGF); epidermal growth factor receptor (EGFR); epithelial membrane antigen (EMA); fibroblast growth factor receptor (FGFR); fetal bovine serum (FBS); human breast cancer (HBC); hydrocortisone (HC); human mammary epithelial (HME); insulin (I); lymph node (LN); lysophosphatidic acid (LPA); progesterone (P); pleural effusion (PE); primary tumor (PT).

INTRODUCTION

Over the past 10 years, our laboratory has been working to develop improved methods for the isolation and long-term culture of human breast cancer cells (HBC). For many years

Stephen P. Ethier, Cheryl A. Ammerman, and Michele L. Dziubinski   **Department of Radiation Oncology, University of Michigan Ann Arbor, Michigan 48109-0984.**

Methods in Mammary Gland Biology and Breast Cancer Research, edited by Ip and Asch. Kluwer Academic/Plenum Publishers, New York, 2000.

now, we and others have successfully cultured normal human mammary epithelial (HME) cells from reduction mammoplasty specimens. A number of media have been developed in different laboratories, and various forms of these media support growth of HME cells of different lineages (1–5). The growth of HME cells of the luminal lineage is most important for studies related to breast cancer cell biology, because luminal mammary epithelial cells of the terminal duct lobular unit are the cells from which the vast majority of breast cancers arise (3).

Despite the great improvements in our ability to culture HME cells, similar improvements have not been made in the methods used to culture human breast cancer cells. Nevertheless, our group as well as others have, over the past few years, developed several new HBC cell lines from primary and metastatic breast cancer specimens. Our laboratory has developed 13 breast cancer cell lines from primary breast cancer specimens, chest wall recurrences, and pleural effusion metastases. Several papers have been published on the isolation of these cell lines and on various aspects of their cellular and genetic characteristics (6–12). A brief summary of the SUM series of HBC cell lines is given in Table 18-1. As can be seen from the table, our HBC cell line panel is heterogeneous with respect to the type of specimen from which the cell lines were derived and with respect to their molecular and cellular characteristics. Thus, the methods used in our laboratory for the isolation and culture of breast cancer cells do not select for one particular subset of breast cancers. Indeed, different HBC cell lines in our panel exhibit amplification and overexpression of most of the currently known breast cancer oncogenes, including ERBB-2, c-MYC, CCND1, FGFR-1, and FGFR-2. In addition,

Table 18-1. Molecular Characteristics of "SUM" HBC Cell Lines

Cell line	Oncogene amp	EGFR exp	p^{53} (IHC)[c]
SUM-44 PE	FGFR-1[a] CCND1[a] c-MYCc[b]	—	+(c)
SUM-52 PE	FGFR-1[a] FGPR-2[a] CCND1[b]	—	+(c)
SUM-16LN	EGFR	++++	+(n)
SUM-102 PT	ND	+++	—
SUM-149 PT	ND	+++	+(n)
SUM-159 PT	c-MYC[b]	++	+(n)
SUM-1315 MO2	ND	+	+(n)
SUM-185 PE	ND	+	NE
SUM-190 PT	ERBB-2[a] CCND1[a]	+	+(n)
SUM 206 cwn	ND	+	+(n)
SUM 224	NE	—	NE
SUM 225 cwn	ERBB-2[a] c-MYC[b]	—	NE
SUM-229 PE	ND	+++	NE

[a]High-level amplifications detected by Southern blot and by FISH. Southern blots were probed for amplification of FGFR1, FGFR-2, ERBB-2, C-MYC, and CCND1.
[b]Low-level amplifications (two- to threefold) detected by FISH only. Cells were probed by FISH for ERBB-2, C-MYC, and CCND1.
[c](c) = cytoplasmic staining; (n) = nuclear staining; ND = no amplifications of the selected oncogenes were detected; NE = not examined.

several of our cell lines overexpress the EGFR in the absence of gene amplification, a characteristic associated with poor prognosis (13–16). Finally, several of our cell lines do not have amplifications of any of the most common breast cancer oncogenes, but do have areas of gene amplification, as detected by comparative genomic hybridization (CGH) (9). Furthermore, the CGH patterns that we have detected in our cell lines are similar to those detected in uncultured breast cancer cells, further confirming the relevance of this panel of cell lines to the spectrum of clinical disease (17, 18).

In this chapter we outline the methods routinely used in our laboratory to isolate and culture breast cancer cells from biopsy specimens. During the course of development of our panel of HBC cell lines, we have learned a great deal about the requirements of breast cancer cells for *in vitro* growth. Some factors that we have found to be important, and which are discussed in detail in the last section, include the cell density dependence of breast cancer cells for growth, the slow proliferation rate of breast cancer *in vivo* which is maintained after transferring the cells into culture, the different hormone and growth factor requirements of breast cancer cells from different patients, and the importance of factors secreted by normal cells that negatively influence the proliferation of breast cancer cells. All of these factors, and others, combine to make primary culture and long-term growth of breast cancer cells *in vitro* a much more difficult challenge than the culture of normal mammary epithelial cells.

This chapter outlines the methods that have allowed us to develop a diverse panel of human breast cancer cells lines. We also discuss some of the approaches that have failed to yield continuously proliferating breast cancer cell cultures. Having an understanding of what is known to work, and what is known not to work in culturing HBC cells is important to anyone who may be trying to use our method, or similar methods, to culture HBC cells from biopsy specimens.

MATERIALS AND INSTRUMENTATION

See Table 18-2 for a materials list.

METHODS

In this section the detailed approaches and formulations that we have used to develop our current panel of cell lines are presented. In addition to the information detailed instructions, formulations, and updates on new methods are provided on our SUM-line website the URL for which is http://p53.cancer.med.umich.edu/clines/elab/ethier.html.

Reagents and Reagent Preparation

See Table 18-3 for hormone and growth factors for the HME and HBC.

Reagents and Solutions List

- Medium 199 with 5 µg/ml gentamicin
- 200 U/ml collagenase in Medium 199
- Freezing medium: Medium 199 + 15% FBS + 5% DMSO
- Counting Solution: 0.5% formaldehyde in 0.9% NaCl
- Nuclei isolation solution: 0.01 M HEPES + 0.015 M $MgCl_2$

Table 18-2. Mateials List for Culturing HBC Cells

Item	Catalog	Company	Location
Media			
Medium M-199	M4530	Sigma	St. Louis, MO
10× Hank's balanced			
salt solution	14180-061	Life Technologies	Gaithersburg, MD
Ham's F-12	51-65178	JRH Biosciences	Lenexa, KS
Antibiotics/antifungal agents			
Gentamicin	15710-064	Life Technologies	Gaithersburg, MD
Fungizone	15290-018	Life Technologies	Gaithersburg, MD
Serum/serum derivatives			
Fetal bovine serum	F2442	Sigma	St. Louis, MO
Bovine serum albumin	85041	JRH Biosciences	Lenexa, KS
Growth factors			
Insulin	I5500	Sigma	St. Louis, MO
Hydrocortisone	H4001	Sigma	St. Louis, MO
Epidermal growth factor	E4127	Sigma	St. Louis, MO
Cholera toxin	C3012	Sigma	St. Louis, MO
Estradiol	E2758	Sigma	St. Louis, MO
Progesterone	P0130	Sigma	St. Louis, MO
Lysophosphatidic acid	L7260	Sigma	St. Louis, MO
Serum replacement factors			
Ethanolamine	E0135	Sigma	St. Louis, MO
HEPES	H3375	Sigma	St. Louis, MO
Apotransferrin	T2252	Sigma	St. Louis, MO
3,3′,5-Triiodo-L-thyronine	T5516	Sigma	St. Louis, MO
Sodium selenite	S9133	Sigma	St. Louis, MO
HBC dissociation/purification reagents			
Collagenase	LS004183	Worthington Biochemical	Freehold, NJ
Percoll	P1644	Sigma	St. Louis, MO
Dynabeads M-450			
Sheep anti-mouse IgG	110.01	Dynal, Inc.	Lake Success, NY
Common acute lymphoblastic			
Leukemia antigen CD10	M0727	DAKO Corporation	Carpinteria, CA
Epithelial membrane antigen	M0613	DAKO Corporation	Carpinteria, CA
Dynal MPC-E	120.04	Dynal, Inc.	Lake Success, NY
Nuclear isolation reagents for coulter counting			
Ethylhexadecyldimethyl			
ammonium bromide	21187-1000	Fisher Scientific/Acros	Fairlawn, NJ
Glacial acetic acid	A38-212	Fisher Scientific	Pittsburgh, PA
Formaldehyde	H121	Mallinckrodt	Paris, KY
Freezing reagent			
Dimethyl sulfoxide	D5879	Sigma	St. Louis, MO

Table 18-3. Hormone and Growth Factors for HME and HBC Media

Ingredient	Stock conc.	Working conc.	500 ml	SFIH[a]	5% IH[b]
Insulin (I)	1 mg/ml	5 µg/ml	2.5 ml	X	X
Hydrocortisone (HC)	1 mg/ml	1 µg/ml	500 µl	X	X
Epidermal growth factor (EGF)	10 µg/ml	10 ng/ml	500 µl		
Cholera toxin (Ct)	100 µg/ml	100 ng/ml	500 µl		
Estradiol (E2)	10E-5 M	10E-8 M	500 µl		
Ethanolamine		5 mM	155 µl	X	
HEPES	1 M	10 mM	5.0 ml	X	
Transferrin	2.5 mg/ml	5 µg/ml	1.0 ml	X	
3,3′,5-Triiodo-L-thyronine (T3)	20 µg/ml	10 µM	167 µl	X	
Sodium selenite (Se)	20 µg/ml	50 µM	217 µl	X	
Lysophosphatidic acid (LPA)	2.4 mM	10 µM	2.085 ml		
Fungizone (F)		0.5 µg/ml	5.0 ml	X	X
Gentamycin (G)		5 µg/ml	250 µl	X	X

[a]For serum-free media (SF), supplement Ham's F-12 with bovine serum albumin (1 mg/ml).
[b]For serum-containing media (5%), add 5% FBS to Ham's F-12.
[c]For complete serum-free media, make up SFIH media and add EGF, E2, and ±LPA.
[d]For luminal cell growth, make up 5% IH media and add EGF, Ct, and ±LPA.

- Lysis solution for nuclei isolation: 5% ethylhexadecyldimethylammonium bromide in a 3% solution of glacial acetic acid
- Percoll solution: 1.09 g/ml Percoll in Hank's BSS

Detailed Procedures

ISOLATION OF HUMAN BREAST CANCER CELLS FROM PRIMARY TUMOR SPECIMENS

1. Weigh tumor specimen in a sterile tissue culture dish. Resuspend collagenase (Worthington Biochemical Corporation, CLS3 type) at 200 U/ml in Medium-199 (M-199) plus gentamycin (5 µg/ml). Prepare 20 ml of collagenase solution for the first gram of tissue and 10 ml for each additional gram.
2. Use aseptic technique for all subsequent steps. Sterile-filter collagenase solution before pouring into a sterile 250-ml Erlenmeyer flask with a sterile cap.
3. Transfer the tumor to an open 100-mm tissue culture dish in a laminar flow hood. Crosscut the tumor, using no. 22 sterile scalpels, being careful to cut the tumor and not to tear it. Mince the specimen into 1-mm³ pieces.
4. Transfer the minced tumor into the flask containing the sterile collagenase solution. Replace the sterile top and fasten securely.
5. Incubate the tumor suspension overnight in a 37°C shaking water bath at 65 rpm.
6. The next day, mix the suspension with rapid pipetting 20 to 25 times, using a 10-ml sterile pipette. Transfer the suspension to sterile 50-ml centrifuge tubes and centrifuge the cells at $225 \times g$ for 5 min at room temperature.
7. Resuspend the cell pellet in 10 ml of M-199 plus gentamycin. Transfer to a 15-ml centrifuge tube. Centrifuge as before. Repeat twice.
8. Epithelial cell aggregates are separated from single cells by differential sedimentation. Resuspend the cells in 10 ml of M-199 and agitate the tube by hand. Let the tube stand for 15 min. Cell aggregates will settle and form a loose pellet.
9. Carefully remove the supernatant above the loose cell pellet and set aside.

10. Repeat steps 8 and 9. Resuspend the loose pellet in 10 ml of M-199.
11. Take a 50-μl aliquot of both the supernatant and the cell pellet for cell counting. Isolate nuclei by resuspending the cells in 500 μl of a solution containing 0.01 M HEPES and 0.015 M $MgCl_2$. Agitate for 5 min at room temperature. Add 50 μl of Bretol (Kodak) solution (5% ethyl hexadecyldimethylammonium bromide in a 3% solution of glacial acetic acid). Agitate for 10 min at room temperature. Finally, bring the volume up to 20 ml with counting solution (0.5% formaldehyde in 0.9% NaCl). Count the nuclei using a Coulter Counter to determine the cell number in each sample.
12. Plate the cells in Ham's F-12 media containing 5% fetal bovine serum, insulin, and hydrocortisone (see Table 18-3 for concentrations) at desired density, usually 10^6 cells per 35-mm plate. Freeze cells that are not plated at $5–10 \times 10^6$ cells per ampule in 750 ml freezing medium, containing 15% FBS and 5% DMSO in M-199 and gentamycin.

ISOLATING CANCER CELLS FROM PLEURAL EFFUSION OR ASCITES FLUID

1. Pipette the pleural effusion or ascites fluid into 50-ml centrifuge tubes.
2. Centrifuge the cells at $225 \times g$ for 5 min. Combine the cell pellets from 1 L of fluid and resuspend the cells in 20 ml of M-199 medium. Centrifuge the cells again at $225 \times g$ for 5 min.
3. At this point, the pellet may contain red blood cells that can be visualized against the white color of the cancer cells. Two methods can be used to remove the red blood cells from the cell suspension.
   a. *Water lysis method*
      (i) Add 9 ml of sterile deionized water to the pellet. Resuspend quickly by pipetting up and down a few times. Immediately add 1 ml 10× Hank's balanced salt solution to readjust the salt concentration to its proper level.
      (ii) Centrifuge the cells at $225 \times g$ for 5 min. If the pellet is still red, repeat the lysis one more time.
      (iii) Proceed to step 4.
   b. *Percoll method*
      (i) Resuspend the cell pellet in 1 ml of media.
      (ii) Add 2 ml of Percoll (1.09 g/ml) to a 15-ml centrifuge tube.
      (iii) Carefully layer the 1-ml cell suspension over the Percoll.
      (iv) Centrifuge at $225 \times g$ for 5 min. The red blood cells will penetrate the Percoll and form a pellet at the bottom of the tube. The other cells will form a layer between the medium and the Percoll.
      (v) Carefully pipette the cells from the interface.
      (vi) Proceed to step 4.
4. Once the red blood cells have been removed, wash the cells twice with M-199 by centrifuging the cells at $225 \times g$ for 5 min. Proceed to the differential sedimentation step (step 8) in the tumor digestion protocol.

CELL SEPARATION USING ANTIBODY-BOUND MAGNETIC BEADS. In all cases the likelihood of successful breast cancer cell culture is increased greatly by enriching the population for breast cancer cells and eliminating stromal cells and normal mammary epithelial cells. In some cases incubating the primary cell suspension can accomplish this, resulting in cultures less likely to be overgrown by normal cells. Antibodies that we have used in our lab to coat magnetic beads for cell separation include

1. Common acute lymphoblastic leukemia antigen (CALLA), CD10, which binds fibroblasts and myoepithelial cells.
2. Epithelial membrane antigen (EMA), which binds luminal epithelial cells. The magnetic beads can be purchased with covalently attached anti-mouse or rabbit antibodies. Thus, incubation of the primary antibody-bound beads with CALLA or EMA antibodies for 30 min at room temperature yields beads that can be used to bind specific cell types.

The protocol for isolating cells using antibody-coated magnetic beads is as follows:

1. Resuspend the cells to be separated in 1 ml of M-199 media. Add magnetic beads coated with antibodies at 10^7 beads per 10^7 cells. Agitate at room temperature for 2 h.
2. Place the tube in a magnetic tube holder for 1–2 min to separate the beads bound to cells from the unbound cells. Transfer the liquid containing unbound cells to a fresh tube. Repeat step 2.
3. Wash the beads plus cells in 1.0 ml M-199. Put the mixture back at room temp with agitation for 30 min.
4. Repeat steps 2 and 3 twice for a total of 3 washes.
5. Centrifuge the cells at $225 \times g$ for 5 min.
6. Resuspend cells in media and plate at desired density.

Note that when using magnetic beads coated with EMA, cells bound to the beads are retained and plated into culture (positive selection), whereas when using CALLA-coated beads the nonbound cells (negative selection) are enriched for luminal cells and should be plated.

COMMENTS AND CRITICAL ISSUES

It is a myth that breast cancer cells grow rapidly. In order to isolate and culture human breast cancer cells from patient-derived biopsy specimens, it is vitally important to know what to expect in terms of the initial growth rate of the cells. Many laboratories are accustomed to working with established cell lines of rodent or human origin, and, in most cases, these cell lines have been in culture for many years. As a result, researchers are often accustomed to working with cell lines, especially transformed cell lines, that grow quite rapidly. In such established cell lines, population doubling times of 15 to 24 h are very common. In addition, it is often widely assumed that cancer cells, by their very nature, are rapidly growing cells. Indeed, countless textbooks generalize about the neoplastic process by saying that cancer is a disease of rapid cell growth, but, especially with regard to adult human malignancies, that statement is simply not true. The human solid malignancies most often studied, such as breast cancer, prostate cancer, colon cancer, etc., are diseases that progress *in vivo* for 15 to 30 years before becoming clinically apparent. Kinetic data obtained from breast cancer biopsy specimens indicate that these cells grow with cell cycle times of hundreds of hours. Furthermore, the tumors themselves expand with volume doubling times of many months (19–21). Indeed, breast cancer cells rarely have S-phase fractions greater than 10%, and S-phase fractions of less than 5% are not uncommon in primary breast cancers (22, 23). These observations clearly demonstrate that human breast cancer is not a disease of rapid proliferation, *per se*. Thus, breast cancer cells that grow with rapid doubling times *in vitro*, and which yield large tumors *in vivo* in a matter of days or weeks, are not necessarily good models for the natural history of breast cancer as it occurs in patients. All of this is important when it comes to establishing primary cultures of human breast cancer cells because one must expect, and plan for, extremely slow growth rates of these cells. In our hands, HBC cell cultures that yield breast cancer cell lines are routinely maintained in primary culture for 2 to 4 months before they are subcultured for the first time. Considering the kinetic data for HBC cell growth *in vivo*, these long doubling times are not an artifact of poor culture conditions but, reflect the true growth potential of the cancer cells.

Because it takes so long for successful HBC cultures to yield cell numbers sufficient for subculture, one must take special precautions to guard against overgrowth of normal cells that can rapidly overtake a culture dish long before the HBC cells have had a chance to expand. Thus, it is essential to use selective media that do not support rapid and extensive growth of normal cells, be they stromal cells or normal mammary epithelial cells, both of which grow quite rapidly under growth-factor-enriched conditions. The culture media that we have developed are designed to reduce overgrowth of the culture dishes by normal cells over extended periods of time, and have allowed for the isolation of the cell lines described. It is for this reason, too, that any methods that can be used to purify breast cancer cells from normal cells before they are seeded into culture dramatically improve one's chances for establishing a breast cancer cell line.

In summary, successful isolation and culture of human breast cancer cells *in vitro* requires, more than anything else, patience. HBC cells expand very slowly in the patient, and they expand at the same slow rate after being explanted into culture. Indeed, in our experience, the growth rate of primary breast cancer cells is not significantly influenced by the presence of exogenous growth factors in the medium, whereas the growth rate of contaminating normal cells is dramatically affected. Thus, the slow expansion of breast cancer cells in primary culture is a fact of the biology of these cells that has to be dealt with in order to work with primary HBC cells *in vitro*.

Importance of Cell Density on HBC Cell Growth *In Vitro*

Cell density is another factor that we have found to be important for the isolation and growth of breast cancer cells. In our experience, early-passage breast cancer cells simply do not grow well at low density and do not grow at all at clonal densities. We discovered this in the course of isolating our very first HBC cell line, SUM-44PE. Whereas normal HME cells arc routinely passaged at 1:10 split ratios about once per week, secondary cultures of SUM-44PE cells did not proliferate when subcultured in a similar manner. In contrast, passaging the cells at a 1:3 split ratio resulted in good growth of the cells, even though it took them 2 weeks to become confluent again. Thus, SUM-44PE cells grow with a population doubling time of about 200 h, and their growth was found to be highly dependent on their density. Conditioned medium experiments demonstrated that low-density SUM-44PE cells could be successfully cultured in conditioned medium obtained from high-density cultures. Furthermore, the factor(s) responsible for this effect were dialyzable and passed through membranes with cutoffs as low as 1000 Da. Based on these results, we hypothesized that the inability of HBC cells to grow under low-density conditions is the result of their relative inability to undergo gap junctional intercellular communication, which is defective in many types of human cancer cells (24–26). Thus, breast cancer cells must obtain critical small molecules by pinocytosis from the medium rather than by direct exchange with neighboring cells, and this process is likely to be very inefficient when cells are at low density. Whatever the exact mechanism, we have consistently observed that HBC cells must be maintained at high densities, even after many *in vitro* passages. We routinely subculture many of our HBC cell lines at 1 : 3 split ratios about every 2 weeks.

The density dependence of HBC cells for *in vitro* growth means that, in initiating these cultures, one must seed cells at high density in a medium that will allow for their slow expansion. The slow growth rate of these cells, coupled with the requirement for using slow split ratios, puts an even higher premium on patience in establishing and working with early-passage human breast cancer cells.

Growth Factor Requirements of HBC Cells

As mentioned, several years ago we developed a culture medium that would support the rapid expansion of normal HME cells of the luminal lineage (6). This culture medium contains many of the hormones and growth factors that we and others have used in our serum-free formulations to grow normal HME cells. However, we found that the addition of 5% FBS to medium supplemented with insulin, hydrocortisone, EGF, cholera toxin, and progesterone stimulated rapid proliferation of small, tightly packed cuboidal epithelial cells that stained positively for the luminal cytokeratin, keratin-19. We have since found that in primary HME cell cultures LPA can replace the serum to support proliferation of these keratin-19–positive cells. Based on these observations, we reasoned that, since HBC cells are almost uniformly keratin-19 positive, factors required for luminal cell proliferation would also be required to culture HBC cells.

Based on this hypothesis, we performed a series of experiments aimed at using a hormone, growth factor, and serum-containing medium to culture HBC cells from primary tumor specimens and pleural effusion metastases. These experiments failed. When used with cells obtained from primary tumor specimens, the enriched culture medium stimulated the rapid emergence of normal luminal mammary epithelial cells. The cells that proliferated, even though they were tumor-derived, exhibited none of the cellular or genetic characteristics of breast cancer cells. These cells were growth factor dependent, mortal, diploid, and exhibited none of the oncogene or tumor suppressor gene alterations present in the primary tumor. Other investigators have made similar observations (27–29). Thus, when using highly-growth-factor-enriched media, one must guard against assuming that any epithelial cells that grow out of a tumor specimen are cancer cells. Of all the breast cancer cell lines that have been developed to date, only two have been isolated by using a highly-growth-factor-enriched culture media (30, 31).

In an attempt to avoid problems associated with the presence of highly-growth-factor-responsive normal HME cells present in primary tumor specimens, we attempted to use the same culture medium to grow HBC cells from pleural effusions. Once again, these experiments failed. This serum and growth-factor-supplemented medium stimulated rapid growth of mesothelial cells and fibroblasts present in these cultures, and breast cancer cells were not responsive to the factors present in this medium. Taken together, these results indicate that enriched culture media, specifically designed for growth of normal human mammary epithelial cells, do not, in most cases, support the growth of breast cancer cells.

Based on these observations, we performed a series of experiments using serum-containing media that were devoid of many of the growth factors required by normal cells.

In these experiments, we found that a relatively simple medium, supplemented only with 5% FBS, insulin, and hydrocortisone (5% IH medium), resulted in the slow emergence of breast cancer cells. These slowly growing cells ultimately gave rise to our first two cell lines, SUM-44PE and SUM-52PE. Indeed, we have now isolated nine cell lines from primary and metastatic sites, using this same growth medium.

At this point, it is appropriate to make additional comments on the basic growth conditions that we have used to isolate our breast cancer cell lines. In addition to the supplements that are added to our medium, it is important to indicate that our base medium for all of our studies is Ham's F-12. We have tested the F-12 medium against many others, including 50:50 mixes of F-12 and DME, and the various MCDB media, and have always found F-12 to be superior for our applications. In addition, we always culture our cells in an atmosphere of 10% CO_2. We observed a number of years ago, in our studies on growth of rat mammary carcinoma cells (32, 33), that breast cancer cells do better under the slightly more acidic conditions achieved using the higher CO_2 concentration. Thus, all of our breast cancer cell lines were isolated by using Ham's-F12-based media and minimal growth factor supplementation, and our cells are always maintained in an atmosphere of 10% CO_2. These culture conditions do not support the growth of normal mammary epithelial cells and result in only limited growth of contaminating fibroblasts and mesothelial cells. As indicated, the slow emergence of breast cancer cells requires that contaminating normal cells have limited proliferative capacity.

In addition to the so-called 5% IH medium described, we have isolated some of our breast cancer cell lines in media containing other additives. In particular, SUM-102 and SUM-206 cells were isolated in 5% IH media that also contained progesterone. For both of these cell lines, the presence of progesterone was essential for the initial outgrowth of the cells. Two cell lines were originally isolated in serum-free medium with insulin and hydrocortisone. In addition, most of our cell lines can be routinely cultured in serum-free medium even though they were originally isolated using serum-containing media. In one instance (SUM-190), the addition of LPA to the serum-free medium was critically important for the emergence of the neoplastic cells. These breast cancer cells, which were isolated from a primary inflammatory breast cancer, were quiescent in culture for several weeks and did not begin proliferating until LPA was added to the culture medium. Thus, when initiating cultures of cells from breast cancer specimens, it is important to use as many different starting conditions as possible.

Growth Inhibitory Activities Present in Mixed Cultures

In at least two cases, the successful isolation of breast cancer cell lines required that HBC cells be purified from contaminating normal cells. The SUM-206 cells were isolated from normal cells by virtue of their relatively slow attachment to the substrate. This allowed the cancer cells to be moved to fresh culture dishes after the normal cells had attached. In the case of the SUM-229 cells, transferring cells into serum-free medium allowed the breast cancer cells to emerge in the absence of normal cells. For these cell lines, performing cell isolation procedures was critically important for their continuous proliferation, since the cancer cells from both specimens failed to grow in the presence of normal cells. Indeed, conditioned medium obtained from mixed cultures of SUM-225 and SUM-229 cells was able to partially inhibit growth of the respective purified breast cancer cells. The development of these breast cancer cell lines after their isolation from normal cells provides data for one hypothesis regarding why some breast cancer cells are difficult to culture *in vitro*. We have observed on many occasions that breast cancer cells fail to proliferate when large numbers of normal cells are present. This even occurs with pleural effusion-derived specimens in which mesothe-lial cells proliferate to some extent in the 5% IH medium. We have often observed cancer cells that failed to grow even after many months in culture. Cells from such specimens even-tually lose viability, and the results obtained with the SUM-206 and SUM-229 cells suggest that, at least in some cases, inhibitory activities present in the medium of mixed cultures can actively block breast cancer cell proliferation *in vitro*.

Unknown Growth Factor Requirements of Breast Cancer Cells

Even under the optimized conditions described, it is not always possible to develop a breast cancer cell line. Indeed, we have often obtained breast cancer specimens from which large numbers of breast cancer cells were isolated and seeded into culture at high density under different growth conditions. In many of these instances, we have not been able to culture the breast cancer cells and develop a cell line. In some cases, we have frozen as many as 30 ampules of cells from a single specimen and then retrieved cells periodically in an attempt to define appropriate growth conditions for those particular cells. The SUM-224PE cell strain is a good example of a breast cancer specimen that we have failed to develop into a cell line despite repeated efforts. Listed in Table 18-4 are the growth factors that we have used in an attempt to develop a cell line from this specimen. SUM-224 cells were obtained from a pleural effusion specimen and, thus, were clearly aggressive breast cancer cells in the patient. Despite that, we have so far been unable to maintain these cells in culture and develop an established cell line from them, even after plating them at high density. Results with specimens like the SUM-224PE suggest that, despite our extensive understanding of the hormonal and growth factor requirements of normal and neoplastic mammary epithelial cells, some breast cancer cells require growth factors that are undefined or that require precise growth factor combi-nations that have yet to be elucidated. The latter possibility is particularly troubling because if precise hormone, growth factor, and cytokine combinations are required to stimulate growth of some breast cancer cells, determining what those combinations are for cells from individ-ual patients is going to be a daunting task. In this regard, gene profiling strategies that are becoming more and more available may offer the ability to examine the pattern of growth

Table 18-4. Hormones and Growth Factors Used with SUM-224 Cell Culture[a]

Fibroblast growth factor acidic (FGF-a)
Fibroblast growth factor basic (FGF-b)
Fibroblast growth factor 4 (FGF-4)
Fibroblast growth factor 5 (FGF-5)
Fibroblast growth factor 6 (FGF-6)
Hepatocyte growth factor (HGF)
Keratinocyte growth factor (KGF of FGF-7)
Granulocyte-macrophage colony-stimulating factor (GM-CSF)
Prolactin (M)
Progesterone (P)
Estradiol (E_2)
Crude human plasma
Lysophosphatidic acid

[a]Media were prepared using the listed hormones and growth factors individually and in various combinations.

factor receptor expression by particular breast cancer cell populations. This, in turn, may offer the possibility of tailoring culture media to cells of individual patients.

Confirmation that Cultured Cells Are Really Breast Cancer Cells

Although it would not seem to be a difficult issue to address, being sure that cells cultured from breast cancer specimens are truly neoplastic is of utmost importance. Cell morphology is not a good indicator of whether epithelioid cells derived from tumor specimens are breast cancer cells. The morphologies of the breast cancer cell lines we have derived are highly varied. Some cells grow as loose clusters of epithelioid cells, whereas others form tightly packed aggregates of cells. In some cases, the tight clusters adhere firmly to the dish, in other cases they form loosely attached cell aggregates. Finally, some cells have polygonal morphologies, which distinguish them from the more cuboidal-appearing cells of other cell lines. Photographs of each of the SUM breast cancer cell lines can be seen at the following website: http://p53.cancer.med.umich.edu/clines/clines.html.

Thus, a number of criteria should be used to ensure that cells isolated from biopsy specimens are, indeed, breast cancer. First, the cells must be obtained from a specimen histologically confirmed as being breast cancer. Second, the putative breast cancer cells should be cytokeratin positive and, moreover, should express the luminal cytokeratins 8, 18, and 19. Next, breast cancer cells, even primary cultures and early-passage cells, have chromosomal abnormalities that can be observed in a karyotype or by flow cytometry when DNA content per cell is determined, and this needs to be determined as early as possible. Luminal mammary epithelial cells from a histologically confirmed breast cancer, which exhibit clonal chromosomal abnormalities are, without question, breast cancer cells. In addition to these basic features, bona fide breast cancer cells often exhibit other cellular and genetic characteristics that distinguish them from normal mammary epithelial cells. Most, but not all, breast cancer cells are immortal *in vitro*, whereas normal HME cells uniformly senesce after multiple *in vitro* passages. This property of breast cancer cells, however, does not appear to be universal. Two cell lines that we have derived, SUM-16LN and SUM-206PT, are not immortal. The SUM-16LN line was derived from a metastatic lymph node of a breast cancer patient. The cells had an amplification of the EGFR gene and also overexpressed mutant p53. These cells proliferated for about 20 passages before undergoing senescence (34). Similarly, the SUM-206 cell line fulfills all of the criteria of breast cancer cells we have described, yet these cells reproducibly cease to proliferate after about passage 20. Thus, 2 of the 13 breast cancer cell lines that we have developed are not immortal *in vitro*.

In addition to their altered proliferative life span, breast cancer cells frequently proliferate in media that do not support growth of normal breast epithelial cells. Thus, growth factor independence is a common feature of breast cancer cell lines. However, given that breast cancer cells from many patient specimens still cannot be cultured, it is impossible to know at this time if growth factor independence is a universal property of breast cancer cells.

Finally, breast cancer cells isolated from patient specimens will sometimes, but not always, exhibit specific genetic changes, such as mutations in p53 or amplifications and overexpression of well-known oncogenes such as ERBB-2. However, the lack of these particular molecular markers does not necessarily mean that the cells are not cancer cells. In these cases, more generalized analyses for genomic integrity need to be performed to determine the normal or neoplastic nature of the cells.

In summary, any cells that are isolated from a human biopsy specimen and cultured *in vitro* should be subject to rigorous cellular and genetic experiments to confirm that the cells are truly breast cancer cells.

SUMMARY

Isolation and culture of human breast cancer cells from patient biopsy specimens is different, in many ways, from the routine tissue culture methods to which many laboratories are accustomed. As has been discussed, establishing breast cancer cell lines requires the ability to obtain cell populations enriched for breast cancer cells that can be seeded at high density and maintained for long periods of time without the overgrowth of contaminating normal cells. The use of approaches outlined here will result in the successful isolation of HBC cells from some specimens. In addition, these approaches provide a good starting point for experiments aimed at defining novel conditions and approaches to stimulate growth of breast cancer cells that otherwise would not proliferate.

REFERENCES

1. M. R. Stampfer, R. C. Hallowes, and A. J. Hackett (1980). Growth of normal human mammary epithelial cells in culture. *In Vitro.* **16**:415–425.
2. S. L. Hammond, R. G. Ham, and M. R. Stampfer (1984). Serum-free growth of human mammary epithelial cells: rapid clonal growth in defined medium and extended serial passage with pituitary extract. *Proc. Natl. Acad. Sci. USA* **81**:5435–5439.
3. J. T. Papadimitriou, M. Stampfer, J. Barter, A. Lewis, M. Boshell, E. B. Lane, and I. M. Leith (1989). Keratin expression in human mammary cells cultured from normal and malignant tissue: relation to *in vivo* phenotypes and influence of medium. *J. Cell Sci.* **94**:403–413.
4. V. Band and R. Sager (1989). Distinctive traits of normal and tumor derived human mammary epithelial cells expressed in a medium that supports long-term growth of both cell types. *Proc. Natl. Acad. Sci. USA* **86**:1249–1253.
5. S. P. Ethier, R. M. Summerfelt, K. C. Cundiff, and B. B. Asch (1990). The influence of growth factors on the proliferative potential of normal and primary breast cancer-derived human breast epithelial cells. *Breast Cancer Res. Treat.* **17**:221–230.
6. S. P. Ethier, M. L. Mahacek, W. J. Gullick, T. J. Frank, and B. L. Weber (1993). Differential isolation of normal luminal mammary epithelial cells and breast cancer cells from primary and metastatic sites using selective media. *Cancer Res.* **53**:627–635.
7. S. P. Ethier, K. E. Kokeny, J. E. Ridings, and C. A. Dilts (1996). erbB family receptor expression and growth regulation in a newly isolated human breast cancer cell line. *Cancer Res.* **56**:899–907.
8. C. I. Sartor, M. L. Dziubinski, C.-L. Yu, R. Jove, and S. P. Ethier (1997). Role of epidermal growth factor receptor and STAT3 activation in autonomous proliferation of SUM-102PT human breast cancer cells. *Cancer Res.* **57**:978–987.
9. R. Garcia, C.-L. Yu, A. Hudnall, R. Catlett, K. L. Nelson, T. Smithgall, D. J. Fujita, S. P. Ethier, and R. Jove (1997). Constitutive activation of Stat3 in fibroblasts transformed by diverse oncoproteins and in breast carcinoma cells. *Cell Growth Diff.* **8**:1267–1276.
10. L. Flanagan, K. VanWeelden, C. Ammerman, S. P. Ethier, and J. Welsh (1999). SUM-159PT cells: A novel estrogen independent human breast cancer model system. *Breast Cancer Res. Treat.* **58**:193–204.
11. K. M. Ignatoski and S. P. Ethier (1999). Constitutive activation of pp125fak in newly isolated human breast cancer cell lines. *Breast Cancer Res. Treat.* **54**:173–182.
12. F. Forozan, R. Veldman, C. A. Ammerman, N. Z. Parsa, A. Kallioniemi, O. Kallioniemi, and S. P. Ethier (1999). Establishment, phenotypic characterization, and a survey of genetic changes in 11 new breast cancer cell lines. *Brit. J. Cancer* **81**:1328–1334.
13. S. Nicholson, J. R. C. Sainsbury, G. K. Needham, P. Chambers, J. R. Farndon, and A. L. Harris (1988). Quantitive assays of epidermal growth factor receptor in human breast cancer: cut-off points of clinical relevance. *Int. J. Cancer* **42**:36–41.
14. S. Nicholson, P. Halcrow, J. R. Farndon, J. R. C. Sainsbury, P. Chambers, and A. L. Harris (1989). Expression of epidermal growth factor receptors associated with lack of response to endocrine therapy in recurrent breast cancer. *Lancet* (**8631**):182–185.
15. S. Nicholson, J. Richard, C. Sainsbury, P. Halcrow, P. Kelly, B. Angus, C. Wright, J. Henry, J. R. Farndon, and A. L. Harris (1991). Epidermal growth factor receptor (EGFr)—results of a six year follow-up study in operable breast cancer with emphasis on the node negative subgroup. *Br. J. Cancer* **63**:146–150.

16. A. L. Harris, S. Nicholson, R. Sainsbury, C. Wright, and J. Farndon (1992). Epidermal growth factor receptor and other oncogenes as prognostic markers. *J. Natl. Cancer Inst. Monogr.* **11**:181–187.

17. T. Nishizaki, K. Chew, L. Chu, J. Isola, A. Kallioniemi, N. Weidner, and F. M. Waldman (1997). Genetic alterations in lobular breast cancer by comparative genomic hybridization. *Int. J. Cancer* **74**:513–517.

18. F. Courjal and C. Theillet (1997). Comparative genomic hybridization analysis of breast tumors with predetermined profiles of DNA amplification. *Cancer Res.* **57**:4368–4377.

19. V. Collins, R. K. Loeffler, and H. Tivey (1956). Observations on growth rates of human tumors. *Am. J. Roentgenol.* **76**:988–1000.

20. J. Gershon-Cohen, S. M. Berger, and H. S. Klickstein (1963). Roentgenography of breast cancer moderating concept of biological predeterminism. *Cancer* **16**:961–964.

21. D. V. Fournier, E. Weber, W. Hoeffken, *et al.* (1980). Growth rate of 147 mammary carcinomas. *Cancer* **45**:2198–2207.

22. A. Dawson, A. Norton, and D. S. Weinberg (1990). Comparative assessment of proliferation and DNA content in breast carcinoma by image analysis and flow cytometry. *Am. J. Pathol.* **136**:1115–1124.

23. P. Vielh, S. Chevillard, V. Mosseri, B. Donatini, and H. Magdelenat (1990). Ki67 index and S-phase fraction in human breast carcinomas. *Am. J. Clin. Pathol.* **94**:681–686.

24. C. Tomasetto, M. J. Neveu, J. Daley, P. K. Horan, and R. Sager (1993). Specificity of gap junction communication among human mammary cells and connexin transfectants in culture. *J. Cell Biol.* **122**:157–167.

25. J. W. Holder, E. Elmore, and J. C. Barrett (1993). Gap junction function and cancer. *Cancer Res.* **53**:3475–3484.

26. K. K. Hirschi, C. E. Xu, T. Tsukamoto, and R. Sager (1996). Gap junction genes Cx26 and Cx43 individually suppress the cancer phenotype of human mammary carcinoma cells and restore differentiation potential. *Cell Growth Differ.* **7**:861–870.

27. R. B. Owens, H. S. Smith, W. A. Nelson-Rees, and E. L. Springer (1976). Epithelial cell cultures from normal and cancerous tissues. *J. Natl. Cancer Inst.* **56**:843–849.

28. H. S. Smith, A. J. Hacket, J. L. Riggs, M. W. Mosesson, J. R. Walton, and M. R. Stampfer (1979). Properties of epithelial cells cultured from human carcinomas and non-malignant tissues. *J. Supramol. Struct.* **11**:147–166.

29. S. R. Wolman, H. S. Smith, M. Stampfer, and A. J. Hackett (1985). Growth of diploid cells from breast cancers. *Cancer Genetics Cytogenetics* **16**:49–64.

30. O. W. Petersen, B. van Deurs, K. V. Nielsen, M. W. Madsen, I. Laursen, I. Balslev, and P. Briand (1990). Differential tumorigenicity of two autologous human breast carcinoma cell lines, HMT-3909S1 and HMT-3909S8, established in serum-free medium. *Cancer Res.* **50**:1257–1270.

31. P. Meltzer, A. Leibovitz, W. Dalton, H. Villar, T. Kute, J. Davis, R. Nagle, and J. Trent (1991). Establishment of two new cell lines derived from human breast carcinomas with HER-2/neu amplification. *Br. J. Cancer* **63**:727–735.

32. S. P. Ethier, A. Kudla, and K. C. Cundiff (1987). The influence of hormone and growth factor interactions on the proliferative potential of normal rat mammary epithelial cells *in vitro*. *J. Cell Physiol.* **132**:161–167.

33. S. P. Ethier and K. C. Cundiff (1987). Importance of extended growth potential and growth factor independence on *in vivo* neoplastic potential of primary rat mammary carcinoma cells. *Cancer Res.* **47**:5316–5322.

34. M. L. Mahacek, D. G. Beer, T. S. Frank, and S. P. Ethier (1993). Finite proliferative lifespan *in vitro* of a human breast cancer cell strain isolatd from a metstatic lymph node. *Breast Cancer Rest. Treat.* **28**:267–276.

Part IV

Molecular Analysis and Gene Transfer Techniques

Chapter 19

mRNA *In Situ* Hybridization in the Mammary Gland

Steven Weber-Hall and Trevor Dale

Abstract. The localization of mRNA expression in the mammary gland is technically challenging due to the unique structural problems posed by breast tissues. These include closely interdigitated and sparse layers of tissue, high levels of extracellular matrix, and large quantities of adipose tissue. This chapter describes an *in situ* hybridization method using radiolabeled oligonucleotides that was developed to allow the detection of the rarest of messenger RNAs in many types of breast sample.

Abbreviations. bromochloroindolyl phosphate/nitro blue tetrazolium (BCIP/NBT); diethyl pyrocarbonate (DEPC); digoxigenin (DIG); expressed sequence tag (EST); *in situ* hybridization (ISH); paraformaldehyde (PFA); phosphate buffered saline (PBS); transforming growth factor (TGF); 0.15 M sodium chloride/sodium citrate pH 7.0 (SSC).

INTRODUCTION

The ability to localize mRNA expression is an essential tool in studies ranging from human breast pathology to analyses of ductal and lobular development. Although many standard *in situ* hybridization techniques have been successfully applied to the mammary gland (1–4), experimenters may encounter problems that are unique to the tissue. The purpose of this Chapter is to highlight potential difficulties and solutions.

For an mRNA target of given abundance, the main factor that influences success is the cellularity of the breast tissue. Cellularity varies dramatically during mammary gland development and between different pathological samples (5, 6). Fetal breast tissues are an easy target for *in situ* hybridization, because the epithelial bud and the underlying mesenchymes have an even distribution of similar-sized cells in which expression can be compared over tens to hundreds of cells per section (7). During lactation, the homogeneous repeating nature of the lactating alveoli again makes *in situ* hybridization analysis relatively easy. However, between these stages, the high fat content of the breast causes problems.

Ductal development is the most difficult stage of mouse mammary development to analyze, and many human pathological specimens share characteristics with this tissue. The

Steven Weber-Hall and Trevor Dale   Institute of Cancer Research, The Breakthrough Toby Robins Breast Cancer Centre, London, SW3 6JB, England.

Methods in Mammary Gland Biology and Breast Cancer Research, edited by Ip and Asch. Kluwer Academic/Plenum Publishers, New York, 2000.

reasons for the difficulty are that the epithelium is sparsely distributed through large areas of fatty tissue (5). Ducts can consist of a single layer of luminal epithelial cells surrounded by a sheath of thin myoepithelial cells. The target area for hybridization is thus small and has a high concentration of nonspecific probe binding sites relative to the surrounding fat-filled adipocytes. These differences in cellularity generate an intrinsic background signal that is greater over the epithelial component and can be mistaken as epithelial-specific mRNA expression. Finally, the interface between the fibroblasts and adipocytes of the stroma and the epithelium is rich in extracellular matrix components, which tend to trap nucleic acid probes.

For any tissue, the twin technical goals for *in situ* hybridization are the maximization of signal and the minimization of nonspecific background. In this Chapter we describe an *in situ* hybridization method that has been optimized for analyzing rare mRNA expression during ductal mammary gland development. This method has been successfully applied to other developmental stages and to pathological specimens. In addition, adaptations of existing *in situ* hybridization protocols are described as they apply to the analysis of fetal, pregnant, and lactating mammary tissues (8–12).

METHODS

The details of our optimized method for *in situ* hybridization (ISH) are given in Table 19-1 and refer to the use of paraffin-embedded sections hybridized with ^{33}P-labeled oligonu-

Table 19-1. Preparation of Sections

Preparation of sections
1. Immerse tissues as soon as possible after isolation in fresh 4% paraformaldehyde–PBS for 3 h. For the mouse, use either the 4th or 2nd mammary glands.
2. Dehydrate glands in 70%, 95%, and 100% ethanol by incubation for 20 min each; then embed in paraffin.
3. Cut 5-μm sections onto aminoalkyl-silicane-treated slides (Sigma).
4. Bake at least 30 min at 60°C on hot plate.
5. Dewax sections in Histoclear (xylene substitute) 2 × 10 min immediately before use, then rehydrate in 100%, 95%, 75% ethanol for 1 min each before transferring to protease solutions.

Pretreatments
1. *Proteinase K digestion* (paraffin only)
   a. Treat with prewarmed, proteinase K (20 μg/ml) in PBS for 45 min. Rinse in PBS 2 × 1 min.
   b. Fix in 4% paraformaldehyde in PBS for 2 min at room temperature.
   c. Rinse in PBS 2 × 5 min.

2. *Acetylation* (frozen and paraffin)
   a. Add the slides to 400 ml 0.1 M triethanolamine in a container with a magnetic stirrer.
   b. Add 1 ml acetic anhydride (97%) and stir for 10 min at room temperature.
   c. Rinse in PBS 2 × 5 min.
   d. Dehydrate through graded ethanol series (75%, 95%, 100%) 5 min each and allow the slides to air-dry. Proceed to prehybridization.

3. *RNAse controls*
   These steps must be carried out in containers dedicated to RNAse-treated slides.
   a. Treat control slides in 20 μg/ml RNAse for 10 min at room temperature.
   b. Rinse in PBS 2 × 5 min at room temperature.
   c. Dehydrate through a graded ethanol series (75%, 95%, 100%) for 5 min each, then allow to air-dry. Proceed to prehybridization.

cleotides. Variations on this technique, such as the use of frozen sections and nonradioactive probes, are discussed within the text.

Materials

SLIDE PREPARATION.   Paraformaldehyde (Sigma P6148); silicanization with 3-amino-propyltriethoxy silane (Sigma A3648); histoclear from National Diagnostics; Proteinase K (Boehringer Mannheim 745 723); triethanolamine (Sigma T1377); acetic anhydride (Sigma A6404); RNAse A (Sigma R 5503).

HYBRIDIZATION.   Formamide AR (BDH 10326 6T); Denhardts (Sigma D2532); dextran sulfate 500,000 mw (Sigma D6001) poly A + RNA (Amersham Pharmacia Biotech 27-4110-01).

WASHES AND DETECTION.   K5 emulsion (Ilford 1355127); Giemsa (Sigma); DPX mounting medium (Fisons D/5319/05); NBT/BCIP (Gibco/BRL 540-8280SA).

Tissue Preparation

PRELIMINARY CONSIDERATIONS.   A vital point that will not be considered in detail here is the prevention of exogenous RNAse contamination. Diethylpyrocarbonate (DEPC)-treated water should be used throughout, and all glassware should be baked at 200°C to destroy pre-existing RNAses. Stock solutions for RNA work should be set aside from normal laboratory use to prevent inadvertent contamination. Detailed methods to prevent RNAse contamination of buffers can be found in Sambrook *et al*. (12). Note that DEPC-treated water should not be used in the labeling reactions because trace amounts of residual DEPC can inactivate the enzymes involved.

FIXATION AND EMBEDDING.   Mouse mammary tissues should be fixed and embedded in paraffin, as described in Table 19-1, or prepared for frozen sections. *In situ* hybridization conditions that proved optimal for paraffin-embedded mouse tissues were found to work well with archival human breast tissue (14). To obtain longitudinal sections through mouse mammary ducts and end buds, use the second mammary glands of 4- to 5-week-old Balb/C mice. In these glands, the ductal network has to grow in a flat plane due to the thinness of the fat pad. When postnatal tissues for frozen sections are prepared, the fourth abdominal mammary glands should be dissected, embedded in Tissuetek OCT compound, and frozen in isopentane cooled by liquid nitrogen. Frozen blocks should be stored at −70°C. In general, tissues should be processed as soon as possible after collection to reduce the degradation of mRNAs by endogenous RNAses. Embryonic mammary glands should be microdissected and grouped in random orientation within a paraffin block. Because fetal mammary glands may not be easily identified, tissue blocks should be prepared that contain a truncated forelimb and a subtending 2-mm circle around the base of the limb. This area will contain mammary primordia for glands 2 and 3. If sufficient glands are processed, tissue blocks can be prepared in which every section should present a cross section of the fetal gland (Figure 19-1).

CUTTING SECTIONS.   Paraffin-embedded sections should be prepared as described in Table 19-1. Frozen 5-μm sections should be cut in the cryostat at −20°C. The fatty content of mammary tissue, especially in glands from virgin mice, can cause sections to crumble. To overcome this problem, vary the temperature at which the sections are cut in steps up to

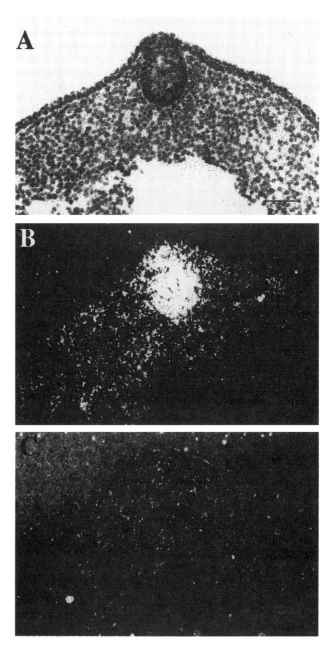

Figure 19-1. Msx-1 expression in 12.5-day fetal mammary gland. (A) Light field. (B) Antisense ^{33}P-labeled riboprobe. (C) Sense ^{33}P-labeled riboprobe. Exposure time 6 weeks. Counterstained with dilute Giemsa. Bar = 80 µM.

−12°C. Frozen sections should be mounted onto ice-cool poly-L-lysine coated slides, then immediately transferred to 4% fresh paraformaldehyde (PFA) for 1 h on ice. Fresh PFA should be used to reduce the formation of cross-linked forms. To aid dissolving, PFA solutions may need brief heating to 50°C prior to cooling and use. Following fixation, slides should be rinsed twice in ice-cold PBS, dehydrated through RNAse-free ethanol, air-dried, and stored at −20°C. In our experience, frozen sections gave poorer morphology and equivalent levels of signal to paraffin-embedded tissues; however, the use of frozen sections may be required if labile protein epitopes are to be simultaneously detected by immunohistochemistry.

PRETREATMENTS.   Although formalin-fixed, paraffin-embedded glands provide high-quality sections and morphology, the target mRNAs are trapped in a cross-linked protein matrix that needs to be partially disrupted to allow access to the probe. The most common method to achieve this end is the partial proteolysis of the section (Table 19-1). Fortunately, the defined size of oligonucleotide probes (compared to ribonucleotide probes) removes an additional variable that can affect access to the mRNA target (10). Following protease digestion, sections should be briefly postfixed in 4% PFA for 5 min to inactivate the proteinase. As a final pretreatment, sections should be acetylated to reduce electrostatic charges, which may contribute to nonspecific background signal.

CONTROLS.   The most important control slide that should be used in all studies is an RNAse-treated slide(s). By removing the specific RNA signal, the true extent of background binding can be assessed. Particular care needs to be taken to use separate containers for the treatment of slides with RNAse A to avoid contamination. If possible, a positive control tissue should be used. Mid-gestation embryos make good controls, as many different tissues are present within a single section. To allow the rapid evaluation of reagent quality and technique, β-casein expression can be simultaneously followed in lactating tissue (Figure 19-2). The β-casein signals should be so strong that they can be monitored with the aid of a hand-held geiger counter.

Hybridization

PREHYBRIDIZATION.   Prehybridization exposes the section to every hybridization component except the labeled antisense probe. Our detailed analysis of prehybridization mixes showed that a close match between prehybridization and hybridization components was essential for low nonspecific signal. This match was particularly important when the nucleic acid content of the mixes was matched. Bulk nucleic acid components such as yeast tRNA lowered background, but were not sufficient to lower background to the level required for rare mRNA detection. The best-matched nucleic acid was found to be random 30mer oligonucleotides [poly(dN)30], possibly because of their identical access to nonspecific binding sites.

PROBE DESIGN.   The number of oligonucleotides used for the hybridization is a primary determinant of the sensitivity of the ISH technique. Oligonucleotide probes of 30 bases in length can be designed to cover the entire length of the target RNA in a nonoverlapping manner. Given recent improvements in oligonucleotide production technology, the synthesis of many oligonucleotides is not prohibitively expensive, particularly as very small quantities of each nucleic acid are required. In practice, we have used cocktails of 12 oligonucleotides against a single target. The concentration of the oligonucleotide mix suggested in the protocol (Table 19-2) was determined by studies using anti-β-casein oligonucleotides against mid-

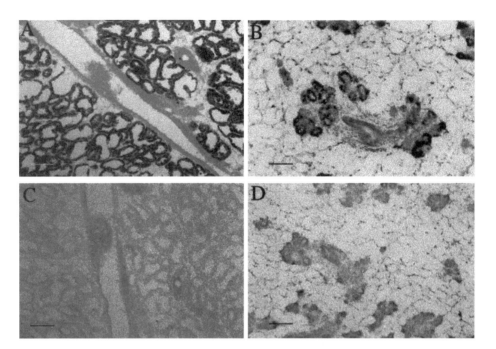

Figure 19-2. Using β-casein to optimize *in situ* hybridization in the mammary gland. Tissues: (A, C) Lactating mammary gland, counterstained with Orange G; (B, D) Mammary tissue from 8-day pregnant animal. Hybridization: (A, B) Cocktail of 2 digoxigenin-labeled antisense β-casein oligonucleotides (sequence: GAGTTTATGAGGCGGAGCACAGTTTCAGAG; GATGCTGGAGTGAAC-TTTAGCCTGGAGCAC); (C, D) Digoxigenin-labeled p(dN)30. Detection: NBT/BCIP. Counterstained with dilute Giemsa. Bar = 150 μM. (For a color representation of this, see figure facing page 216.)

pregnant mammary tissue (Figure 19-2A) The sequences of putative oligonucleotides should be screened to minimize the range of melting temperatures (T_m) between each of the oligonucleotides. In individual studies, we confined the T_m range within 10°C, although the overall T_m range of oligonucleotides used spanned 74–88°C. Melting temperatures were determined by the nearest-neighbor technique (15). To rapidly screen oligonucleotides, a program such as Oligo (National Biosciences Inc, Plymouth, MN) may be useful. This program can also be used to identify oligonucleotides with inverted repeats that might form stem–loop structures, although we have no particular evidence that these structures may contribute to background. Finally, it has been noted by Hougaard *et al.* (9) that probes containing a high percentage of G should be avoided because they bind nonspecifically to cellular components. Importantly, probes with a high C content did not create such problems. These authors recommended probes with levels of G lower than 33% and the avoiding of runs of 4 or more Gs in a row. With the increasing amounts of data now available in sequence databases, panels of oligonucleotides should be screened to remove those showing strong complementarity to expressed sequence tags (ESTs), since ESTs define a subset of nucleic acids that are known to be transcribed into mRNA.

CONTROLS.   Control oligonucleotide probes should ideally be matched for melting temperature, length, and base distribution with the experimental probe(s). In practice, we have found that the random p(dN)30 oligonucleotide used in the prehybridization behaves as a good control probe. In experiments in which this probe was tested directly against individually

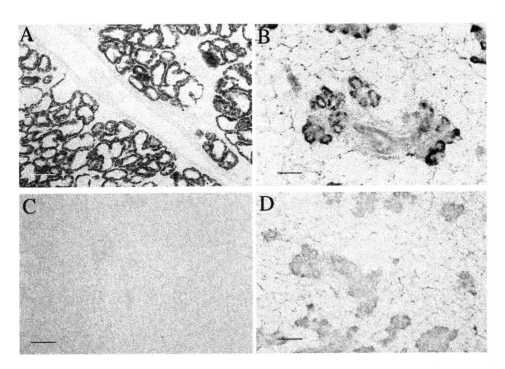

Figure 19-2. Using β-casein to optimize *in situ* hybridization in the mammary gland. Tissues: (A, C) Lactating mammary gland, counterstained with Orange G; (B, D) Mammary tissue from 8-day pregnant animal. Hybridization: (A, B) Cocktail of 2 digoxigenin-labeled antisense β-casein oligonucleotides (sequence: GAGTTTATGAGGCGGAGCACAGTTTCAGAG; GATGCTGGAGTGAAC-TTTAGCCTGGAGCAC); (C, D) Digoxigenin-labeled p(dN)30. Detection: NBT/BCIP. Counterstained with dilute Giemsa. Bar = 150 μM.

Table 19-2. Prehybridization and Hybridization

Prehybridization

1. Calculate the volume of prehybridization solution required for the experiment; this will depend on the size and number of the sections. Allow 25 µl under a 22-mm square coverslip or 50 µl under a 50 × 22-mm coverslip. This number should then be doubled to allow for hybridization and post-prehybridization washes, and then doubled again to allow for losses during filtering.
2. Make up prehybridization solution: 6 × SSC, 50% formamide (deionized), 5 × Denhardts (Sigma), 10% dextran sulfate, p(dN)30 oligonucleotide 20 µg/ml and poly A+ RNA 20 µg/ml. Filter through 0.8-µm filter.
3. With a tissue carefully wipe dry the region around the section to prevent the prehybridization solution from running.
4. Cover the section with minimum prehybridization solution (approximately 100 µl) and gently cover with coverslip.
5. Incubate slides at 37°C for 3 h in sealed chamber supported above blotting paper soaked in 6 × SSC, 50% formamide to humidify the chamber in order to reduce drying.

Probe preparation

To maximize the specific activity of the probe, experiments can be coordinated with the radionucleotide supplier to obtain ^{33}P nucleotides immediately after production. dATP (800 Ci/mMol was supplied by Boehringer Manheim Cat. No. 1028707).

1. Set up terminal transferase reaction.

Oligonucleotide cocktail 25 ng	× µl
1 mM CoCl$_2$	3 µl
5 × buffer (Boehringer terminal transferase)	4 µl
Terminal transferase	1 µl
P33 dATP (25☐Ci 33P)	2.5 µl
Water	to final 20 µl

    Incubate at 37°C for 30 min; dilute reaction with 30 µl of 1 × terminal transferase buffer.
2. Remove unincorporated nucleotides by two passes over a spin-gel filtration column (Chromaspin 10 columns; Promega).
3. Monitor incorporation by scintillation counting 1☐l probe, and the length of the tails by running a 1-µl aliquot on a 12% urea polyacrylamide gel.

Identical levels of oligonucleotide were used for digoxigenin labeling (Boehringer Cat. No. 1417231). Some oligonucleotide-producing companies now directly supply digoxigenin–labeled probes. T4 polynucleotide kinase and [γ^{32}P]-ATP can be used to 5′-end-label the digoxigenin oligonucleotides to allow probe tracking during washes.

Hybridization

1. Add labeled probe to prehybridization solution to a final concentration of 50–100 ng/µl. (Assume 80% recovery from the gel filtration columns.) This mix can be assumed to be 2 × hybridization mix.
2. Add an equal volume of probe mixture to the prehybridization solution already present on the section from the prehybridization stage. Mix gently with pipette 2–3 times. Take care not to disturb the sections; they are easily removed from this point on.
3. Incubate overnight in a 6 × SSC, 50% formamide humidified chamber at 45°C.

designed control probes that were matched for G/C content and T_m, we saw slightly higher background with the p(dN)30 probe, possibly due to the presence of individual oligonucleotides with a high G content among the complex mixture.

PROBE LABELING. ^{33}P, in preference to ^{35}S, was used to label probes because it resulted in lower background signals with similar levels of resolution (Figure 19-3). ^{33}P-oligonucleotide probes were labeled with ^{33}PdATP using terminal transferase as described in Table 19-2. The length of the added tails was estimated by comparison with 5′-end-labeled oligonucleotide using denaturing urea polyacrylamide gel electrophoresis. Preparations routinely contained

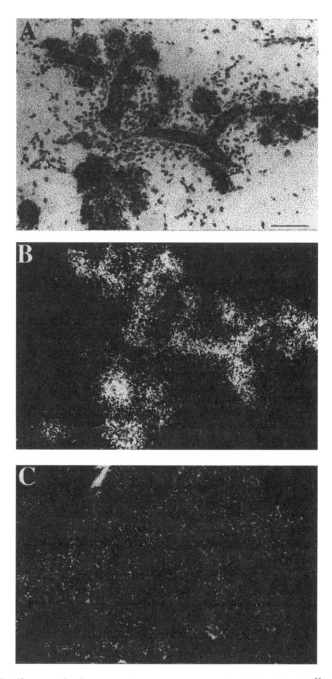

Figure 19-3. *Wnt-5b* expression in pregnant mouse mammary gland detected with ^{33}P-labeled oligonu-cleotides. (A) Light field. (B) ^{33}P-labeled oligonucleotide probe comprising 16-oligonucleotide cock-tail. (C) ^{33}P-labeled control oligonucleotides [p(dN)30]. Exposure time 8 weeks. Counterstained with dilute Giemsa stain. Bar = 80 μM.

tails from 5–12 nucleotides in length (mean 8 nucleotides). In principle, the use of multiple oligonucleotides (<12) should generate a label density equivalent to that of long ribonucleotide probes, and in practice the tailing of oligonucleotide probes is simpler and less prone to variablility than ribonucleotide probes. An example of a ^{33}P-labeled riboprobe ISH of Msx-1 expression in the fetal mammary gland is shown in Figure 18-1.

HYBRIDIZATION AND WASHES. The protocol for addition of ^{33}P-labeled oligonucleotide probes is described in Table 19-2, and protocols for washes are described in Table 19-3. Digoxigenin-labeled oligonucleotides should be treated identically. [33]P riboprobes can also be processed by the same hybridization protocol; however, for detailed descriptions of posthybridization RNAse treatments, see Poulsom *et al.* (10).

Table 19-3. Washes and Detection

Washes and detection

Sections hybridized with oligonucleotide probes

1. Rinse the labeled probe off the sections by very gently dripping $5 \times$ SSC across the sections.
2. Add 50 μl (or sufficient to cover section) of prehybridization solution to the sections.
3. Incubate at 37°C, 30 min.
4. Repeat steps 1 to 3.
5. Gently rinse in $5 \times$ SSC at room temperature for 5 min.
6. Rack up slides and wash in $5 \times$ SSC, 60% formamide for 1 h at room temperature.
7. Wash in $5 \times$ SSC, 60% formamide at 37°C for 1 h; repeat and monitor for probe levels using a hand-held Geiger counter.
8. Air-dry and monitor for counts using autoradiographic film or a phosphorimager as required. If RNAse-treated slides have very low levels of counts, proceed with slide-coating autoradiography.

Autoradiography

1. Melt 15 ml Ilford K5 emulsion in 25 ml distilled water at 45°C.
2. Dip slides vertically, drain 10 s, wipe back of slides, allow to dry 3 h.
3. Store in lightproof box at 4°C with dessicant. Ensure no radioactive samples are stored within the same 4°C area. Exposure time must be determined for each probe. Duplicate slides may be produced and developed periodically. For abundant messages 1–2 weeks may be sufficient. For the rarest targets, 8 weeks may be necessary.
4. Develop using Kodak D19 at 19°C for 4 min.
5. Rinse in 0.5% acetic acid for 1 min.
6. Rinse in tap water for 1 min.
7. Fix in 30% sodium thiosulfate 2×4 min.
8. Counterstain using dilute (1 : 5) Giemsa solution 3 min (the dilute counterstain allows visualization of the cellular morphology but also makes possible visualization of the silver grain deposits using transmitted light. Wash in tap water.
9. Air-dry; mount in 50 μl DPX and apply coverslip.

Digoxigenin

Digoxigenin detection was carried out using a DIG nucleic acid detection kit (Boehringer Cat. No 1175041).

1. Soak in blocking reagent 1 h (we also used 10% milk powder in PBS).
2. Add 100 μl anti-DIG-coupled alkaline phosphatase 1 U/ml in blocking agent to the sections.
3. Incubate 1 h at room temperature.
4. Rinse in PBS 2×5 min.
5. Add 100 μl detection reagents NBT/BCIP prepared according to manufacturer's instructions. Leave 15 min at room temperature. Positive signal should be seen within a few minutes for highly expressed messages.
6. Slides may be counterstained with dilute Giemsa as above or acridine orange.
7. Air-dry and mount for analysis.

A key step in the reduction of background levels for oligonucleotide probes was found to be a "postprehybridization" step. In this stage, prehybridization mix (containing unlabeled 30mer oligonucleotides) was incubated with the section after the labeled probe has been removed. The rationale for this was that unlabeled oligonucleotides would compete away non-specifically bound, labeled oligonucleotides more effectively than nucleic-acid-free salt washes. Although the exact mechanism is not clear, the step was found to reduce nonspecific binding fivefold (data not shown) and was critical for the detection of the rarest mRNAs (Figure 19-3). Throughout the washing stages, the slides should be monitored with a Geiger counter. If counts are detected on the control RNAse A–treated sections, the final washes should be repeated.

DETECTION. Standard methods for detecting ^{33}P- and digoxigenin-labeled probes are described in Table 19-3. In our experience, digoxigenin-labeled oligonucleotide probes generated higher levels of background than radioactive probes. This level of background was too high to allow detection of the rarest messages, but allowed the localization of TGFβ-3 and β-casein mRNAs in early pregnant mammary tissue (data not shown; Figure 19-2B). For a detailed description of oligonucleotide-based nonradioactive detection methods including staining controls see Hougaard et al. (9).

COMMENTS AND CRITICAL ISSUES

A variety of ISH methods have been described in the literature, some of which will reproducibly detect mRNA in a variety of tissues (8, 9, 11, 12, 16). In our experience, however, these techniques fail when the distribution of rare mRNAs is studied in tissues with a variable cellularity. We have investigated in detail the factors determining signal level and background in the mouse mammary gland and have developed a highly sensitive method based on radioactive oligonucleotides. This method has been successfully applied to archival breast tissue (14, 17).

The methods described were optimized for maximal sensitivity by using two antisense β-casein oligonucleotides and mouse mammary gland sections (Figure 19-3). For novice experimenters, the use of β-casein as a positive control is highly recommended because it allows all aspects of the ISH to be optimized. For example, sections of the lactating gland can be used to rapidly optimize protease digestion conditions using autoradiographic exposures to X-OMAT AR film or phosphorimager analysis to detect radioactive signals. Tissues from pregnant breast can also be used to measure signal sensitivity, because β-casein is expressed at a range of levels during pregnancy. Northern analysis of the gene of interest can help to estimate expression levels and can be performed with the same labeled oligonucleotides used for ISH. If the size of the message is known, northern hybridization can test for the possibility that the probe might cross-hybridize to unrelated messages. However, absolute exclusion of cross-hybridization to unrelated sequences requires the use of a different probe against the same sequence. A practical approach may be to split the panel of oligonucleotides in half and compare the pattern of hybridization with each. In the future, the availability of information from the genome mapping programs should eliminate the guess-work from the design of nucleic acid probes and may enable the automation of techniques, including in situ hybridization.

ACKNOWLEDGMENTS. We would like to thank Neville Young for useful comments, Hiran Jayatilake for preparing tissues, and the Cancer Research Campaign for funding this work.

REFERENCES

1. T. A. Buhler, T. C. Dale, C. Kieback, R. C. Humphreys, and J. M. Rosen (1993). Localization and quantification of Wnt-2 gene expression in mouse mammary development. *Dev. Biol.* **155**:87–96.
2. S. D. Robinson, G. B. Silberstein, A. B. Roberts, K. C. Flanders, and C. W. Daniel (1991). Regulated expression and growth inhibitory effects of transforming growth-factor-beta isoforms in mouse mammary-gland development. *Development* **113**(3):867–875.
3. K. T. Barker, J. E. Martindale, P. J. Mitchell, T. Kamalati, P. M. J. Page, D. J. Phippard, T. C. Dale, B. A. Gusterson, and M. R. Crompton (1995). Discoidin domain receptor expression in breast tumours. *Oncogene* **10**:569–575.
4. J. J. Wysolmerski, W. M. Philbrick, M. E. Dunbar, B. Lanske, H. Kronenberg, and A. E. Broadus (1998). Rescue of the parathyroid hormone-related protein knockout mouse demonstrates that parathyroid hormone-related protein is essential for mammary gland development. *Development* **125**(7):1285–1294.
5. C. W. Daniel and G. B. Silberstein (1987). In M. C. Neville and C. W. Daniel (eds.), *The Mammary Gland: Development, Regulation and Function*, Plenum Press, New York, pp. 3–36.
6. I. A. Forsyth (1991). The mammary gland. *Balliere's Clin. Endocrinol. Metabol.* **5**(4):809–832.
7. M. Farquharson, R. Harvie, and A. M. McNicol (1990). Detection of messenger RNA using a digoxigenin end labelled oligonucleotide probe. *J. Clin. Pathol.* **43**:424–428.
8. A. Giaid, Q. Hamid, C. Adams, D. R. Springall, G. Terenghi, and J. M. Polak (1989). Non-isotopic RNA probes. Comparison between different labels and detection systems. *Histochemistry* **93**:191–196.
9. D. M. Hougaard, H. Hansen, and L. I. Larsson (1997). Non-radioactive *in situ* hybridisation for mRNA with emphasis on the use of oligodeoxynucleotide probes. *Histochem. Cell. Biol.* **108**:335–344.
10. R. Poulsom, J. M. Longcroft, R. E. Jeffery, L. A. Rogers, and J. H. Steel (1998). A robust method for isotopic riboprobe *in situ* hybnridisation to localise mRNAs in routine phatology specimens. *Eur. J. Histochem.* **42**:121–132.
11. D. G. Wilkinson (1992). In D. G. Wilkinson (ed.), *In situ hybridisation: A practical approach*, IRL Press, Oxford, pp. 75–83.
12. J. Sambrook, E. F. Fritsch, and T. Maniatis (1989). In N. Ford (ed.), *Molecular Cloning: A Laboratory Manual*, Cold Spring Harbor Laboratory Press, pp. 7.3–7.5.
13. T. C. Dale, S. J. Weber-Hall, K. Smith, E. L. Huguet, H. Jayatalike, B. A. Gusterson, G. Shuttleworth, M. O'Hare, and A. L. Harris (1996). Compartment switching of WNT-2 expression in human breast tumours. *Cancer Res.* **56**:4320–4323.
14. K. J. Breslauer, R. l. Frank, H. Blocker, and L. A. Markey (1986). Predicting DNA duplex stability from base sequence. *Proc. Natl. Acad. Sci. USA* **83**:3746–3750.
15. J. H. Steel, R. E. Jeffery, J. M. Longcroft, L. A. Rogers, and R. Poulsom (1998). Comparison of isotopic and non-isotopic labelling for *in situ* hybridisation of various mRNA targets. *Eur. J. Histochem.* **42**:143–150.
16. S. J. Weber-Hall, D. Phippard, C. Niemeyer, and T. C. Dale (1994). Developmental and hormonal regulation of Wnt gene expression in the mouse mammary gland. *Differentiation* **57**:205–214.
17. J. M. Rosen, E. Bayna, and K. F. Lee (1989). Analysis of milk protein gene expression in transgenic mice. *Mol. Biol. Med.* **6**(6):501–509.

Chapter 20

Application of *In Situ* PCR to Studies of the Mammary Gland

Russell C. Hovey and Barbara K. Vonderhaar

Abstract. The ability to detect low numbers of target nucleic acid sequence provides a powerful tool to investigate the molecular events that underlie development and disease in organs such as the mammary gland. Recent development of the polymerase chain reaction *in situ* (IS-PCR) now enables the intracellular amplification of DNA by PCR and its subsequent localization in preparations of fixed cells and tissue. This chapter outlines the procedure and materials required for the localization of integrated mouse mammary tumor virus proviral DNA in mouse mammary tissue by an indirect IS-PCR method. Also discussed are several aspects critical to the success of this emerging technique, particularly regarding tissue pretreatment and the importance of appropriate controls. In addition, various potential applications of this technique to studies of the mammary gland are considered.

Abbreviations. diethylpyrocarbonate (DEPC); dithiothreitol (DTT); *in situ* PCR (IS-PCR); Moloney murine leukemia virus (MMLV); mouse mammary tumor virus (MMTV); phosphate buffered saline (PBS); polymerase chain reaction (PCR); reverse transcriptase polymerase chain reaction (RTPCR); recombinant *Thermus thermophilus* DNA polymerase (r*Tth*); sodium chloride/sodium citrate (SSC).

INTRODUCTION

The advent of the polymerase chain reaction (PCR) represented a major technical advance in the field of molecular biology, enabling single copies of nucleic acid sequence to be amplified in solution. The limitation of PCR in this form, however, is its inability to describe the spatial distribution of target sequences at the cellular level; although conventional *in situ* hybridization affords such localization, its sensitivity is limited to approximately >10 copies/cell and represents a major limitation for low-abundance nucleic acids.

The marriage of these technologies has led to the development of PCR *in situ* (IS-PCR). Since being first described by Haase *et al.* (1) in 1990, the methodology, equipment, and range of applications for IS-PCR has improved considerably (2). The IS-PCR technique has been successfully employed to localize a variety of viruses in a range of tissue types (3, 4) as well as intracellular bacterial infections (5). Furthermore, the ability to reverse-transcribe intracellular mRNA to cDNA before its subsequent amplification by PCR (IS-RTPCR) affords the opportunity to detect mRNAs expressed at low abundance (6). Although IS-PCR is

Russell C. Hovey and Barbara K. Vonderhaar   Laboratory of Tumor Immunology and Biology, National Cancer Institute, National Institutes of Health, Bethesda, Maryland 20892.

Methods in Mammary Gland Biology and Breast Cancer Research, edited by Ip and Asch. Kluwer Academic/Plenum Publishers, New York, 2000.

beginning to find widespread utility, some limitations of this technique remain, particularly its ability to generate false positive results, the low efficiency of amplification *in situ*, and the diffusion of PCR products from within cells (7, 8).

Mammary tissue represents a heterogeneous collection of cell types that can be a particularly challenging material for any form of cytomolecular analysis. The spatial assessment of gene expression within the mammary gland to date has generally relied on *in situ* hybridization. However, the sensitivity limitations of this technique coupled with a recognition that many genes are expressed at low levels within the mammary gland (possibly only within a small subpopulation of cells) lends support to the potential application of IS-PCR to such studies. Our objective here is to describe an IS-PCR protocol that has been developed and successfully used in our laboratory to localize mouse mammary tumor virus (MMTV) proviral DNA and, in doing so, to demonstrate the potential application of IS-PCR to studies of the mammary gland.

MATERIALS AND INSTRUMENTATION

Reagents

The following reagents are required to perform the IS-PCR technique, in addition to various standard laboratory buffer and salt solutions (prepared nuclease free).

1. Paraformaldehyde, acetic anhydride, triethanolamine, salmon sperm DNA, bovine serum albumin, yeast-soluble tRNA, and RNAse A are all available from Sigma (St. Louis, MO).
2. The GeneAmp *in situ* PCR core kit is from Perkin–Elmer Applied Biosystems (Foster City, CA); it includes Taq polymerase, nucleotide mix, $MgCl_2$, $10 \times$ PCR buffer. Amplicover slides, disks, and clips for the GeneAmp system are also from Perkin–Elmer. Proteinase K (RNA grade) and DTT are from Life Technologies (Gaithersburg, MD).
3. The Maxiscript *in vitro* transcription kit is from Ambion (Austin, TX). Emulsion autoradiography is performed using NTB2 emulsion and developing chemicals from Eastman Kodak (Rochester, NY). Nonradioactive *in situ* hybridization uses reagents from the DIG RNA labeling kit combined with the DIG nucleic acid detection kit (both from Boehringer Mannheim, Indianapolis, IN). Nuclear fast red is from Vector Laboratories (Burlingame, CA).

Tissues and Sections

As with any cytological technique, care must be exercised when fixing and processing tissue for IS-PCR analysis. We routinely fix mouse mammary tissues with 4% paraformaldehyde for 16h at 4°C. Paraformaldehyde fixative is prepared fresh (to avoid macromolecular cross-linking of formaldehyde) by dissolving paraformaldehyde in PBS with heating to 60°C followed by the addition of 1–3 drops of 10 N NaOH to complete dissolution; once cooled the pH is adjusted to pH 7.4. Cross-linking fixatives such as formalin and paraformaldehyde are generally preferred for IS-PCR amplification because they effectively preserve cellular integrity while allowing cell permeability to be manipulated during tissue pretreatment. Acid–alcohol fixatives tend to give poorer cytological preservation that can result in the diffusion of amplification products. In contrast, strong cross-linking fixatives (such as glutaraldehyde) can cause the tissue to become impermeable to PCR reagents. Samples are subsequently processed to, and embedded in, low-melting-point paraffin. It is desirable to use the lowest possible temperatures during embedding to prevent extensive heat-induced damage of DNA.

Sections of 4–5 μm are cut onto slides suited to the IS-PCR thermal cycler available. Precautions to minimize the contamination of samples (gloves, DEPC-treated water, etc.) are also employed. For the Perkin–Elmer GeneAmp system, three sections are arranged on a 1.2-mm-thick, presilanized slide designed to accommodate the special PCR reagent containment disks. Our experience indicates that sections can be stored in a dry, dust-free box for several months before IS-PCR analysis.

Thermal Cycler

The first-described method for IS-PCR of cells or tissues involved the placement of glass slides directly on the block of a conventional thermal cycler, with the reagents contained under a coverslip sealed with nail polish and mineral oil. Given the number of unappealing features surrounding this approach, several thermal cyclers have been developed along with the IS-PCR technique. Certain models still incorporate an oil-sealed coverslip to contain the reagents during thermal cycling of slides in a horizontal position. Our experience is with the Perkin–Elmer GeneAmp 1000 IS-PCR system. This purposebuilt thermal cycler holds 10 slides vertically against vanes of a thermal cycler block, with PCR reagents contained over the individual sections by an airtight silicon disk held in place by means of a metal clip clamped onto the slide prior to thermal cycling. This design has some minor disadvantages, but it has proven in our hands to be a suitable apparatus for IS-PCR.

METHODS

Reagent Preparation

The basic reagents and reaction conditions for solution PCR apply to IS-PCR, although several modifications are necessary. Careful primer selection is critical for successful IS-PCR. Aside from satisfying standard requirements (similar T_m, GC-enriched 3′-ends, generation of a single band in solution PCR), an important consideration in designing primers for IS-PCR is the size of the resultant amplicon. Short products may easily diffuse from within cells, leading to diffuse or diminished signal. Conversely, the efficiency of IS-PCR is substantially reduced when one attempts to generate large products. A widespread consensus is that primers that generate PCR products of 150–300 bp are most suitable for IS-PCR. In mammary tissue we have successfully amplified a genomic sequence of up to 540 bp. An alternative approach adopted by several investigators is to use overlapping primer pairs that generate a concatamerized product; this will be of particular utility where the diffusion of PCR products is a concern. The following primers are used to amplify a 220 bp MMTV *gag* sequence:

5′   gttcgtcttgtattgtctctt
3′   aattctattgcactgctctcc

The PCR Cocktail

Amplification of MMTV by IS-PCR is performed in the presence of the cocktail described here. As with normal PCR, parameters such as the concentration of MgCl₂ and primers need to be optimized for each primer pair, whereas IS-PCR typically calls for a higher final concentration of reagents such as primers, Taq polymerase, and $MgCl_2$. We use reagents provided with the GeneAmp PCR core kit (Perkin–Elmer). The final volume for each section is 50 μl:

	Stock	Volume (μl)	Final conc.
PCR buffer	10×	5	1×
PCR nucleotide mix	10 mM each	1.7	0.34 mM
5′-primer	10 pmol/μl	2	0.4 μM
3′-primer	10 pmol/μl	2	0.4 μM
Bovine serum albumin	2%	1.7	0.07%
$MgCl_2$	25 mM	7.5	3.75 mM
Taq polymerase	20 U/μl	0.5	0.2 U/μl
Water		29.6	
		50	

DETAILED PROCEDURES

A wide variety of factors, including tissue type, tissue preparation, and the gene(s) of interest influence the exact protocol and conditions used for IS-PCR. The following protocol is relevant for paraffin-embedded mouse mammary tissue.

Tissue Preparation and Pretreatment

1. Deparaffinize in xylenes, 2 × 10 min.
2. Delipidate in chloroform, 10 min.
3. Rehydrate, 5 min each in 100%, 95%, 70% ethanol.
4. Water, 2 min.
5. 0.02 M HCl, 20 min.
6. Rinse PBS.
7. 0.01% Triton X-100 in PBS, 90 s.*
8. 1–20 μg/ml proteinase K in 0.1 M Tris, 50 mM EDTA pH 8.0, 30 min at 37°C.
9. Wash in 0.1 M glycine in PBS, 5 min.[†]
10. Microwave slides in proteinase K buffer to achieve boiling for 10 s.[‡]
11. Immerse in ice-cold 20% acetic acid, 15 s.
12. Rinse PBS.
13. Acetylate, 2 × 5 min with 0.25% acetic anhydride in 0.1 M triethanolamine buffer, pH 8.0.[§]
14. Rinse PBS.
15. Dehydrate to 100% ethanol, air-dry.

---

*Treatment with Triton X-100 as a means to permeabilize cell membranes can be considered optional in addition to HCl treatment.

[†] Glycine is used to inactivate protease activity; although some researchers suggest this is unnecessary, our preference is for its inclusion to avoid any risk of protease carryover.

[‡] Microwave pretreatment substantially improves nucleic acid amplification by IS-PCR. The means by which it achieves its effect is unknown, although it may act to unmask DNA-histone complexes.

[§] Acetylation has been reported to improve the specificity of subsequent primer annealing.

PCR Amplification

Once samples have been pretreated, the PCR mix is contained over the sections by means of a silicon disk clamped in place by using the GeneAmp assembly tool. One benefit of this method is that it allows PCR to be initiated under hot-start conditions by means of a heating element contained in the assembly tool. Our approach is to prepare a cocktail of PCR reagents that is heated to and held at 70°C in a heating block until the cocktail is applied to all sections.

Once a given slide has been assembled, it is transferred to the thermal cycler on a 70°C soak file until all slides are complete.

The following cycling parameters are used for the amplification of MMTV proviral DNA:

1. 15-min soak delay, 70°C
2. 5 min at 94°C, then 90 s at 55°C
3. 50 cycles of 94°C for 1 min, 52°C for 1 min, 72°C for 2 min
4. Final extension at 72°C for 10 min
5. Soak hold at 4°C

Post-PCR

Once thermal cycling is complete, the containment disks are removed and the sections washed in 2 × SSC for 5 min at room temperature. The sections are then postfixed in 2% paraformaldehyde for 5 min to fix amplicons within the cells before subsequent detection by *in situ* hybridization. Following fixation, sections are dehydrated to 100% ethanol and air-dried.

In Situ Hybridization

In contrast to the direct method whereby amplicons are detected due to their incorporation of a labeled nucleotide, the indirect method detects PCR products by *in situ* hybridization. Although both methods can yield successful results, we have adopted the indirect approach for reasons discussed later in more detail. An additional consideration for this method is choice of probe; our approach has been to use a sense-strand riboprobe (labeled with radioactive or nonradioactive nucleotide). The synthesis and labeling of riboprobes has been discussed elsewhere (9) and can be accomplished by using several commercially available kits.

The final concentration of reagents used in the hybridization cocktail is 50% formamide, 5 × SSC, 10% dextran sulfate, 5 × Denhardt's solution, 2% SDS, 100 μg/ml denatured salmon sperm DNA, 1 mg/ml yeast-soluble transfer RNA, and 100 mM DTT. For radioactive riboprobes a final activity of between 40,000 and 100,000 cpm/μl has proven effective, and digoxigenin-labeled probes are used at a final concentration of 1 μg/ml.

Prior to adding the probe to sections, PCR products generated within cells must be denatured to facilitate annealing of the probe. Denaturing is achieved simply by placing the slides in the IS-PCR thermal cycler at 95°C for 5 min, followed by rapid cooling to 4°C.

The probe cocktail (typically 10 μl) is added to the dry sections (prehybridization is unnecessary because background levels are generally reduced following IS-PCR, possibly due to heat denaturation of protein structure) and covered with a parafilm coverslip. Slides are then transferred to a humidified chamber (humidified with 50% formamide, $2 \times$ SSC) and incubated overnight at a temperature compatible with the annealing temperature of the probe (typically 48–60°C).

Posthybridization

The following wash conditions are used after hybridization to remove nonspecifically bound probe (10 mM DTT is included in washes for ^{35}S probes):

1. Remove coverslips in $2 \times$ SSC, 50% formamide, 20 min at room temperature.
2. Wash in $2 \times$ SSC, 50% formamide, 30 min at 60°C with shaking.
3. Wash in 0.1 M TrisHCl, 0.4 M NaCl, 0.05 M EDTA (pH 7.5), 10 min at 37°C with shaking.
4. RNAse digestion: 20 μg/ml RNAse A, 30 min at 37°C in 10 mM Tris, 1 mM EDTA, 500 mM NaCl (pH 8.0).
5. Wash in $2 \times$ SSC, 15 min at 37°C.
6. Wash in $0.1 \times$ SSC, 15 min at 45°C.
7. Dehydrate through graded alcohols to 100% ethanol, all including 300 mM ammonium acetate; air-dry.

Sections hybridized with a radiolabeled probe are exposed to X-ray film to determine exposure time then dipped in emulsion for autoradiographic detection. Nonradioactive probes are visualized with a method appropriate for the label used. Sections can be counterstained with an appropriate stain, such as nuclear fast red. Results obtained following the isotopic and nonisotopic localization of IS-PCR-amplified MMTV sequence in lactating mouse mammary tissue are shown in Figure 20-1. In particular, the intracellular distribution of the amplified sequence should be noted; as expected, proviral DNA localizes primarily to the nucleus as the result of chromosomal integration.

COMMENTS AND CRITICAL ISSUES

Protease Digestion

Protease digestion during pretreatment is one of the most critical steps for the success of IS-PCR, necessitated as the result of protein cross-linking during fixation. However, the optimum extent of digestion represents a balance. Although it is essential for the permeabilization of cell membranes and the unmasking of fixed proteins to permit reagent penetration, excessive digestion leads to the diffusion of PCR amplicons and the destruction of tissue integrity. Figure 20-2 illustrates the influence of proteinase K digestion on the amplification of MMTV in mouse mammary tissue by IS-PCR. In the absence of protease digestion there is minimal amplification. Digestion with concentrations of proteinase K up to 10 μg/ml improves PCR amplification, but at 15 μg/ml the signal intensity is reduced due to excessive amplicon diffusion from cells. Furthermore, we recommend that even before performing IS-PCR, tissue integrity following digestion with various protease concentrations at different time intervals be assessed by routine counterstaining. Hence, the optimization of protease digestion (a function of protease concentration and time) is imperative for successful IS-PCR and depends on factors such as type of fixative, fixation time, and tissue type.

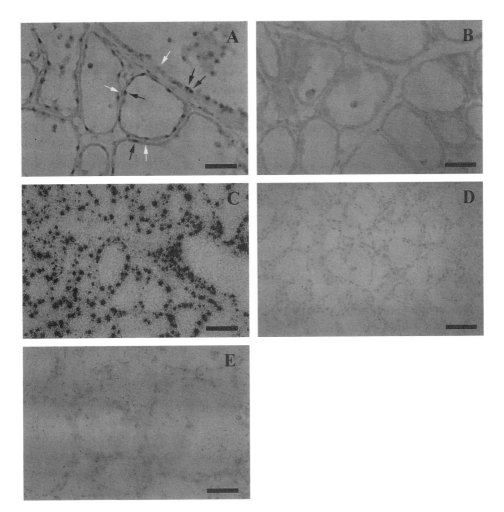

Figure 20-1. Localization of MMTV proviral DNA in infected Czech II lactating mouse mammary tissue by indirect IS-PCR. (A) PCR products generated by IS-PCR were detected by *in situ* hybridization using a DIG-labeled cRNA probe and NBT/BCIP chromogenic detection. Black arrows point to MMTV-positive cells, white arrows point to MMTV-negative cells. (B) Negative control for (A) where primers were excluded during IS-PCR. (C) Sections were subjected to IS-PCR and *in situ* hybridization as in (A) except that the cRNA probe was labeled with ^{35}S and the signal detected by emulsion autoradiography. (D) Negative control for (C) in the absence of primers during IS-PCR. (E) Confirmatory negative result for (C) obtained with lactating mammary tissue from Czech II mice negative for MMTV. (A, B, E) scale bar = 50 μm; (C, D) scale bar = 100 μm.

Direct versus Indirect IS-PCR

A widely discussed aspect of IS-PCR concerns the most appropriate method for detecting PCR products generated *in situ*. For the direct approach a labeled nucleotide (typically digoxigenin- or biotin-11-dUTP) is included in the PCR reaction and is incorporated into the PCR product to enable its direct detection. The major advantages of this approach are a reduced number of steps and a fast turnaround time. However, a significant drawback of the

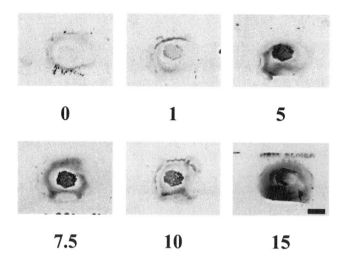

0   **1**   **5**

7.5   **10**   **15**

Figure 20-2. Effect of proteinase K digestion on the ability of IS-PCR to subsequently amplify MMTV proviral DNA. After initial pretreatment, sections of infected Czech II lactating mammary tissue were digested with the indicated concentrations of proteinase K (µg/ml) for 30 min at 37°C. Sections were then subjected to IS-PCR as described, and PCR products detected using a ^{35}S-labeled riboprobe. The images shown were achieved by exposing the probed slides to X-ray film for 10 h. Note that in addition to the signal originating from the sections there is a halo of signal surrounding the sections; the halo represents PCR product that has diffused from cells and has remained captured in the silicon containment disk. Scale bar = 5 mm.

direct method in the hands of ourselves and others (2, 8) is a high incidence of false positives. This occurs as the result of DNA repair during PCR, where nicks and gaps formed as the consequence of tissue preparation, apoptosis, etc., are repaired by Taq polymerase, even in the absence of primers.

An alternative approach that has become the method of choice for several laboratories is the indirect method. Although more laborious and time consuming, this method utilizes *in situ* hybridization to detect PCR-generated amplicons. Although riboprobes are tedious to synthesize and handle, in our hands they have proven to be particularly useful for this application. Riboprobes can be synthesized to incorporate a high proportion of labeled nucleotide (radioactive or nonradioactive). Further, by their sequence specificity and by use of a sense-strand probe, the likelihood of detecting nonspecific PCR-generated artifacts is greatly reduced. Also, the greater strength of RNA–DNA hybrids and the inclusion of an RNAse digestion step during the posthybridization washing steps help minimize background signal.

Alternatively, double-stranded DNA and oligonucleotide probes can be used, although self-annealing and lower probe activity, respectively, are important considerations. Finally, a modification of the direct approach that may find increased application to IS-PCR is the use of labeled primers, where each strand of synthesized DNA contains a labeled nucleotide. However, this approach does not eliminate the possibility of detecting non-specifically-generated PCR products.

Negative Controls

Another consideration that is critical for successful IS-PCR is the inclusion of appropriate negative controls. Several types of negative control include

1. Gene-negative tissue/cells
2. Omission of primer(s) or the inclusion of mis-sense primer(s)
3. Omission of Taq polymerase or $MgCl_2$
4. Predigestion of samples with DNAse

It is strongly recommended that several forms of negative control be evaluated when testing gene-specific primers. An ideal negative control for our studies of MMTV integration has been tissue from infected and uninfected Czech II mice, a strain devoid of endogenous genomic MMTV sequence (10). It is also not necessarily feasible to include all negative controls in a given IS-PCR run. Our approach for routine analyses using the indirect method is to dedicate one of three sections on each slide as a negative control in the absence of primers. When modifications of the IS-PCR technique are being employed, other appropriate controls must be included; for example, for IS-RTPCR these include the omission of RT enzyme and the digestion of negative control tissue sections with RNAse.

POTENTIAL APPLICATIONS OF IS-PCR TO THE MAMMARY GLAND

In this chapter we detailed a technique for IS-PCR and its specific application for the detection of integrated MMTV provirus in mouse mammary tissue. This technique holds a variety of other potential applications for studies of mammary gland biology. In addition to localizing all proviral DNA, cells harboring oncogenic MMTV insertions could be identified by using primers designed that span specific MMTV–oncogene junctions. A further application is the use of IS-PCR to identify mammary cells *in vitro* or *in vivo* that have been infected by different vectors (including retrovirus, adenovirus, adenoassociated virus) for the purpose of gene transfer (11, 12), an approach that is finding application in several other gene transfer systems (13, 14). An extension of IS-PCR that shows utility for localizing low-abundance mRNAs is IS-RTPCR, where mRNA is reverse-transcribed to cDNA prior to its amplification by IS-PCR. Reverse transcription is typically primed by an antisense 3′-primer or random hexamers in the presence of MMLV reverse transcriptase, although a one-step RTPCR method using the r*Tth* enzyme has also been described (15). We are presently optimizing this methodology for gene expression analyses within the mammary gland.

CONSIDERATIONS AND PITFALLS

Although IS-PCR and associated procedures represent powerful methods for the spatial analysis of gene expression, it represents a still-emerging technology beleaguered by technical constraints that are continually being resolved. These difficulties should be fully appreciated and not underestimated, and their associated time and financial burden carefully understood before committing to establish IS-PCR in the laboratory.

ACKNOWLEDGMENTS. The authors wish to thank Dr. Gil Smith and Dr. Robert Callahan, NIH, for kindly providing discussion and Czech II mouse tissues. The assistance provided by Dr. Alfredo Martinez, NIH, in establishing this technique is also appreciated.

REFERENCES

1. A. T. Haase, E. F. Retzel, and K. A. Staskus (1990). Amplification and detection of lentiviral DNA inside cells. *Proc. Natl. Acad. Sci. USA* **87**:4971–4975.

2. A. A. Long (1998). *In-situ* polymerase chain reaction: foundation of the technology and today's options. *Eur. J. Histochem.* **42**:101–109.

3. G. J. Nuovo (1998). Current concepts in pathologic diagnosis: viral diseases. *J. Histotechnol.* **18**:233–240.

4. C. Boshoff, T. F. Schulz, M. M. Kennedy, A. K. Graham, C. Fisher, A. Thomas, J. O'D. McGee, R. A. Weiss, and J. J. O'Leary (1995). Kaposi's sarcoma-associated herpesvirus infects endothelial and spindle cells. *Nature Med.* **1**:1274–1278.

5. T. Schlott, G. Ruda, M. Hoppert, H. Nagel, S. Reimer, I. K. Schumacher-Lütge, and M. Droese (1998). The *in situ* polymerase chain reaction for detection of *Chlamydia trachomatis*. *J. Histochem. Cytochem.* **46**:1017–1023.

6. G. Morel, M. Berger, B. Ronsin, S. Recher, S. Ricard-Blum, H. C. Mertani, and P. E. Lobie (1998). *In situ* reverse transcription-polymerase chain reaction. Applications for light and electron microscopy. *Biol. Cell* **90**:137–154.

7. I. A. Teo and S. Shaunak (1995). Polymerase chain reaction *in situ*: an appraisal of an emerging technique. *Histochem. J.* **27**:647–659.

8. A. A. Long, P. Komminoth, E. Lee, and H. J. Wolfe (1993). Comparison of indirect and direct *in-situ* polymerase chain reaction in cell preparations and tissue sections. *Histochem.* **99**:151–162.

9. D. G. Wilkinson (ed.) (1993). *In Situ Hybridization: A Practical Approach*, IRL Press at Oxford University Press, New York, 163 pp.

10. D. Gallahan and R. Callahan (1987). Mammary tumorigenesis in feral mice: identification of a new Int locus in mouse mammary tumor virus (Czech II)-induced mammary tumors. *J. Virol.* **61**:66–74.

11. M. Li, K-U. Wagner, and P. A. Furth (2000). Transfection of primary mammary epithelial cells by viral and non-viral methods. Chapter 21, this volume.

12. J. Yang, T. Tsukamoto, N. Popnikolov, R. C. Guzman, X. Y. Chen, J. H. Yang, and S. Nandi (1995). Adenoviral-mediated gene transfer into primary human and mouse mammary epithelial cells *in vitro* and *in vivo*. *Cancer Lett.* **98**:9–17.

13. C. Catzavelos, C. Ruedy, A. K. Stewart, and I. Dubé (1998). A novel method for the direct quantification of gene transfer into cells using PCR *in situ*. *Gene Ther.* **5**:755–760.

14. J. Yin, M. G. Kaplitt, A. D. Kwong, and D. W. Pfaff (1998). *In situ* PCR for *in vivo* detection of foreign genes transferred into rat brain. *Brain Res.* **783**:347–354.

15. B. K. Patterson, M. Till, P. Otto, C. Goolsby, M. R. Furtado, L. J. McBride, and S. M. Wolinsky (1993). Detection of HIV-1 DNA and messenger RNA in individual cells by PCR-driven *in situ* hybridization and flow cytometry. *Science* **260**:976–979.

Chapter 21

Transfection of Primary Mammary Epithelial Cells by Viral and Nonviral Methods

Minglin Li, Kay-Uwe Wagner, and Priscilla A. Furth

Abstract. Primary mammary epithelial cells have been used widely to study basic biology in mammary gland development and breast oncogenesis. A variety of technologies have been developed to deliver genes into these cells in order to increase their utility for the study of gene expression and function. Both viral and nonviral methods are available. This chapter presents a protocol for preparation of normal mouse primary mammary epithelial cells and three techniques that can be used to introduce exogenous genes into them. Procedures for the application of calcium phosphate precipitation, jet injection, and adenoviral vectors for gene transfer into primary mammary epithelial cells *in vitro* are described.

Abbreviations. [N,N-bis(2-hydroxyethyl)-2-aminoethane sulfonic acid]-buffered saline (BES); ethylenediaminetetraacetic acid (EDTA); fetal bovine serum (FBS); N-(2-hydroxyethyl) piperazine-N'-(4-butane sulfonic acid) (HEPES); polyethylene glycol (PEG); phosphate buffered saline (PBS).

INTRODUCTION

Mammary gland development and malignant transformation of mammary epithelial cells are complex processes. Multiple factors are involved, including hormones, growth factors, and products of oncogenes and tumor suppressor genes (1). The precise role of individual factors is not easily discriminated in intact organisms because of the complexity of *in vivo* interactions. Instead, primary cultures of mammary epithelial cells can be used to investigate specific factors. These systems have expanded our understanding of fundamental events, including growth, morphogenesis, differentiation, apoptosis, migration, interaction, and malignant transformation (2–5).

Mammary epithelial cells can be prepared by enzymatic digestion of normal mammary tissue from different developmental stages (e.g., virgin, pregnancy and lactation) as well as

Minglin Li   Institute of Human Virology and Division of Infectious Diseases, Department of Medicine, University of Maryland Medical School, Baltimore, Maryland 21201.   Kay-Uwe Wagner   Laboratory of Genetics and Physiology, National Institute of Diabetes, Digestive, and Kidney Diseases, National Institutes of Health, Bethesda, MD 20892; *Current address*: Eppley Center for Research in Cancer and Allied Diseases, University of Nebraska Medical Center, Omaha Nebraska 68198-6805.   Priscilla A. Furth   Institute of Human Virology and Division of Infectious Diseases, Department of Medicine and Department of Physiology, University of Maryland Medical School, Baltimore, Maryland 21201.

Methods in Mammary Gland Biology and Breast Cancer Research, edited by Ip and Asch. Kluwer Academic/Plenum Publishers, New York, 2000.

cancers from human and animal tissue (6–10). Isolated epithelial cells can be grown in serum-containing or serum-free media on different substrata, including plastic, collagen, feeder cells, and reconstituted extracellular matrices (11–14). Normal mammary epithelial cells can have different requirements for specific components in the media compared to transformed mammary epithelial cells (15). Primary epithelial cells are used for many different kinds of studies, including cell proliferation, differentiation, or establishment of cell lines. This chapter gives a detailed protocol for preparation of primary mammary epithelial cells from pregnant mice based on the protocols described by Lee *et al.* (12) and Smith (16).

An advantage of tissue culture is that isolated cells can be manipulated under relatively well controlled experimental conditions. Introduction of nucleic acid vectors into these cells enables study of the regulation and function of specific genes. Both transfection and infection can be employed. Transfection is a nonviral method using chemical reagents, such as DEAE, calcium phosphate, and liposomes, or physical methods, including direct microinjection, electroporation, microparticle-mediated gene transfer, and jet injection (17, 18). Infection is a viral method and includes the use of adenoviral and retroviral vectors (19, 20). Infection of primary epithelial cells with retrovirus vectors *in vitro* and subsequent transplantation into an epithelium-free fat pad enables *in vitro* genetic manipulation of mammary epithelium for *in vivo* study (21). In this chapter, two non-viral-based protocols and one viral-based procedure for gene transfer into primary mammary epithelial cells in culture are discussed.

PREPARATION OF PRIMARY CELL CULTURE

Materials and Instrumentation

- Pregnant mice such as BALB/c and CD1 (22)
- Biosafety hood for sterile removal of mammary glands
- Dissection instruments
- Rotary shaker
- Centrifuge
- Incubator with CO_2 supply
- Microscope
- Beakers, culture dishes, pipettes, and needle syringes
- F-10 medium (Gibco Life Technologies, Grand Island, NY, Cat. No. 12390-035)
- F-12 medium (Gibco Life Technologies, Cat. No. 11765-054)
- Collagenase A (Sigma, St. Louis, MO, Cat. No. C2674)
- Trypsin (Sigma, Cat. No. T5276)
- Fetal bovine serum (FBS) (Gibco Life Technologies, Cat. No. 10082-147)
- Fetuin (Sigma, Cat. No. F2379)
- Insulin (Sigma, Cat. No. I5500)
- Hydrocortisone (Sigma, Cat. No. H4001)
- Prolactin (Sigma, Cat. No. L6520)

Reagents and Their Preparation

1. Autoclave all dissection instruments and sterilize hood with 70% ethanol.
2. Digestion medium: F-10 medium containing collagenase A (0.3%), trypsin (0.15%), FCS (5%), and gentamicin (50 μg/ml). Before adding FCS and gentamicin, sterilize the collagenase A- and trypsin-containing medium by using a 0.2-μm filter.

3. Wash medium I: F-10 medium containing FCS (10%).
4. Wash medium II: F-12 medium containing FCS (10%).
5. Serum–fetuin solution: F-12 medium containing fetuin (2 mg/ml) and FCS (20%). Fetuin is presterilized by using a 0.2-μm filter.
6. Culture medium: F-12 medium containing FCS (10%), fetuin (1 mg/ml), insulin (5 μg/ml), hydrocortisone (5 μg/ml), prolactin (5 μg/ml), gentamicin (50 μg/ml). Fetuin, insulin, hydrocortisone, and prolactin are presterilized by using a 0.2-μm filter.

Procedure for Preparing Primary Mammary Epithelial Cell Culture from Pregnant Mice

1. Euthanize day 15 pregnant mice by cervical dislocation. Dip the mice in 70% ethanol for 1 second and fix them on a Styrofoam dissection board by pinning all four paws. Expose all mammary glands with a vertical abdominal incision. Remove all glands, but avoid muscle and tendons. Place glands in F-10 medium in a 100-mm petri dish. Total weight of the glands should be 1–1.5 g per mouse.
2. Mince the tissue to an estimated fragment size of 1.0–2.0 mm³ with two scalpels in the petri dish. Transfer the minced tissue with a Pasteur pipette into a 50-ml conical tube. Remove the entire F-10 medium and add collagenase- and trypsin-containing digestion medium (4 ml/g tissue). Place on rotary shaker, ~200 rpm, 60 min, 37°C to digest tissue.
3. While the tissue is digesting, prepare fetuin-treated culture dishes by adding 5 ml serum–fetuin solution to each 100-mm petri dish. Gently shake the dish to make sure that all surface is covered. Keep the dish at 37°C for at least 2 h. Before plating cells remove the solution and wash the disk with PBS solution. These dishes will be used in step 7.
4. Centrifuge the conical tube at $15 \times g$ for 30 s. Remove the floating fat and collect the supernatant in a new 50-ml conical tube. Add the same amount of new digestion medium to the original tube in order to suspend the pellet. Incubate the tube at 37°C for another 60 min on a rotary shaker. Centrifuge the supernatant-containing tube at $100 \times g$ for 10 min. Collect the pellet and discard the supernatant. The supernatant largely contains a population of single cells such as fibroblasts and blood cells. Resuspend the pellet with the same amount of wash medium I and keep the pellet-containing tube on ice. The pellet is predominantly an organoid composed of epithelial cells.
5. Gently pipette the digested mixture through a 10-ml pipette until no tissue clumps are seen by visual inspection. Centrifuge at $15 \times g$ for 30 s and at $100 \times g$ for 10 min and collect the organoid-containing pellet as described in step 4. If there is still a significant amount of undigested tissue after centrifugation at $15 \times g$, the tissue can be further digested with new digestion medium and the procedure repeated.
6. Pool all organoid-containing pellets and suspend them with wash medium II (5 ml/g tissue). Gently push the cell suspension through a sterile 19-gauge needle. Centrifuge at $100 \times g$ for 10 min and collect the pellet. Wash the pellet two more times by repeating suspension and centrifugation. Resuspend the final pellet with culture medium (see item 6 in "Reagents and Their Preparation") into a concentration of approximately 2.5×10^4 organoids/ml. Estimate the concentration of the organoid particles by using a hemocytometer or Coulter counter, as described by Smith (16).

7. Plate 10 ml suspension into the serum–fetuin pretreated 100-mm petrie dish (step 3). Incubate plate at 37°C in a CO_2 incubator. Cells will be ready for transfection between 24 and 48 h. During this period the plate should not be moved so as to obtain the best attachment of the organoids to the plate surface.

Important Notes

In the final pellet there will be significant contamination with nonepithelial particulate matter, including nonfragmented blood vessels, skeletal muscle, and nerve. They will be removed by subsequent medium changes. The contaminating fibroblasts, which do not attach to the plate as tightly as the epithelial cells do, should be removed before transfection by short trypsin digestion (1× trypsin-EDTA) for 5 min as described by Smith (16).

TRANSFER OF GENES INTO PRIMARY MAMMARY EPITHELIAL CELLS

Genes can be transferred into primary mammary epithelial cells by nonviral methods, such as calcium phosphate precipitation, lipofection, electroporation, biolistic gene transfer, and microinjection, and by retroviral and adenoviral vectors (17–20). In this chapter protocols for the use of calcium phosphate precipitation, jet injection, and adenoviral vectors are presented. The advantage and disadvantage of each method are briefly discussed.

Gene Transfer Using Calcium Phosphate Precipitation

Calcium phosphate coprecipitation is used widely to transfect a variety of mammalian cells because the components are easily available and the protocol is simple. Primary mammary epithelial cells from different sources can be transfected *in vitro* using this method (9, 23–25). The protocol described here is based on the method of Chen and Okayama (26) with some modifications.

MATERIALS AND INSTRUMENTATION.   Biosafety hood; incubator with CO_2 supply; microscope for evaluation of culture.

REAGENTS AND THEIR PREPARATION
1. 2.5 M $CaCl_2$ stock solution. Sterilize solution by using a 0.2-μm filter and store at −20°C.
2. 2 × BES containing 50 mM BES (pH 6.95), 280 mM NaCl, 1.5 mM Na_2HPO_4. Adjust pH with HCl at room temperature. Sterilize solution by 0.2-μm filter and store at −20°C.
3. Plasmid DNA: DNA isolated using either Qiagen plasmid preparation Kit (Qiagen, Valencia, CA) or other methods should be free from protein, RNA, and chemical contamination. Precipitated DNA should be resuspended in sterile water to a concentration of 0.2–1 mg/ml.

PROCEDURES
1. Prepare a primary culture of mouse mammary epithelial cells as described earlier. Use exponentially growing cells for transfection. Cells become confluent about 48 h after plating. Remove the medium 4 h before transfection and replace with 10 ml fresh medium.

2. Thaw all solutions at room temperature. Prepare DNA mixture in the following order: Add 20–30 μg of DNA into appropriate volume of sterile water (DNA solution and water total 400 μl) and mix well; add 100 μl of 2.5 M of CaCl$_2$ and mix well. Prepare 500 μl of 2 × BES in a separate Eppendorf tube. Slowly add the CaCL$_2$–DNA solution into the 2 × BES solution, and vortex after each addition. Incubate the mixture for 20 min at room temperature. Precipitates containing the DNA will form.

3. Add the 1.0-ml mixture to the plate of cells. Swirl the plate gently to ensure an even distribution of the precipitates. The precipitates can be observed under the microscope. Return the plate to the 37°C CO$_2$ incubator and incubate for 4–24 h.

4. After 4–24 h remove the medium and wash the cells twice with fresh medium.

5. After the initial 4–24 h transfection procedure, the cells can be returned to the incubator or transferred onto different substrata, such as reconstituted basement membrane (23).

IMPORTANT NOTES.   The length of the incubation with calcium phosphate should be optimized based on the sensitivity of cells to calcium phosphate and transfection efficiency. In general, primary cells should not be incubated with calcium phosphate more than 24 h in order to avoid cell death.

Gene Transfer by Biolistic Methods

Primary mammary epithelial cells have been successfully transfected by two biolistic methods: jet injection and microparticle bombardment (27–31). Advantages and disadvantages of the two techniques have been compared previously (32). Cells are transfected through the use of a physical force with both methods. A jet is a pressurized column of fluid. When jet injection is used, transfected cells lie around the path of the DNA solution delivered through the tissue by jet injection. The passage of the DNA solution as a jet stimulates the uptake of plasmid DNA into the cells. Transfected cells can lie from a few millimeters to 2 cm distant from the site of injection, depending on the type of jet injector utilized. When particle bombardment is used, the DNA or other genetic material is complexed onto particles, usually gold or tungsten. These particles are then accelerated into cells. Penetration through tissue is relatively limited with this technology. Cells that are transfected generally lie within 500 μm of the injection site.

Both technologies should be considered developmental. In both cases relatively few cells are transfected with each injection, but multiple injections can be used to increase transfection efficiency. Either technique can be used to transfect differentiated mammary epithelial cells in organ culture. The jet injection technique has been used successfully *in vitro* in pregnant and lactating gland tissue without significant differences in transfection efficiency. *In vivo* we have noted that breast adenocarcinoma tissue from a transgenic mouse model of breast cancer progression is more readily transfectable than either pregnant or lactating mammary gland tissue, but the reasons for this difference have not yet been defined (Ren, Li, and Furth, unpublished data). The higher proliferative rate of the adenocarcinoma tissue is one possibility. Preliminary studies have demonstrated that jet injection can also be used to transfect adherent or suspension cells in culture. However, since the transfection efficiency is low, we recommend that other methods, such as calcium phosphate transfection, be tried first, reserving jet injection for cell lines resistant to other methods. Equipment for particle bombardment mediated delivery of nucleic acids into cells is commercially available. Commercially available equipment for jet injection was designed originally for the delivery of proteins into tissue. However, new jet injectors optimized for delivery of nucleic acids into cells are being developed (33, 34).

A protocol for the use of jet injection for transfection of primary mammary epithelial cells is presented here. For particle bombardment, protocols designed for the marketed device should be followed. The jet injection protocol is based on a general protocol for transfection of somatic tissues by jet injection (35). It can be used with commercially available jet injectors and with any of the newer injectors under development (33–36).

MATERIALS AND INSTRUMENTATION

The Jet Injector.   The Ped-O-Jet injector (Stirn Industries, Dayton, NJ) was used in all of the published studies on mammary gland (27, 29, 35). This injector was developed in the 1960s for delivery of protein vaccines into humans. Although rarely used now for human vaccine delivery, it can be utilized for laboratory studies. A few other jet injection systems are on the market for delivery of anesthetic agents, vaccines, or other therapeutic agents into animals or people (34, 36). Some of these may be adaptable to the laboratory. If an investigator decides to use one of the newer systems, transfection efficiency at various different injection pressures and volumes should be tested by using a reporter gene to establish optimal conditions. In general, transfection efficiency is improved and tissue damage is minimized with higher injection velocities. If the injection velocity is too low, there is blunt force injury to the tissue and poor transfection efficiency.

Nucleic Acid and Solutions for Transfection.   In theory, any plasmid DNA expression vector can be used. Expression levels are higher when strong promoters are used in combination with RNA-stabilizing elements and optimized polyadenylation sites. Plasmid DNA can be purified by a variety of methods, including cesium chloride gradient centrifugation, PEG precipitation, and Qiagen columns (Qiagen, Valencia, CA). The DNA concentration of the injected solution should range between 0.35 and 2.0 µg/µl. Within this range, higher DNA concentrations are generally associated with higher transient expression levels. When generating stable cell transfections, lower concentrations may be adequate. As with other transfection protocols, selectable markers should be used when stable transfectants are made. Marker dyes can be added to the solution in order to trace the path of injection. "DiI" (3,3,3′,3′-tetramethyl indocarbocyanine perchlorate) (Molecular Probes, Inc., Eugene, OR) or 1% India ink have been used (28, 29). We have not observed any significant cellular toxicity related to the use of these dyes, but most of the studies were carried out for only 2–5 days before harvesting the transfected tissue. Many different solutions can be used in combination with jet injection. In the past, 0.9 M NaCl, 0.15 M saline–1% India ink; 0.3 M sucrose, 0.05% "DiI"; 1 mM Tris-HCl, 0.1 mM EDTA; and H_2O alone have all been used successfully to transfect somatic cells.

PROCEDURE

Injection.   The gland may be transfected after removal from the animal or *in situ* after it has been exposed in an anesthetized or recently euthanized animal. If the gland is transfected in the animal, it is removed after jet injection and the tissue is subsequently processed by standard methods for explant culture or isolation of primary mammary epithelial cells. If the gland is transfected *in vitro*, it is first removed by standard surgical procedures and placed into a petrie dish or other suitable vessel. It is then jet-injected as an intact gland or after it is minced into 1–2 cm^3 cubes. After jet injection the mammary gland can be processed as before for explant culture or isolation of primary epithelial cells. When the mammary gland tissue is transfected, the jet injector should be held at, or only slightly above, the surface of the tissue. Care should be taken not to contaminate the tissue with infectious agents.

Analysis of Gene Expression. Analysis of gene expression is carried out by standard methods. Tissue can be harvested for RNA or protein assays. Immunohistochemistry can be used to localize expressing cells. Co-transfection with reporter genes is used to help standardize transfection conditions between different samples. For transient transfections, expression is optimally measured between 48 and 72 h following transfection, but the timing can be adjusted for individual experiments. Selection of stable cell lines is carried out by standard methods using selectable markers and is a technique under development in our laboratory.

NOTES. Jet injection can also be used to deliver viral vectors into mammary glands. For example, adenoviral vectors have been successfully introduced into liver cells with this technique. Jet injection has been used in small rodents (mice, rabbits) and large domestic animals (sheep, pigs). The low volume–high force jet injectors currently under development are designed to reduce waste and increase transfection efficiency in target tissues (33).

To date, when mammary gland tissue is transfected *in vivo*, we generally limit the number of separate jet injections to five or less as defined by our current animal protocols. Approximately 200–500 cells may be transfected with each injection. When the gland is removed from the animal and injected *in vitro*, more injections may be performed with a corresponding increase in the total number of cells transfected.

Acceptable levels of transfection vary with the experimental goal and vectors utilized. When testing for a biological effect from the injected vectors, higher levels of transfection may be necessary. Lower levels of transfection efficiency may be sufficient for studies such as gene transcription experiments when simple detection of the expressed mRNA or protein is the experimental goal.

Gene Transfer Using Adenoviral Vector

Adenoviral and retroviral vectors are widely used to transfer genes into mammalian cells, including primary mammary epithelial cells, and have a higher transfection efficiency than calcium phosphate precipitation (8, 16, 37). In comparison to retroviral vectors, adenoviral vectors have a bigger capacity to carry exogenous genes and are able to infect non-proliferating cells.

MATERIALS AND INSTRUMENTATION. The production and purification of recombinant adenovirus require a P2 cell culture facility. The following equipment and instruments should be available: cold room, centrifuge, ultracentrifuge, Slide-A-Lyzer dialysis cassettes (Pierce, Rockford, IL).

REAGENTS AND REAGENT PREPARATION
1. Growth medium: DMEM medium containing 10% FBS and 2 mM glutamine.
2. Infection medium: DMEM medium containing 2% FBS and 2 mM glutamine.
3. 10× buffer for preparation of CsCl solutions: 80 g NaCl, 3.8 g KCl, 30 g Tris, 1.0 g Na$_2$HPO$_4$ in 1 L of distilled water. Adjust pH to 7.5.

4. CsCl solutions with densities of 1.25, 1.33, and 1.40 g/ml in 1× buffer (step 3). Mix 175 ml of 1× buffer (step 3) with 100 g of CsCl and stir. Calibrate 1 ml of water on a scale (1 ml equals 1 g). Weigh out 1 ml of the CsCl solution. Add more 1 × buffer (step 3) or CsCl to the stock until the exact gradient concentration is reached. Autoclave the final stock solutions.
5. Dialysis buffer: 400 ml of 10 × buffer (100 mM Tris, pH 7.4, and 10 mM $MgCl_2$), 3 L of sterile H_2O, 400 ml of sterile glycerol, stir; add H_2O to final 4 L.
6. 293 cells (Quantum Biotechnology, Inc., Quebec, Canada).

DETAILED PROCEDURES

Adenovirus Purification.   Adenovirus purification is a simplified protocol for the propagation and purification of a recombinant adenovirus. For detailed procedures on how to generate a recombinant vector please refer to protocols supplied with the adenovirus expression system kit (Quantum Biotechnology, Inc. Quebec, Canada).

Propagation of Viral Vector

a. Seed 293 cells in 70 to 120 tissue culture plates (diameter of 150 mm; 10^8 cells/plate) and incubate them until they reach 70–80% of confluency. Mix cell lysate or purified recombinant adenovirus with infection medium (1 : 4 v/v if cell lysate is used). Remove all liquids and cover the cells with infection medium containing the recombinant adenovirus. Tilt the plates every 15 min while incubating for 1 h at 37°C in the CO_2 incubator.

b. After the initial 1 h incubation, add a suitable amount of growth media and incubate the cells for at least 24 h at 37°C in the CO_2 incubator. Start harvesting the cells when they round up and lose contact from the surface (cytopathic effect). Detach the cells by pipetting the medium up and down. Collect and pool cell suspensions in a 50-ml conical bottom tube. The cells can be concentrated and then resuspended in 7 ml media or Tris (10 mM, pH 8.0). Store the crude virus stock at −20°C (media) or −70°C (Tris). The virus is released by 5 cycles of freezing and thawing. Spin the crude viral lysate for 10 min at 7000 rpm and transfer the supernatant into a sterile conical bottom tube.

c. Purify the virus by using CsCl gradient centrifugation. Prepare two layers of CsCl with a density of 1.25 and 1.40 (2.5 ml each) in an ultraclear tube and overlay the crude viral lysate. Balance the tubes and centrifuge for 1 h at 35,000 rpm (200,000 × g) in Beckman Ultracentrifuge Rotor SW-41. After centrifugation the virus is located in the middle of the tube to form a white layer in the dark orange background, and the cell debris is at the bottom. Insert a 3-ml syringe with a 21-gauge needle into the virus layer and aspirate the white virus layer through the wall of the tube. The eluted viral solution is further purified over a 1.33 CsCl layer (8 ml). Spin for 18 h at 35,000 rpm in Beckman ultracentrifuge rotor SW-41. Isolate the virus as described earlier, add glycerol to a final concentration of 10%, and vortex briefly. Transfer the viral solution into Slide-A-Lyzer cassettes following the manufacturer's guidelines. Other dialysis methods can be used. However, Slide-A-Lyzer cassettes do not needed to be pretreated and are more convenient for loading and recovery of samples. Wash the cassettes 8 times in 500 ml dialysis buffer. Change the buffer every 30 min. Recover the virus from the dialysis chamber, following the manufacturer's protocol and store the virus at −70°C in 20-, 50-, or 100-µl aliquots.

d. The titer of the virus can be estimated by plaque assay (see special protocol by Quantum Biotechnology, Inc., Quebec, Canada) or, more simply, by spectrophotometry ($1.0\ OD_{260} = 10^{12}$ viral particles/ml). Prepare an adenovirus solution in medium with a final

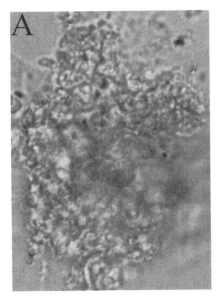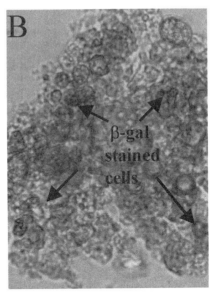

Figure 21-1. β-Galactosidase activity in cultured murine primary mammary epithelial cells 72 h following infection with adenoviral vectors. Murine primary epithelial cells were prepared as described in the text. After 24 h incubation the cells were either singly infected with a recombinant adenoviral vector encoding a reporter gene for Cre activity (Ad-*lox*STOP*lox*-β-*gal*) (A) or dually infected with recombinant adenoviral vectors encoding the Cre recombinase gene (Ad-Cre) and Ad-*lox*STOP*lox*-β-*gal* (B). Cells were tested for β-galactosidase activity 72 h later (39). The presence of β-galactosidase activity is indicated by the presence of blue staining. Since no Cre activity was present in the cells illustrated in (A), there is no blue staining. Blue staining of cells illustrated in (B) demonstrates that the β-galactosidase gene was activated by Cre expression confirming dual infection. Cells were infected at a concentration of ~10^8 viral particles per ml/medium per construct for 90 min. Following infection cells were washed twice in 1 × PBS and maintained in regular growth medium for 72 h before measuring β-galactosidase activity.

concentration of ~10^8 viral particles per milliliter for infection of primary mammary epithelial cells.

Infection of primary mammary epithelial cells

    a. Grow primary mammary epithelial cells using culture medium as described earlier (see "Reagents and Their Preparation"). The confluency of the cells is not critical for adenovirus infection. Adenoviral vectors do not require continuously dividing cells.

    b. Infect cells by laying on a solution of ~10^8 viral particles per milliliter in medium. Two or more adenoviral constructs can be co-infected.

    c. Incubate the viral solution on the cells for 90 min.

    d. After infection wash cells twice in 1× PBS and maintain in regular growth medium afterwards.

    e. Cells may be harvested 24–72 h after infection for studies of gene expression or function.

IMPORTANT NOTES.   Primary mammary epithelial cells may be simultaneously infected with more than one adenoviral vector. Adenoviral vectors encoding two components of the Cre-*lox* system were used to demonstrate that primary mammary epithelial cells can be dually infected (37). Figure 21-1 illustrates cultured murine primary epithelial cells that have been tested for β-galactosidase activity 72 hours after infection with adenoviral vectors. One adenoviral vector contained sequences encoding the Cre recombinase gene (Ad-Cre). The second adenoviral vector contained sequences encoding a reporter gene for Cre recombinase activity (Ad-*lox*STOP*lox*-β-*gal*). The STOP sequence, which lies between the two *lox* sites, prevents transcription of the β-galactosidase gene. When Cre recombinase activity is present, the STOP sequence is removed and the β-galactosidase gene is expressed (38). Cells in Figure 21-1A were infected only with the Ad-*lox*STOP*lox*-β-*gal* vector. Since no Cre was present, the STOP sequence was not removed and there was no blue staining indicating β-galactosidase activity. Cells in Figure 21-1B were co-infected with the Ad-Cre and Ad-*lox*STO-P*lox*-β-*gal* vectors. Therefore, Cre activity was present, the STOP sequence was removed, and blue staining from β-galactosidase activity was present. Approximately 70% of cells showed staining for β-galactosidase. Remember to treat all solutions and buffers as biological waste.

ACKNOWLEDGMENTS.   This work was supported by a National Cancer Institute grant CA-68033 to P.A.F., a research contract from EMS Medical GmbH (Konstanz, Germany) to P.A.F., an American Cancer Society grant # IRG-97-153-01 to M.L., and a DFG grant (Wa-119/1-1) to K.U.W. We thank Dr. Jason J. Coull at the Institute of Human Virology, University of Maryland Baltimore, Baltimore, MD, for his constructive discussion and suggestion. Current address for K.U.W. is Eppley Institute for Research in Cancer and Applied Diseases, University of Nebraska Medical Center, Omaha, Nebraska 68198-6805.

REFERENCES

1. Y. J. Topper, and C. S. Freeman (1980). Multiple hormone interactions in the developmental biology of the mammary gland. *Physiol. Rev.* **60**:1049–1106.
2. U. K. Ehmann, W. D. Peterson, Jr., and D. S. Misfeldt (1984). To grow mouse mammary epithelial cells in culture. *J. Cell Biol.* **98**:1026–1032.
3. B. K. Levay-Young, W. Imagawa, J. Yang, K. E. Richards, R. C. Guzman, and S. Nandi (1987). Primary culture systems for mammary biology studies. In D. Medina, W. Kidwell, G. Heppner, and E. Anderson (eds.), *Cellular and Molecular Biology of Mammary Cancer*, pp. 181–203. New York: Plenum.
4. M. R. Stampfer and J. Bartley (1987). Growth and transformation of human mammary epithelial cells in culture. In D. Medina, W. Kidwell, G. Heppner, and E. Anderson (eds.), *Cellular and Molecular Biology of Mammary Cancer*, pp. 419–436.
5. V. K. Pechenko and W. T. Imagawa (1998). Mammogenic hormones differentially modulate keratinocyte growth factor (KGF)-induced proliferation and KGF receptor expression in cultured mouse mammary gland epithelium. *Endocrinology* **139**:2519–2526.
6. H. A. Hahm, M. M. Ip, K. Darcy, J. D. Black, W. K. Shea, S. Forczek, M. Yoshimura, and T. Oka (1990). Primary culture of normal rat mammary epithelial cells within a basement membrane matrix. II: Functional differentiation under serum-free conditions. *In Vitro Cell Dev. Biol.* **26**:803–814.
7. L. M. Varela and M. M. Ip (1996). Tumor necrosis factor-α: a multifunctional regulator of mammary gland development. *Endocrinology* **137**:4915–4924.
8. J. Yang, T. Tsukamoto, N. Popnikolov, R. C. Guzman, X. Chen, J. H. Yang, and S. Nandi (1995). Adenoviral-mediated gene transfer into primary human and mouse mammary epithelial cells *in vitro* and *in vivo*. *Cancer Lett.* **27**: 9–17.
9. T. A. Thompson, M. N. Gould, J. K. Burkholder, and N. S. Yang (1993). Transient promoter activity in primary epithelial cells evaluated using particle bombardment gene transfer. *In Vitro Cell Dev. Biol.* **29A**:165–170.

10. Q. Gao, S. H. Hauser, X. L. Liu, D. E. Wazer, H. Madoc-Jones, and V. Band (1996). Mutant p53-induced immortalization of primary human mammary epithelial cells. *Cancer Res.* **56:**3129–3133.

11. U. K. Ehmann, R. C. Guzman, R. C, Osborn, L. J. T. Young, R. D. Cardiff, and S. Nandi (1998). Cultured mouse mammary epithelial cells: Normal phenotype after implantation. *J. Natl. Cancer Inst.* **78:**751–756.

12. E. Y. Lee, W. H. Lee, C. H. Kaetzel, G. Parry, and M. Bissel (1985). Interaction of mouse mammary epithelial cells with collagen substrate: regulation of casein gene expression and secretion. *Proc. Natl. Acad. Sci. USA* **82:**1419–1423.

13. C. H. Streuli, N. Bailey, and M. Bissel (1991). Control of mammary epithelial differentiation: Basement membrane induced tissue-specific gene expression in the absence of cell–cell interaction and morphological polarity. *J. Cell Biol.* **115:**1383–1395.

14. M. M. Ip and K. M. Darcy (1996). Three-dimensional mammary primary culture model system. *J. Mammary Gland Biol. Neoplasia* **1:**91–110.

15. S. P. Ethier (1996). Human breast cancer cell lines as models of growth regulation and disease progression. *J. Mammary Gland Biol. Neoplasia* **1:**111–121.

16. G. H. Smith (1996). Experimental mammary epithelial morphogenesis in an *in vivo* model: Evidence for distinct cellular progenitors of the ductal and lobular phenotype. *Breast Cancer Res. Treat.* **39:**21–23.

17. P. L. Felgner (1997). Nonviral strategies for gene therapy. *Sci. Am.* **276:**102–106.

18. T. M. Klein and S. Fitzpatrick-McElligott (1993). Particle bombardment: a universal approach for gene transfer to cells and tissues. *Curr. Opin. Biotechnol.* **4:**583–590.

19. A. D. Miller and G. J. Rosman (1989). Improved retroviral vectors for gene transfer and expression. *Bio. Techniques* **7:**980–990.

20. A. Garnier, J. Cote, I. Nadeau, A. Kamen, and B. Massie (1994). Scale-up of the adenovirus expression system for the production of recombinant protein in human 293S cells. *Cytotechnology* **15:**145–155.

21. P. A. W. Edwards, C. L. Abram, and J.M. Brandbury (1996). Genetic manipulation of mammary epithelium by transplantation. *J. Mammary Gland Biol. Neoplasia* **1:**75–89.

22. M. H. Barcellos-Hoff, J. Affeler, T. G. Ram, and M. J. Bissell (1989). Functional differentiation and alveolar morphogenesis of primary mammary cultures on reconstituted basement membrane. *Development* **105:**223–235.

23. M. Yoshimura and T. Oka (1990). Transfection of β-casein chimeric gene and hormonal induction of its expression in primary murine mammary epithelial cells. *Proc. Natl. Acad. Sci. USA* **87:**3670–3674.

24. A. Kanai, N. Nonomura, M. Yoshimura, and T. Oka (1993). DNA-binding proteins and their cis-acting sites controlling hormonal induction of a mouse beta-casein: CAT fusion protein in mammary epithelial cells. *Gene* **126:**195–201.

25. J. Y. Ahn, N. Aoki, T. Adachi, Y. Mizuno, R. Nakamura, and T. Matsuda (1995). Isolation and culture of bovine mammary epithelial cells and establishment of gene transfection conditions in the cells. *Biosci. Biotechnol. Biochem.* **59:**59–64.

26. C. Chen and H. Okayama (1987). High-efficiency transformation of mammalian cells by plasmid DNA. *Mol. Cell Biol.* **7:**2747–2752.

27. P. A. Furth, A. Shamay, R. J. Wall, and L. Hennighausen (1992). Gene transfer into somatic tissues by jet injection. *Anal. Biochem.* **205:**365–368.

28. P. A. Furth, A. Shamay, and L. Hennighausen (1995). Gene transfer into mammalian cells by jet injection. *Hybridoma* **14:**149–152.

29. D. E. Kerr, P. A. Furth, A. M. Powell, and R. J. Wall (1996). Expression of gene-gun injected plasmid DNA in the ovine mammary gland and in lymph nodes draining the injection site. *Animal Biotechnol.* **7:**33–45.

30. N. S. Yang, J. K. Burkholder, B. Roberts, B. Matinell, and D. McCabe (1990). *In vivo* and *in vitro* gene transfer to mammalian somatic cells by particle bombardment. *Proc. Natl. Acad. Sci. USA* **87:**9568–9572.

31. A. V. Zelenin, A. A. Alimov, V. Titomirov, A. V. Kazansky, S. I. Gorodetsky, and V. A. Kolesnikov (1991). High-velocity mechanical DNA transfer of the chloramphenicol acetyl transferase gene into rodent liver, kidney and mammary gland cells in organ explants and *in vivo*. *FEBS Lett.* **280:**94–96.

32. P. A. Furth (1997). Gene transfer by biolistic process. *Molec. Biotechnol.* **7:**139–143.

33. R. Cartier, S. V. Ren, W. Walther, U. Stein, A. Lewis, P. Schlag, M. Li, and P. A. Furth (2000). *In vivo* gene transfer by low-volume jet injection. *Analytical Biochemistry* **282:**262–265.

34. J. Haensler, C. Verdelet, V. Sanchez, Y. Girerd-Chambaz, A. Bonnin, E. Trannoy, S. Krishnan, and P. Meulien (1999). Intradermal DNA immunization by using jet-injectors in mice and monkeys. *Vaccine* **17:**628–638.

35. P. A. Furth, D. Kerr, and R. Wall (1995). Gene transfer by jet injection into differentiated tissues of living animals and in organ culture. *Molec. Biotechnol.* **4:**121–127.

36. C. L. Baer, W. M. Bennett, D. A. Folwick, and R. S. Erickson (1996). Effectiveness of a jet injection system in administering morphine and heparin to healthy adults. *Am. J. Crit. Care* **5:**42–48.

37. P. A. Furth (1997). Conditional control of gene expression in the mammary gland. *J. Mammary Gland Biol. Neoplasia* **2**:373–383.
38. K. W. Wagner, E. B. Rucker, and L. Hennighausen (1999). Adenoviral and transgenic approaches for the conditional deletion of genes from mammary tissue, Chapter 24, this volume.
39. P. A. Furth, L. St.-Onge, H. Boger, P. Gruss, M. Gossen, A. Kistner, H. Bujard, and L. Hennighausen (1994). Temporal control of gene expression in transgenic mice by a tetracycline-responsive promoter. *Proc. Natl. Acad. Sci.* **91**:9302–9306.

Chapter 22

Direct Gene Transfer into the Mammary Epithelium *In Situ* Using Retroviral Vectors

Todd A. Thompson and Michael N. Gould

Abstract. Insertion of specific exogenous genes into the mammary parenchyma genome has been shown to have many important uses, including production of experimental models and production of commercially valuable proteins in milk. Most transgenic mammary tissue has thus far been produced by germ-line gene transfer. Here we describe a rapid and inexpensive alternative method in which genes of interest are placed directly into the *in situ* mammary ductal epithelium using a "gene-therapy-like" approach. The gene of interest is cloned into a replication-incompetent retroviral vector. The vector is produced to yield very high titers and is then infused into the central mammary duct of mammals ranging from rats to goats. Larger mammals are used mainly for protein production, and rats are used to develop models for the study of mammary biology and carcinogenesis.

Abbreviations. mouse mammary tumor virus (MMTV); long terminal repeat (LTR).

INTRODUCTION

A variety of methods have been developed to study the expression of exogenous genes in selected tissues. To target gene expression to the mammary gland, both germ-line transgenic animal models and infection of the mammary gland with retroviral vectors expressing a gene of interest have been used. In germ-line transgenic animal models, the transgene is present in all the animal's cells, and thus transgene expression may not be limited to the mammary gland, despite efforts to target gene expression to the mammary gland using tissue-specific regulatory elements, such as the mouse mammary tumor virus long terminal repeat (MMTV LTR). In addition, the development of transgenic animal models requires extensive technical expertise and complex instrumentation. In contrast, retroviral-mediated gene transfer allows the introduction of novel genes specifically into the mammary gland by using standard laboratory technologies and equipment.

Retroviruses are RNA viruses that infect mammalian cells based on specific tropisms [e.g., ecotropic (infecting their natural host) and amphotropic (infecting natural host cells as

Todd A. Thompson and Michael N. Gould   **University of Wisconsin Comprehensive Cancer Center and McArdle Laboratory for Cancer Research, University of Wisconsin-Madison, Madison, Wisconsin 53792.**

Methods in Mammary Gland Biology and Breast Cancer Research, edited by Ip and Asch. Kluwer Academic/Plenum Publishers, New York, 2000.

well as cells from other mammals)]. Upon infection, the viral RNA genome is reverse-transcribed to DNA, which becomes stably integrated into the host genome (1). The virally coded genes are then expressed in the infected cell. Modified retroviral vectors have been produced such that regions of the viral genome have been replaced with a wide variety of nonviral genes. Using cell lines that produce the elements necessary for the generation of retroviral particles in *trans* (i.e., packaging cell lines), vectors with modified retroviral genomes have been produced. These modified retroviruses allow infection of cells resulting in expression of the genes present in the retrovirus. The use of retroviruses for gene transduction enables the study of the role of defined genes in cancer development in contrast to the poorly defined events that result in the development of cancer when using chemical carcinogens.

An early example of the use of retroviral vectors to target genes specifically to the mammary epithelium was that of Wang *et al.* (2), who transferred both β-galactosidase and activated *ras* directly to the mammary parenchyma *in situ*. Previous studies support a significant role for the Harvey *ras* gene in rat mammary carcinogenesis (3). To further define the role of the Harvey *ras* gene in rat mammary carcinogenesis, Wang *et al.* (2) produced replication-defective retroviral vectors that expressed the v-H-*ras* gene. Infection of rat mammary parenchyma by intraductal cannulation with these retroviral vectors produced mammary carcinomas that were similar in histopathology and temporal development to mammary carcinomas produced in rats by chemical carcinogens (2). These studies illustrated the effectiveness of retroviral-mediated gene transfer for investigating the action of select genes within the rat mammary gland.

The objective of this chapter is to describe methods to transduce the rat mammary gland with retroviral vectors expressing a gene of interest. The following topics will be reviewed: (1) the generation of replication-defective retroviral vectors from retroviral plasmid constructs; (2) methods for the infusion of retroviral preparations into the rat mammary gland; (3) methods to establish that effective retroviral transduction has occurred in the mammary gland.

METHODS FOR RETROVIRAL PREPARATION

Materials and Instrumentation

Dulbecco's modified Eagle's medium (DMEM), LipofectAMINE reagent, G418, phosphate buffered saline (PBS), and 0.1% trypsin were obtained from Gibco/BRL (Gaithersburg, MD). Polybrene (i.e., hexadimethrine bromide) and sucrose were obtained from Sigma (St. Louis, MO). Fetal calf serum (FCS) was obtained from HyClone (Logan, UT). The ψ-CRE ecotropic retroviral packaging cell line was obtained from Mulligan (4). The PA317 amphotropic retroviral packaging cell line and NIH3T3 cells were obtained from American Type Culture Collection (Manassas, VA). Syringe filters, tissue culture dishes, and tissue culture flasks were obtained from Costar (Corning, NY). Fifty-milliliter polypropylene tubes were obtained from Fisher (Pittsburgh, PA). Cloning rings were obtained from Bellco Glass Co. (Vineland, NJ). The CO_2 cell culture incubators used were from Forma (Marietta, OH). Low-speed centrifugation was performed in an IEC clinical centrifuge (Needham Heights, MA) at setting number 3 (i.e., approximately $150 \times g$). A Beckman (Palo Alto, CA) LE-80 ultracentrifuge was used with Beckman 1×3.5 ultracentrifugation tubes and a Beckman SW28 swinging bucket rotor for retroviral vector concentration.

Reagents and Reagent Preparation

The cell culture medium is prepared as DMEM with 10% FCS and antibiotics (i.e., gentamycin used at 80 µg/ml). Polybrene is prepared as a 100 × stock (0.5 mg/ml) in PBS and filter-sterilized before use. Twenty percent (w/v) sucrose is prepared in PBS.

Procedures for Retroviral Vector Preparation

RETROVIRAL VECTOR BACKBONE CONSTRUCTS.   Many retroviral vector backbones are available that can be used for the introduction of novel genes into the rat mammary gland (5). The studies performed in our laboratory have used the pJR retroviral vector backbone (2), which contains the key features common to many retroviral vectors (Figure 22-1). The pJR vector was derived from the pLNL6 vector (6). To create pJR, the *neo*^{r} region of pLNL6 was replaced with the SV40 early promoter, the Tn5 *neo* gene, and the pBR322 origin of replication, derived from the pBAG vector (7). The gene to be transduced into the rat mammary gland can be subcloned into the cloning site of pJR or other retroviral vector cassettes by using standard molecular subcloning techniques (8).

PRODUCTION OF RETROVIRAL VECTOR EXPRESSING CELL LINES.   The generation of replication-defective retroviral vectors requires only the standard equipment used for most cell culture and eucaryotic cell transfection procedures. Replication-defective retroviral vectors have been modified such that most of the *trans* components (e.g., *gag*, *pol*, *env*) necessary for virus production are absent. Therefore, retroviral packaging cell lines have been developed that provide the *trans* packaging elements necessary to generate infectious viral particles (5). The retroviral plasmid is first transfected into an ecotropic packaging cell line, followed by infection of an amphotropic packaging cell line with virus produced from the ecotropic cell line. Transfection of the ecotropic packaging cell line followed by infection of the amphotropic packaging cell line have been found to generate clones producing high titers (5). This infection scheme can be reversed if ecotropic packaging cells are desired. The retroviral vector plasmid is transfected into the ecotropic packaging cell line (e.g., ψ-CRE; 4) using a suitable eucaryotic cell transfection procedure such as lipofection, calcium phosphate precipitation, or electroporation. We use lipofectAMINE reagent (Gibco/BRL) for the initial transfection. When high titers of ecotropic vectors are being produced (i.e., 1 to 3 days after transfection), medium from these cells is used to infect an amphotropic packaging cell line,

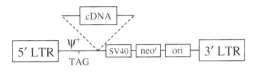

pJR

Figure 22-1. pJR backbone containing key features of retroviral vectors (adapted from Ref. 2). LTR = long terminal repeat; ψ$^+$ = viral packaging signal; TAG = amber mutation in the Pr60^{gag} translational start site from pLNL6 (6); cDNA = site for inserting the gene of interest; SV40 = SV40 immediate/early promoter; *neo*^{r} = bacterial Tn5 neomycin resistance gene conferring resistance to G418; ori = pBR322 origin of replication, which may allow vector rescue following vector incorporation in the host genome. SV40, *neo*^{r}, and ori were derived from pBAG (7). Figure not to scale.

such as PA317 cells (9). To remove debris and contaminating ecotropic cells, medium from the ecotropic packaging cell line is first filtered through a sterile 0.8 μm pore filter before addition to the amphotropic packaging cells. Polybrene, at a final concentration of 5.0 μg/ml, is added to the amphotropic packaging cells to promote viral infection. The filtrate is then added to infect the amphotropic cells at approximately 50% confluence in 60-mm tissue culture dishes. Twenty-four hours after infection, the amphotropic packaging cells are passed to 100-mm plates under selective conditions to obtain independent cell clones. Amphotropic packaging cell line clones expressing neo^r, such as those infected with the JR vector, can be selected using resistance to 400 μg/ml G418. Typically, 10 to 20 clones from each vector are selected after 10–14 days in culture using cloning rings, expanded, and titered. Retroviral vectors that express neo^r are commonly titered by using neomycin resistance with standard titering protocols (see the section on retroviral vector titration). The expanded packaging cell line clones are then independently tested to determine those producing the highest viral titers. To reduce the time required for retrovirus preparation, the medium from polyclonal populations of packaging cells (i.e., infected amphotropic packaging cells grown under selective conditions without expansion for independent clones) can also be used. However, we find that these polyclonal packaging cells generally produce lower retroviral titers than do clones that have been screened for high titer retrovirus production. For vectors that express oncogenes, clones are selected that produce high titers and that are minimally transformed (i.e., that remain adherent to the cell culture dish), so they can be effectively maintained in cell culture.

RETROVIRAL VECTOR CONCENTRATION.   Suitable clones are initially seeded in 162-cm^2 flasks in 30 ml of DMEM containing 10% FCS with 200 μg/ml G418 at 37°C in a 5% CO$_2$ incubator. On reaching 90% confluence, fresh medium without G418 is added and the cultures are transferred to a 5% CO$_2$ incubator at 32°C. A 37°C incubator can be used for the generation of retrovirus, although the virus half-life is reduced at this temperature, and we find that the PA317 cells grown for extended periods of time (i.e., 4 to 5 days) at 37°C produce by-products that interfere with viral concentration by centrifugation. Our conditions favor the generation of high retroviral vector titers due to both the isolation of clones that generate high retroviral titers and the added stability of the retroviral vector at 32°C. The retrovirus-containing medium is placed in a 50-ml polypropylene tube and centrifuged (e.g., using an IEC clinical centrifuge at 150 × g) for 5 min to remove suspended cells and cellular debris. Medium replacement can be continued daily for 3 to 4 days before the viral titer begins to decrease. Virus-containing medium can be stored at −80°C until needed or until further concentrated by centrifugation.

    To further concentrate the retrovirus preparations, 28 ml of the cleared supernatant is added to an ultracentrifugation tube. The remaining viral-containing medium (i.e., approximately 2 ml) is stored at 4°C and used to resuspend the concentrated retrovirus after ultracentrifugation. Four milliliters of 20% sucrose is then carefully added to the bottom of the tube containing the viral preparation using a 5-ml pipette. The viral preparation is then centrifuged (e.g., using a Beckman LE-80 ultracentrifuge) at 122,000 × g (r_{max}) using a swinging bucket rotor for 3 h. Following centrifugation, the supernatant and sucrose cushion are removed by aspiration, taking care not to disturb the small viral pellet. The viral pellet is then resuspended in 300 μl of the original viral preparation. We find this concentration process produces virus titers 20- to 50-fold higher than the original titer. Virus preparations can be stored in polypropylene tubes at −80°C until titered and used for mammary gland infusions.

RETROVIRAL VECTOR TITRATION.   Retroviral vectors are commonly titered by utilizing neomycin resistance with standard titering protocols (5). For example, each viral preparation is serially diluted 1 to 10 with an expected titer of 10^5 to 10^9 colony-forming units (CFU) per milliliter and used to infect NIH3T3 cells at 50% confluence in 60-mm cell culture plates. After 24 h, the infected NIH3T3 cells from each plate are removed with trypsin and transferred to 100-mm tissue culture plates with medium containing 400 μg/ml G418. Plates are maintained undisturbed under selective conditions, using G418 resistance in a 5% CO_2 incubator for 10 to 14 days. Colonies generated from oncogene expressing vectors may adhere poorly to plates and may not withstand standard staining procedures; thus colonies are counted directly on the plates. The presence of helper virus, which would result in the transfer of virus beyond the initial infection, can be tested using the marker rescue assay (10).

METHODS FOR RETROVIRAL INFUSION INTO RAT MAMMARY GLANDS

Materials and Instrumentation

Perphenazine and formaldehyde were obtained from Sigma (St. Louis, MO). Fast green was obtained from Fluka (Ronkonkoma, NY). Oster Golden A5 clippers (Milwaukee, WI) were used to shave rats prior to retroviral infusion. Fine-tipped forceps and scissors were obtained from Fine Science Tools (Foster City, CA). Blunt-ended 27-gauge needles can be made as described here or purchased from Hamilton (Reno, NV). Hamilton syringes were obtained from Fisher (Pittsburgh, PA).

Reagents and Reagent Preparation

Perphenazine is prepared as a stock solution of 6 mg/ml in acidified saline (0.02 N HCl). Frozen viral preparations are thawed on ice. A $100 \times$ stock solution of polybrene (8 mg/ml) in PBS is used for addition to the viral preparation to produce a final concentration of 80 μg/ml polybrene. In addition, a 0.5-mg/ml final concentration of fast green from a $100 \times$ stock solution in PBS is added to assist in the visual determination of infusion efficiency into the mammary ductal structure. Four percent (v/v) formalin is prepared from formaldehyde in PBS.

Procedures for Retroviral Mammary Gland Infusion

Each of the 12 teats of the rat mammary glands can be infused with retroviral preparations into the central duct (Figure 22-2A; 2). For effective infusion, the mammary gland must be sufficiently developed to allow infusion through the teats (i.e., rats must be approximately 40 days of age or older). Since retroviruses require proliferating cells for productive retroviral incorporation into DNA, proliferation of the rat mammary gland is stimulated prior to retroviral infusion. Perphenazine, which indirectly stimulates the release of prolactin from the pituitary, has been used for this purpose (2). Rats receive 3 subcutaneous injections of 3.0 mg/kg perphenazine at 48, 24, and 4 h before viral infusion (2).

Under suitable anesthesia, the thoracic, abdominal, and inguinal regions of the rat are shaved to expose the 12 mammary teats (Figure 22-2A). With fine-tipped forceps and scissors, each teat is clipped (Figure 22-2B), and the remaining orifice is cannulated by using a syringe with a blunt-ended 27-gauge needle. The needle tip is blunted by gripping it with a pair of hemostats and bending the tip back and forth until it severs. Immediately prior to infusion, the area surrounding the teat is wiped with gauze soaked in 70% ethanol, which helps visualize the area surrounding the remaining mammary gland central lacteal and helps detect the spread of tracking dye through the mammary gland. Fifteen microliters of viral preparation, which contains polybrene and the fast green tracking dye, is delivered into the teat while the skin

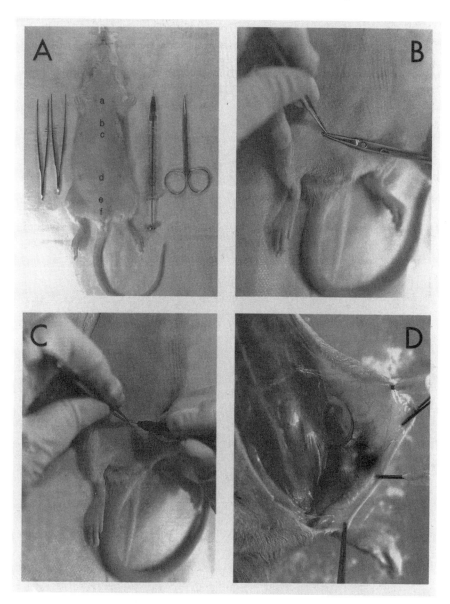

Figure 22-2. Rat mammary gland infusion methodology. (A) The abdominal region of the rat is shaved and washed with 70% ethanol to expose the 12 teats. Equipment used for infusion: 60-μl Hamilton syringe, blunt-ended 27-gauge needle, 2 pair of fine-tipped forceps, scissors, anesthesia cone, and suitable anesthetic. The six pairs of rat mammary glands, as designated by van Zwieten (26), flank the lowercase letters: a. cervical, b. cranial thoracic, c. caudal thoracic, d. abdominal, e. cranial inguinal, and f. caudal inguinal. (B) The teat is first extended from the skin using two pairs of fine-tipped forceps and then clipped as illustrated. The clipped teat area is then washed with 70% ethanol to allow for infusion into the central lacteal. (C) A blunted-ended 27-gauge needle is used to enter the remaining orifice into the central lacteal. Prior to infusion, forceps are used to secure the needle–orifice juncture. During infusion, the spread of dye through the mammary ductal tree can be observed. (D) During practice, rats may be euthanized followed by separation of the skin and mammary fat pad from the abdominal muscle to observe the efficiency of infusion into the mammary ductal structure. (For a color representation of this, see figure facing page 250.)

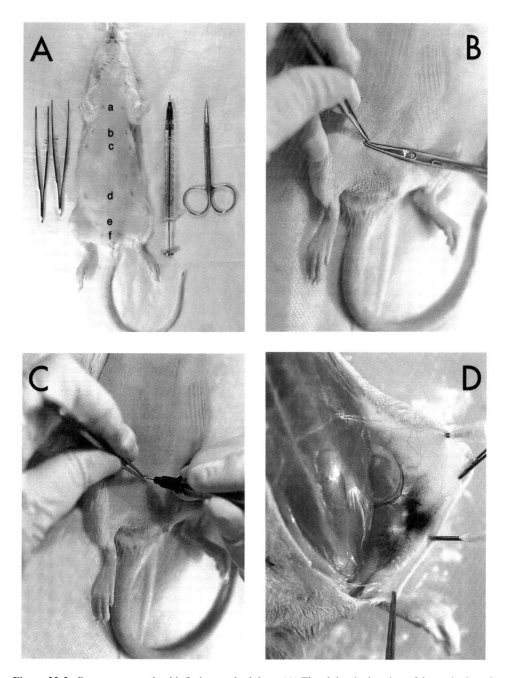

Figure 22-2. Rat mammary gland infusion methodology. (A) The abdominal region of the rat is shaved and washed with 70% ethanol to expose the 12 teats. Equipment used for infusion: 60-µl Hamilton syringe, blunt-ended 27-gauge needle, 2 pair of fine-tipped forceps, scissors, anesthesia cone, and suitable anesthetic. The six pairs of rat mammary glands, as designated by van Zwieten (26), flank the lowercase letters: a. cervical, b. cranial thoracic, c. caudal thoracic, d. abdominal, e. cranial inguinal, and f. caudal inguinal. (B) The teat is first extended from the skin using two pairs of fine-tipped forceps and then clipped as illustrated. The clipped teat area is then washed with 70% ethanol to allow for infusion into the central lacteal. (C) A blunted-ended 27-gauge needle is used to enter the remaining orifice into the central lacteal. Prior to infusion, forceps are used to secure the needle–orifice juncture. During infusion, the spread of dye through the mammary ductal tree can be observed. (D) During practice, rats may be euthanized followed by separation of the skin and mammary fat pad from the abdominal muscle to observe the efficiency of infusion into the mammary ductal structure.

surrounding the needle end is held in place with forceps (Figure 22-2C). After infusion, the teat is held shut for several seconds with the forceps to prevent leakage of the viral preparation. The teat and surrounding area is then wiped again with gauze soaked in 70% ethanol to destroy any uninfused vector. Spread of the viral preparation into the mammary tree is visualized during infusion by following the movement of the infusate that contains the fast green dye. The effectiveness of the infusion is most readily visualized by making a central incision through the abdominal skin following infusion and retracting the skin from the adjoining muscle to observe the mammary gland structure within the fat pad (Figure 22-2D).

Following viral infusions of vectors containing oncogenes, rats are housed on ground corncob bedding in plastic suspended cages and given lab chow and acidified water *ad libitum*. Palpation for mammary tumors is typically initiated 4 to 5 weeks after viral infusions of *ras* expressing vectors, although more potent oncogenes, such as *neu*, may produce palpable tumors within 2 weeks of infusion. Tumor size and location are determined by palpation and recorded weekly. Tumors reaching 10 to 20 mm prior to study termination are surgically resected while the animal is under suitable anesthesia. These rats are returned to the study after resection wounds are cleaned and clipped or sutured. Sections of resected mammary tumor are divided, flash-frozen in liquid nitrogen, and stored frozen at −80°C for later molecular characterization or fixed in 4% formalin for hematoxylin and eosin staining for histopathological analysis.

METHODS FOR ASSESSING RETROVIRAL INTEGRATION IN THE MAMMARY GLAND

Materials and Instrumentation

X-gal (i.e., 5-bromo-4-chloro-3-indolyl-β-D-galactopyranoside) was obtained from Molecular Probes (Eugene, OR). Glutaraldehyde, potassium ferricyanide, potassium ferrocyanide, $MgCl_2$, *N,N*-dimethylformamide, and glycerol were obtained from Sigma (St. Louis, MO).

Reagents and Reagent Preparation

Primary rat mammary cell cultures were fixed by using 0.5% glutaraldehyde in PBS. X-gal staining solution is prepared in PBS and contains 20 mM potassium ferricyanide, 20 mM potassium ferrocyanide, 1.0 mM $MgCl_2$, and 1.0 mg/ml X-gal; add X-gal fresh from a 50-mg/ml stock in *N,N*-dimethylformamide stored at −20°C.

Procedures for Assessing β-Galactosidase Expression in the Rat Mammary Gland

To determine the efficiency of retroviral integration in the mammary gland following infusion, retroviral vectors expressing the reporter gene β-galactosidase (e.g., pJRgal) can be assessed in whole mount mammary glands or primary mammary gland tissue culture (2). Whole mammary glands can be stained for β-galactosidase activity, as described (11). Such staining provides a qualitative analysis of vector incorporation in the mammary structure (Figure 22-3A). Methods for whole mount mouse mammary preparations are presented in Chapter 7 of this volume (12).

Alternatively, vectors expressing β-galactosidase in mammary cells can be assayed in primary tissue cultures (Figure 22-3B), permitting quantification of infected cells in the mammary gland (2). After sufficient time has been allowed for mammary gland infection

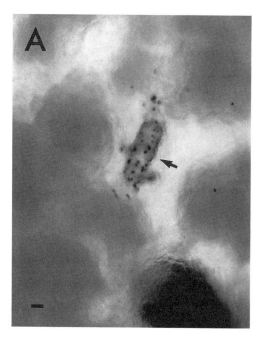
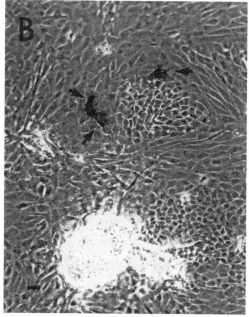

Figure 22-3. Retroviral vector β-galactosidase expression in rat mammary cells. (A) Whole rat mammary gland in fat pad mounted on a glass microscope slide and stained with X-gal 3 months after infusion of a retroviral vector expressing β-galactosidase (i.e., JRgal) at 10^7 CFU/ml. The arrow points to a mammary structure with multiple infected cells expressing β-galactosidase. This mammary gland was not counterstained, allowing better resolution of the X-gal stained (i.e., infected, β-galactosidase expressing) cells. Due to the thickness of the fat pad only the stained cells are clearly resolved in the limited depth of field at this magnification, although other mammary structures (e.g., ductal and alveolar structures) are present surrounding the stained cells. Bar = 120 μm. (B) Expression of β-galactosidase in primary cultures of rat mammary cells removed 24 h after infusion of JRgal. The arrows point to cultured mammary cells expressing β-galactosidase. Rat mammary cells were cultured 4 days before X-gal staining was performed as described in the text. Bar = 25 μm.

(approximately 2 days), primary cultures of rat mammary cells can be prepared as described (13). After cells have spread onto the surface of the tissue culture dish (approximately 4 days after plating), cells are fixed with ice-cold 0.5% glutaraldehyde in PBS for 10 min and then washed 3 times with room-temperature PBS for 15 min per wash. The cells are then overlaid with X-gal staining solution overnight at 37°C. The stained cells are washed 3 times with PBS at room temperature, and a thin layer of glycerol is added to prevent the stained cell preparation from drying out.

COMMENTS

Precautionary safety measures should be used in the handling of all retroviral preparations. Incubators and freezers containing retroviral preparations should be clearly marked, and access to cell cultures containing retroviruses should be limited. During handling of cultures containing retroviral packaging cell lines and viral preparations, gloves, lab coats, and face masks should be worn. During viral infusion in the mammary gland, viral preparations should be used in a positive-pressure hood (e.g., fume hood) and the person administering the viral preparation should wear protective clothing and a protective respirator (e.g., Air Mate, Racal Health and Safety, Inc., Frederick, MD). Bleach and 70% ethanol should be available when handling retroviral preparation in the event of viral spills.

Perfecting the infusion technique for introducing viral preparations into the rat mammary gland requires practice. Spend several weeks practicing this technique, using the fast green tracking dye in PBS, before attempting this procedure with retroviral preparations. Successful infusion is best monitored by surgically opening the skin to view the mammary gland in the fat pad as shown in Figure 22-2D. A defined mammary structure is readily observed with successful infusion of the gland (Figure 22-2D). Prior to performing rat mammary gland infusions using experimental vectors, successful transduction of retrovirus into the mammary gland should be established by using a retrovirus expressing a reporter gene such as β-galactosidase (e.g., JRgal; 2).

Virus titer greatly affects the level of vector incorporation in the mammary gland; therefore it is best to obtain the highest retroviral titer possible and dilute this preparation as needed for the experimental procedure. Mammary gland vector transduction is also affected by viral tropism, with amphotropic vectors being more efficient than ecotropic vectors in the rat (2).

We have noted that retroviral packaging cell lines producing retroviruses that express oncogenes are not easily reestablished after the cell lines are frozen. Therefore, these packaging cell lines may require recloning prior to each experiment. Alternatively, if future experiments for a particular vector are anticipated, large quantities of retroviral stocks can be frozen at −80°C for extended periods of time (e.g., years) without greatly affecting viral titer. Packaging cell lines producing vectors that are not expressing oncogenes can often be reestablished from frozen stocks. These cells are placed on selective conditions for the *trans* components produced by the packaging cell line being used and for the vector being expressed. These cells should be carried through at least 3 cell passages on selective conditions, followed by several passages without selective conditions prior to collecting retroviruses. Determination of the retrovirus titer produced from reestablished retroviral generating cell lines should be performed before using these cells to collect retroviral stocks.

Variations in the mammary teat structure between rat strains have been observed with this procedure. Therefore, it is necessary to practice the infusion procedure with the rat strain to be used in experimentation prior to viral infusion. Also, variations in teats from rats of the same strain are observed. For example, in the Wistar–Furth rat strain, it is common to find the right, and occasionally left, cranial thoracic teat missing, with fusion of this gland to the caudal thoracic gland, in which case the infusion volume into the cranial thoracic gland can be doubled. These two glands may also be merged such that infusion into one gland results in leakage from the adjoining teat. Less common is the absence of the caudal inguinal glands. Infusion of too great a volume may result in rupture of the mammary structure. A 15-µl infusion volume is sufficient for 50-day-old female Wistar–Furth rats. The optimal infusion volume may vary for rats of different strains and ages.

LIMITATIONS

The retroviral genome is limited in size by the amount of RNA that can be packaged into the retroviral particle. Therefore, the size of the cDNA that can be incorporated into a retroviral vector is likewise limited, albeit at a size that will accommodate most genes. The maximum size of cDNA that can be placed in the retroviral vector depends on the retroviral backbone being used (e.g., an approximately 4000 bp limit can be placed in the pJR vector). Once incorporated into the retroviral genome, the insert is usually regulated by viral promoters (e.g., the 5′ LTR). Several modifications of retroviral vectors have been created in an effort to provide better fidelity of gene expression, such as self-inactivating vectors (14), although the region of retroviral incorporation into the host genome can also influence gene expression. Ultimately, the expression from most retroviral vectors is attenuated over time (e.g., by altered methylation of the viral regulatory elements), which has also proven to be a limiting factor in the use of retroviral vectors in gene therapy. Again, a number of modifications have recently been introduced into retroviral vectors that may provide more prolonged expression (15).

In order for the retroviral genome to be incorporated into the host genome, mitosis is required. Thus, static tissues are not easily transduced by retroviral vectors. In the rat mammary gland, proliferation of the mammary gland can be induced through a variety of means, such as perphenazine treatment as described here, although other means may suffice, such as pregnancy. Also, the mammary gland must be sufficiently developed (e.g., approximately 40 days of age) so that the retroviral vector can be effectively introduced into the gland. Therefore, retroviral transduction of the mammary gland in young animals may prove difficult.

CONCLUSIONS

We have presented methods to rapidly establish "transgenic" mammary glands by the infusion of retrovirus vectors that carry genes of interest into the mammary gland via the terminal mammary duct. This approach has been successfully adapted to small mammals, such as the rat (2), and to large mammals, such as goats (16). In rodents, this method has been mainly used to study mammary biology and carcinogenesis. In larger mammals this methodology is used to produce exogenous proteins for commercial or experimental uses.

The current competing method to produce exogenous proteins from the mammary gland is to establish transgenic mammals by using conventional germ-line gene transfers. The germ-line transgenic method may place transgenes into every cell of the organism, including the mammary gland. In contrast, the retrovirus infusion method, at this point, can only transfer genes into approximately 1% of mammary ductal cells (2). The germ-line approach to establish a transgenic mammary gland for protein production thus has the advantage of allowing most mammary cells to produce the protein of interest. Its disadvantage, in this context, is that it takes several years to accomplish and is expensive. In comparison, the retroviral gene delivery method is rapid and inexpensive. In addition, the retroviral method uses anatomical targeting that produces absolute mammary cell gene expression selectivity. The germ-line transgenic methods enrich for mammary targeting using mammary active promoters (e.g., MMTV LTR), which unfortunately are not fully specific for mammary gland expression.

Compared to germ-line transgenic models for retroviral delivery of genes involved in mammary carcinogenesis, such as oncogenes, the viral model has the following advantages and disadvantages: (1) Most transgenes in germ-line transgenic models are targeted to the mammary gland by using hormonally driven promoters, such as the whey acidic protein promoter or the MMTV LTR (17). Use of these promoters leads to two major problems. First, they are not exclusively expressed in the mammary gland. Second, since they are driven by "mammary" effective hormones, the function of the transgene can be confounded by additive, subadditive, or synergistic interactions of these hormones on mammary gland cellular functions and malignant transformation. (2) In general, most cancers develop in a clonal manner where the transformed cell is surrounded by normal interacting cells. The viral model can mimic clonal development by infecting only rare cells, whereas germ-line-produced transgenic mammary gland express the transgenic oncogene in all cells. (3) In a germ-line transgenic mammal, all cells have the same insertion site, leading to confounding effects of transgene positioning in the genome. In contrast, each primary infected cell has a unique and random integration site in the viral model. (4) The retroviral model is rapid and inexpensive in contrast to the germ-line transgenic model. (5) A disadvantage of the retroviral model that is only shared occasionally by germ-line transgenics is the inactivation of the expression of the transgene over time. Thus, both the retroviral and germ-line mammary transgenic mammary models have their respective advantages and disadvantages. It is important to take these limitations into account when choosing a method to establish transgenic mammary glands for the study of carcinogenesis.

The retroviral method of producing transgenic mammary glands has to date mainly been used by our group to study mammary biology and carcinogenesis (2, 18–23). In addition, retroviral-mediated oncogene transfer to the rat mammary gland has been proposed as a model for investigating therapeutic and chemopreventive measures of breast cancer (24). For example, approximately 60% of mammary carcinomas induced with retroviruses expressing the *neu* oncogene are hormonally responsive (22). Thus, breast cancers with aberrant *neu* expression may better model human breast cancer than chemically induced cancer in which most cancers are estrogen receptor positive (25). The retroviral model has also been shown to be useful in chemoprevention studies. For example, the monoterpene limonene has been shown to be effective at inhibiting mammary carcinomas induced with retroviral vectors expressing the viral Harvey *ras* gene (23). Therefore, retroviral-mediated gene transfer to the rat mammary gland combined with a specific treatment regimen may serve as a useful model for studying therapeutic and chemopreventive approaches for breast cancer.

In summary, we have presented detailed methods for transferring genes into *in situ* mammary gland by infusing replication-defective retroviral vectors carrying selected transgenes into the mammary milk lumen. We have also summarized current applications of this model together with its advantages and disadvantages as compared to germ-line transgenic models. When chosen carefully for specific applications, the methodology described here should be useful in studying mammary specific functions of a wide variety of genes, including oncogenes, and in producing exogenous proteins in a cost-effective, rapid manner.

ACKNOWLEDGMENTS. This work was supported by National Institutes of Health Grant CA77527. The authors would like to thank Dr. Debra MacKenzie and Dr. Kwanghee Kim for critical review of this manuscript.

REFERENCES

1. H. M. Temin (1986). Retrovirus vectors for gene transfer: efficient integration into and expression of exogenous DNA in vertebrate cell genomes. In R. Kucherlapati (ed.), *Gene Transfer*, Plenum Press, New York, pp. 149–187.

2. B. Wang, W. S. Kennan, J. Yasukawa-Barnes, M. J. Linstrom, and M. N. Gould (1991). Carcinoma induction following direct *in situ* transfer of v-Ha-*ras* into rat mammary epithelial cells using replication-defective retrovirus vectors. *Cancer Res.* **51**:2642–2648.

3. S. Sukumar, V. Notario, D. Martin-Zanco, and M. Barbacid (1983). Induction of mammary carcinomas in rats by nitroso-methylurea involves malignant activation of H-*ras*-1 locus by single point mutations. *Nature* **306**:658–661.

4. O. Danos and R. C. Mulligan (1988). Safe and efficient generation of recombinant retroviruses with amphotropic and ecotropic host ranges. *Proc. Natl. Acad. Sci. U.S.A.* **85**:6460–6464.

5. M. Kriegler (1990). *Gene Transfer and Expression, a Laboratory Manual*, Stockton Press, New York.

6. M. A. Bender, T. D. Palmer, R. E. Gelinas, and A. D. Miller (1987). Evidence that the packaging signal of Moloney murine leukemia virus extends into the *gag* region. *J. Virol.* **61**:1639–1646.

7. J. Price, D. Turner, and C. Cepko (1987). Lineage analysis in the vertebrate nervous system by retrovirus-mediated gene transfer. *Proc. Natl. Acad. Sci. USA* **84**:156–160.

8. J. Sambrook, E. F. Fritsch, and T. Maniatis (1989). *Molecular Cloning: A Laboratory Manual*, 2nd ed., Cold Spring Harbor Laboratory Press, New York.

9. A. D. Miller and C. Buttimore (1986). Redesigning of retrovirus packaging cell lines to avoid recombination leading to helper virus production. *Mol. Cell. Biol.* **6**:2895–2902.

10. A. D. Miller, D. R. Trauber, and C. Buttimore (1986). Factors involved in production of helper virus-free retrovirus vectors. *Somat. Cell. Mol. Genet.* **12**:175–183.

11. E. C. Kordon, R. A. McKnight, C. Jhappan, L. Hennighausen, G. Merlino, and G. H. Smith (1995). Ectopic TGFβ1 expression in the secretory mammary epithelium induces early senescence of the epithelial stem cell population. *Dev. Biol.* **168**:47–61.

12. S. B. Rasmussen, L. J. Young, and G. H. Smith (2000). Preparing mammary gland whole mounts from mice, Chapter 7, this volume.

13. M. N. Gould, D. R. Grau, L. A. Seidman, and C. J. Moore (1986). Interspecies comparison of human and rat mammary epithelial cell-mediated mutagenesis by polycyclic aromatic hydrocarbons. *Cancer Res.* **46**:4942–4945.

14. A. Fassati, A. Bardoni, M. Sironi, D. J. Wells, N. Bresolin, G. Scarlato, M. Hatanaka, S. Yamaoka, and G. Dickson (1998). Insertion of two independent enhancers in the long terminal repeat of a self-inactivating vector results in high-titer retroviral vectors with tissue-specific expression. *Hum. Gene Ther.* **9**:2459–2468.

15. P. B. Robbins, D. C. Skelton, X-J. Yu, S. Halene, E. H. Leonard, and D. B. Kohn (1998). Consistent, persistent expression from modified retroviral vectors in murine hematopoietic stem cells. *Proc. Natl. Acad. Sci. USA* **95**:10182–10187.

16. J. S. Archer, W. S. Kennan, M. N. Gould, and R. D. Bremel (1994). Human growth hormone (hGH) secretion in milk of goats after direct transfer of hGH gene into the mammary gland by using replication-defective retrovirus vectors. *Proc. Natl. Acad. Sci. USA* **91**:6840–6844.

17. M. A. Webster and W. J. Muller (1994). Mammary tumorigenesis and metastasis in transgenic mice. *Semin. Cancer Biol.* **5**:69–76.

18. B. Wang, W. S. Kennan, J. Yasukawa-Barnes, M. J. Linstrom, and M. N. Gould (1991). Overcoming the activity of mammary carcinoma suppressor gene in Copenhagen rats by v-Ha-*ras* oncogene transfer into mammary epithelial cells *in situ*. *Cancer Res.* **51**:5298–5303.

19. T. A. Thompson, K. Kim, and M. N. Gould (1998). Harvey *ras* results in a higher frequency of mammary carcinomas than Kirsten *ras* after direct retroviral transfer into the rat mammary gland. *Cancer Res.* **58**:5097–5104.

20. B. Wang, W. S. Kennan, J. Yasukawa-Barnes, M. J. Lindstrom, and M. N. Gould (1991). Frequent induction of mammary carcinomas following *neu* oncogene transfer into *in situ* mammary epithelial cells of susceptible and resistant rat strains. *Cancer Res.* **51**:5649–5654.

21. Y. T. Tai and M. N. Gould (1997). The genetic penetrance of the activated *neu* oncogene for the induction of mammary cancer *in vivo*. *Oncogene* **14**:2701–2707.

22. B. Wang, W. S. Kennan, J. Yasukawa-Barnes, M. J. Lindstrom, and M. N. Gould (1992). Difference in the response of *neu* and *ras* oncogene-induced rat mammary carcinomas to early and late ovariectomy. *Cancer Res.* **52**:4102–4105.

23. M. N. Gould, C. J. Moore, R. Zhang, B. Wang, W. S. Kennan, and J. D. Haag (1994). Limonene chemoprevention of mammary carcinoma induction following direct *in situ* transfer of v-Ha-*ras*. *Cancer Res.* **54**:3540–3543.

24. M. N. Gould (1993). The introduction of activated oncogenes to mammary cells *in vivo* using retroviral vectors: a new model for the chemoprevention of premalignant and malignant lesions of the breast. *J. Cell. Biochem.* **17G:**66–72.

25. S. Nandi, R. C. Guzman, and J. Yang (1995). Hormones and mammary carcinogenesis in mice, rats, and humans: a unifying hypothesis. *Proc. Natl. Acad. Sci. USA* **92:**3650–3657.

26. M. J. van Zwieten (1984). *The Rat as Animal Model in Breast Cancer Research*, Martinus Nijhoff, Boston.

Chapter 23

Intraductal Injection into the Mouse Mammary Gland

Duy-Ai Nguyen, Neal Beeman, Michael Lewis, Jerome Schaack, and Margaret C. Neville

Abstract.   The mammary epithelium is continuous with the skin through a teat canal leading to a single primary duct in the mouse. Using fire-polished micropipettes 60 to 75 μm in diameter, it is possible to inject any desired substance directly through the teat into the lumen of the mammary gland. If the primary duct of the gland is exposed surgically, hypodermic needles can also be used for injection. Both techniques can be used to investigate the state of tight junctions in the mammary gland by examining transepithelial movement of radioactive sugars or fluorescent-labeled proteins. The intraductal or up-the-teat injection of adenoviral and plasmid vectors provides a convenient means of altering gene expression in the luminal epithelium. Finally, injected fluorescent probes as well as adenovirus-transduced green fluorescent protein can be directly visualized in the mammary gland in the living mouse by using confocal microscopy.

Abbreviations.   green fluorescent protein (GFP); bovine serum albumin (BSA); fluorescein (FITC); a blue nuclear stain (DAPI).

The mammary epithelium is accessible from the exterior of the animal through the teat canal. This unusual characteristic is technically advantageous and was exploited nearly 30 years ago by James Linzell and his colleagues for assessing the transepithelial permeability of the mammary gland to a variety of substances in the pregnant and lactating goat (1–3). Falconer injected ^{125}I-prolactin intraductally in rabbits to assay its distribution. More recently, intraductal injection of the mammary gland has been used in the rat for transduction of the epithelium with retroviruses (Chapter 22 this volume) and adenovirus (4, 5). Intraductal injection of antitumor agents has been proposed for breast cancer therapy in women, but reports of its efficacy do not seem to be available in the literature. This powerful technique has not been much exploited in the mouse, because of the small size of the teats and major mammary duct. This difficulty can be overcome with the use of appropriately sized micropipettes inserted directly into the teat canal through the nipple (up-the-teat injection) or with the use of large-gauge needles inserted into the primary duct of the surgically exposed mammary gland. In this laboratory the technique has been used to assess the status of the tight junctions between

Duy-Ai Nguyen, Neal Beeman, Michael Lewis, Jerome Schaack, and Margaret C. Neville   **Department of Physiology, University of Colorado Health Sciences Center, Denver, Colorado, 80262.**

Methods in Mammary Gland Biology and Breast Cancer Research, edited by Ip and Asch. Kluwer Academic/Plenum Publishers, New York, 2000.

epithelial cells by measuring the permeability of the mammary epithelium to radioactive sucrose and to fluorescent-labeled proteins. It has also been used for adenoviral transduction and transfection with plasmids and for visualization of the mammary gland *in vivo*.

In this chapter we describe fabrication of the micropipettes used for up-the-teat injection. For the injection we utilize a dissection microscope and a drawn micropipette mounted on a micromanipulator to enter the teat canal. An alternative technique uses surgical exposure of the third or fourth mammary gland and injection with a Hamilton syringe directly into the primary duct. We illustrate the use of up-the-teat injection to measure transepithelial permeability, using [^{14}C]-sucrose and fluorescently labeled proteins. Transduction of the luminal epithelium with an adenoviral vector and visualization of the mammary lumen with the confocal microscope in the living mouse are also described briefly.

MATERIALS

General

- Anesthetic: pentobarbital, 60 μg/gm body weight with 10 to 20 μg/gm as follow-up dose or as specified by your Institutional Animal Care and Use Committee
- Dissecting microscope
- Fiber-optic light source

Fabrication of Micropipettes for Up-the-Teat Injection

- Bunsen burner with flame spreader
- Fine forceps (old ones that can be put in the flame)
- 10-μl or 25-μl glass micropipettes (Drummund precision disposable micropipettes on 10 or 25 μl or Wiretrol calibrated micropipettes with stainless steel plunger, up to 100 μl)
- Compound microscope with calibrated ocular reticle and adjustable stage
- Micromanipulator
- Platinum wire electrode
- Variable power source

Up-the-Teat Injection

- Prepared micropipette with 60 to 75 μM tip (see above)
- Drummond digital pipette (10 or 100 μl)
- Micromanipulator
- Blunt-tipped forceps
- High-intensity fiber-optic light
- Electric light to keep mouse warm

Intraductal Injection

SURGICAL
- Dissecting microscope and fiber-optic light source
- Cork board (4 inch × 6 inch)
- Straight pins

- Surgical tape
- 70% ethanol
- Opening scissors
- Forceps—mouse tooth and smooth
- Cotton-tipped wooden applicators
- Wound clips or suturing supplies
- Recovery chamber, warm
- Black "Sharpie" or magic marker (optional)

EXPERIMENTAL

- Injectable substance (viruses, plasmids, tracer dyes, etc.)
- 30G1/2 needle or higher (Becton Dickinson & Co., Franklin Lakes, NJ 07417)
- Hamilton syringe with hub for removable needles (50 µl) or similar
- Tracer dye (optional), e.g., 0.1–0.5% trypan blue or Evan's blue in 1× PBS or 0.9% saline

Measurement of Transepithelial Permeability

- ^{14}C-sucrose (2×10^6 cpm/8 µl)
- Drummond digital microdispenser set to 8.8 µl
- Injection apparatus as above

Observation of the Mammary Alveolus in a Living Mouse

- Inverted confocal microscope with removable stage diaphragm
- Heating pad
- Large coverslips
- Duct or surgical tape
- Anesthetic (pentobarbitol, 5 mg/ml; inject 0.01 ml/g body weight)
- Fine scissors
- Forceps
- Blunt probe
- Gauze pads
- Ringer's solution

METHODS

Fabrication of Micropipettes for Up-the-Teat Injection

The goal is to pull a calibrated micropipette (Drummund Precision Disposable micropipettes, 10 or 25 µl) so that it has a strong, tapered, and polished tip 60 to 75 µm in diameter. The trick in achieving proper tip size and conformation is to pull each pipette in two stages. The first pull is slow and reduces the diameter by a factor of 2; the second pull is rapid and results in a gradual taper to a diameter less than 75 µm. The pipette is then broken under the microscope and fire-polished in a microforge.

DETAILS.   Attach a flame spreader to a large Bunsen burner or fashion a flame spreader from heavy foil. Adjust the flame to 1 inch. Insert one tine of the forceps into the lumen of the dispensing end of the pipette and grasp the glass gently. Hold the plunger end with the fingertips. Hold the dispensing end of the pipette at the top of the flame with the pipette level and perpendicular to the band of flame. Maintain light tension only so that the wall thickness is unchanged and the glass melts to form an hourglass shape (Figure 23-1A, pipette 1). When the dispensing end begins to move, remove the pipette from the flame as rapidly as possible while keeping the glass tube as straight as possible. Dip the dispensing end in water to cool. Water will be drawn up into the pipette. The external diameter at the waist of the pulled section is about one-half the original diameter of the tube (Figure 23-1A, pipette 1).

For the second pull hold the pipette as before, but exert tension horizontally throughout the pull. Expose the pipette to the flame as before, with the band of flame at the waist of the hourglass. The water in the lumen may boil but this will not affect the correct pull. As the pipette becomes plastic, both hands begin to move apart rapidly. At this point remove the pipette immediately from the flame while maintaining horizontal tension and dip the dispensing end in water to cool. Water should be drawn into the pipette past the waist of the elongated hourglass. The waist of the hourglass should be 75 µm or less in external diameter at its narrowest point; the wall of the pipette at this point is very thin, and often flexible (Figure 23-1A, pipette 2). If water is not drawn into the pipette, it has been sealed. The end of the pipette is often pulled off accidentally during this step. These pipettes and the sealed ones should be examined under the microscope to determine whether the lumen is patent. If not, discard them.

The pulled tubes are broken with fine forceps under a dissecting microscope to obtain a tip of proper diamenter. The ocular reticle of a *compound* microscope is used to locate the region of the pipette with an external diameter between 60 and 75 µm. The shape of this target region is carefully noted and the pipette is placed flat on the stage of a *dissecting* microscope. The pipette is grasped just below the target diameter with fine forceps held flat against the stage. The forceps are rotated gently to force the dispensing end upwards and snap it off. If the forceps are maintained at the level of the stage and perpendicular to the pipette, the dispensing end will snap off at the desired diameter and a reasonably smooth break will be obtained (Figure 23-1A, pipette 3). Once a pipette of ideal tip diameter is obtained it can be used as a guide in breaking other tips correctly under the dissecting scope.

The broken pipettes are polished on the stage of the *compound* microscope with a platinum wire electrode (or microforge) held in a micromanipulator (Figure 23-1B). The broken pipette is placed flat on the microscope stage so that the tip is just visible with a 10× objective. Using the micromanipulator, advance the tip of the microforge into the other side of the field of view (M, Figure 23-1B). The variable power source is used to adjust the power gradually upward until the wire just begins to glow in the microscope field. The wire loop will extend forward slightly as it is heated. When the pipette tip and the tip of the microforge are brought within 3 to 4 µm of each other, a smoothly broken tip will be polished rapidly and should be removed as soon as the tip appears smooth. More jaggedly broken tips can often be polished smoothly if they are positioned carefully near the electrode so that jagged projections are closer to the heat source. It is often necessary to reposition such a tip several times during polishing. Polished tips do not have to be perfectly regular. Two finished tips are shown in Figure 23-1C.

Before attempting an injection, always test the pipette to make certain that fluid can be drawn up and expelled freely. A pipette can be used until it is broken or clogged. For cleaning, the pipette can be attached to a vacuum apparatus (Figure 23-1D) and large volumes of fluiddrawn rapidly through it. To clean pipettes, 70% ethanol followed by sterile water is recommended.

Up-the-Teat Injection

ANIMAL PREPARATION. For injection into the lumen of the mouse mammary gland through the teat canal (up-the-teat injection), the mouse is positioned on a platform beneath a

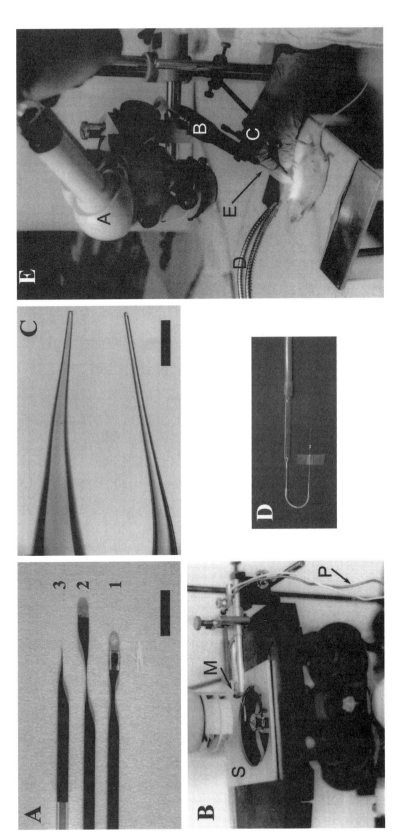

Figure 23-1. Fabricating and using micropipettes for up-the-teat injection. (A) Stages in pulling micropipettes. After a slow pull the heated portion of the pipette has an hourglass shape and the wall has not appreciably thinned (bottom pipette). When the pipette is pulled a second time, the waist of the indentation narrows to less than 75 μm (middle pipette) or breaks entirely (top pipette). (Pipettes are filled with dye solution to facilitate photography.) (B) Microforge (M) positioned over movable stage (S) of a compound microscope with wires to a variable power source (P). The platinum heating wire can be seen above the objective in the opening on the movable stage. For fire-polishing, a freshly broken micropipette is placed on the left-hand side of the stage with the tip about 4 μm from the platinum wire. (C) Tips of two fire-polished pipettes. Bar is 100 mm. (D) A Pasteur pipette attached to a piece of flexible tubing and a micropipette for cleaning. (The micropipette was taped down for the purposes of the photograph.) (E) Setup for teat canal injection using a Drummond microdispenser (B) mounted on a micromanipulator (C) beneath a dissecting microscope (A). The micropipette (E) is inserted into the teat canal by manipulating the tissue surrounding the nipple with a pair of fine forceps.

dissecting microscope (Figure 23-1E, A). A micropipette (E) inserted into a Drummond digital microdispenser (B) held in a micromanipulator (C) is positioned above the second, third, or fourth nipple that has been prepared as will be described. A fiber-optic light (D) is convenient for visualizing the field. The tip of the micropipette is inserted into the lumen of the canal, and 8 to 25 µl of solution is injected. For larger volumes a Wiretrol micropipette (5 to 100 µl) can be held in the micromanipulator with a length of narrow-bore rubber tubing to fit the pipette to the micromanipulator, and the solution can be dispensed with the accompanying stainless steel plunger.

The first step is to prepare the nipple for injection. Removing the hair around the nipple to obtain a clear unobstructed work area can facilitate the injection procedure. For lactating mice, the opening for the teat canal is readily apparent at the center of the teat, and the capillary tip will readily slip in when pushed against the nipple at this location. Staining the teat with trypan blue will make the opening more visible in the beginning. In nonlactating mice, the opening to the teat canal is often covered with a layer of dead skin that must be removed by repeated gentle grabbing and pulling with a pair of microscissors. Although the layer of dead skin can also be removed by cutting off a thin layer of skin at the tip of the nipple, excessive cutting can deform the nipple and makes the task of locating the opening more difficult.

INJECTION.   To insert the tip of the capillary tube into the teat canal, the tube is first positioned immediately adjacent to the base of the nipple with the micromanipulator. The center of the nipple is then positioned under the tip of the capillary by manipulating the skin around the nipple with a pair of blunt forceps. Direct manipulation of the nipple is possible, but can result in damage. Next, the center of the nipple is pushed upward against the tip of the capillary by using the natural elasticity of the nipple or a light upward motion of the forceps. If correctly performed the tip of the capillary should enter the teat canal easily. If it does not, then the tip may not be positioned properly at the opening of the teat canal or the opening is still covered by skin. A delicate touch is critical to these procedures.

Finally, the material in the capillary tube is injected into the lumen of the mammary gland. Since the tip of capillary was initially positioned at the level of the base of the nipple, the nipple will be under compression and exert an upward force against the capillary tip. This upward push helps to prevent the capillary tip from slipping out of the teat canal during slight movements of the mouse, such as breathing. The nipple and the inserted capillary tip should be observed carefully throughout the injection because even slight movement can dislodge the tip from the teat canal.

Intraductal Injection

For younger or nulliparous virgin mice, injection through the teat canal is difficult. In this case the gland can be exposed surgically and the primary duct just below the teat injected with a Hamilton syringe.

ANIMAL PREPARATION.   The mouse is anesthetized and affixed on its back to a cork board with surgical tape or straight pins through the paw webbing. The ventral fur is wetted with 70% ethanol to reduce fur entry into the wound. If the animal has a light coat color (e.g., BALb/c, CD1) the nipple region may be "painted" with a black magic marker to provide better visualization of the nipple and primary duct.

A 1.5–2 cm mid-ventral incision is made beginning just above the pubic area. Two additional incisions are made from the base of the incision at an angle toward the midpoint of the hind legs. The angled cuts should be well behind the nipple for the number 4 mammary gland.

The triangular patch of skin and the attached number 4 mammary gland are peeled back gently with mouse-tooth forceps and a cotton-tipped wooden applicator and pinned to the cork board such that the skin is tight and the gland is roughly flat.

INJECTION.   Locate the nipple under the dissecting microscope: it will appear as a grayish circular spot against a lighter background of the skin. The nipple should be near the corner created by the two incisions but not so close that the pin will interfere with the injection.

Next, locate the primary duct of the mammary gland. The primary duct extends from the nipple back toward the no. 4 fat pad. If necessary, use the smooth forceps to wiggle the fat pad gently. The location of the primary duct should become apparent since it is attached to the nipple and will move with the fat pad.

Load the syringe with approximately 25–30 μl of the injectable substance; there will be some dead airspace in the syringe. Using an oblique angle of attack in the same orientation as the length of the primary duct, carefully insert the tip of the needle a few millimeters into the lumen of the primary duct near the nipple. The skin may need to be held with forceps to facilitate needle penetration. Take care not to penetrate the back wall of the duct. Slowly inject 10–20 μl of the substance into the gland. If done correctly, the entire mammary ductal tree will fill with the injected fluid. The exact volume tolerated by the gland before the terminal end buds or duct termini burst varies with the age of the animal and the extent of gland development and should be determined empirically by using a tracer dye on a few test animals.

After injection, wait about 5 s for the back pressure to reduce; then use smooth forceps to gently squeeze the fat pad around the needle and slowly pull the needle out of the duct. Pinch the duct with the forceps as the needle passes the tip and hold to prevent leakage of the injected substance. Close the animal with wound clips or sutures and allow recovery in a warm chamber or fresh cage. Repeat for the contralateral gland.

Injection of Adenovirus

ADENOVIRUS PREPARATION.   Adenovirus preparation has been described in detail in Li et al. (Chapter 21 this volume).

For these experiments adenovirus containing green fluorescent protein (GFP) or lacZ under control of the cytomegalovirus major immediate early promoter (CMV promoter) was used. Adenoviral E1A and E1B genes within the left end of the adenovirus chromosome were deleted so that the virus was replication defective, although replication was not completely eliminated (6).

TRANSDUCTION OF THE MAMMARY EPITHELIUM IN VIVO.   We have found that adenovirus transduction is more efficient when the virus is injected into the gland of the pregnant animal. Presumably the presence of large amounts of milk in the lumen interferes with infectivity in the lactating animal. For observations during lactation we carry out the injections on day 19 of pregnancy, injecting 5–8×10^7 pfu (plaque-forming units) of virus particles diluted with Ringer's solution containing 10% calf serum. In general, we inject a volume of 50–200 μl. Although we often assay the mouse at 3 days of lactation, GFP expression has been found to persist through late lactation.

Observation of the Mammary Alveolus in a Living Mouse

Fluorescent probes can be injected up the teat or intraductally to visualize the mammary lumen in the live mouse. Adenovirally encoded fusion proteins containing GFP can also be visualized *in vivo*. The fourth mammary gland is the easiest to visualize with the anesthetized mouse placed on the stage of an inverted microscope equipped for laser or digital confocal fluorescence microscopy.

PREPARATION OF THE ANIMAL.   The microscope stage is warmed with a stage heater (ideal) or heating lamp. If a heat lamp is used it must be turned off while taking micrographs. The stage insert is removed from the microscope and placed with a 50-ml centrifuge tube of Ringer's solution on a heating pad to warm. A coverslip is taped over the aperture in the insert.

The mouse, anesthetized as described, is placed on its back on a warm heating pad. A 2-cm mid-ventral incision is made beginning midway between the fourth and fifth teats. A second incision is made from the base of the mid-ventral incision at an angle toward the mid-point of the hind legs, passing over the junction of the fourth and fifth mammary glands. A third incision is made at the anterior end of the midline incision angled laterally between the third and fourth mammary glands, leaving a wide margin of skin around the fourth mammary gland. A blunt probe or cotton-tipped applicator is worked along the length of the three inci-sions and is used to lift the ventral two-thirds of the fourth mammary gland entirely free of the body wall while preserving mammary circulation.

The mouse is now placed prone on the warmed stage insert and the deflected flap of skin is arranged on the secured coverslip over the aperture. The mammary gland should be visible through the aperture. In general, most fluorescent probes can also be seen with the naked eye, an aid in positioning the animal. Tape the flap of skin lightly to the insert, taking care not to compress the gland. A flaccid fold of skin between the mouse and the taped area helps to reduce the transmission of breathing movements to the visualized tissue. Place a gauze pad dampened with warm Ringer's solution beneath the mouse, making sure that the gauze contacts all exposed tissues. The edge of the gauze pad should extend over the edge of the coverslip but not across the aperture. A film of saline will spread between the coverslip and the visualized tissue and prevent drying.

VISUALIZATION OF THE MAMMARY GLAND.   The stage insert bearing the mouse is placed on the stage of the inverted microscope and the mammary gland is visualized through the objective. To prolong visualization of a living gland, keep the gauze pad well moistened with Ringer's solution and maintain body temperature of the mouse. A microscope with a heated stage is ideal for this experiment. Alternatively, a heat lamp may be placed over the microscope stage to keep it warm but must be be switched off while taking micro-graphs. The stage should remain warm to the touch but not allowed to become hot. A dark redness of the ears, feet, and tail indicates overheating. Etiolation or whitening of these areas indicates underheating. If the anesthetic begins to wear off, small doses may be injected intraperitoneally through the ventral body wall by simply rolling the mouse toward the tape.

Throughout the experiment red blood cells should be seen coursing through the vas-culature of the gland, indicating adequate circulation. Although it is occasionally possible to obtain usable images with a 100× oil emersion objective, because most structures lie more deeply in the tissue a long working distance 60× objective is generally more satisfactory. In addition, best results are obtained in a mouse that has been lactating for 10 days or more because the thickness of the adipose layer that generally surrounds the parenchyma is reduced at this time. More detailed discussion of the use of digital or laser confocal microscopy is beyond the scope of this chapter.

RESULTS AND DISCUSSION

In this section we give examples of the application of up-the-teat injection to studies of mammary function.

Measurement of Transepithelial Permeability

The teat canal injection procedure can be applied to the assessment of permeability of tight junctions between the mammary epithelial cells *in vivo*. Tracer injected into the lumen of the mammary gland will remain there if the tight junctions are closed. However, if they are open the injected tracer will leak out of the lumen and into the interstitial space. Since small molecules such as sucrose can readily transfer across the endothelium of the capillaries and enter the bloodstream, the peak level in the blood mirrors the leakage rate of such molecules. In our study, we injected the tracer [^{14}C]-sucrose into the lumen of the mammary glands during pregnancy and lactation. During pregnancy, [^{14}C]-sucrose appeared in the bloodstream almost immediately after injection, as the tracer leaked across the permeable tight junctions (Figure 23-2). The level in the bloodstream then fell with a half-time of about 20 min as the nonmetabolizable sugar was cleared by the kidneys. During lactation, injected [^{14}C]-sucrose was not detectable in blood samples, because it was confined to the lumen by the impermeable tight junctions of lactation.

The movement of large tracer molecules, such as proteins that might not cross the capillary endothelium, can be followed by using fluorescently labeled proteins and fluorescent microscopy. Figures 23-3A, B show the results of an experiment in which FITC–BSA was injected into the lumen of the mammary glands of deeply anesthetized mice during pregnancy (A) and lactation (B). The probe was followed immediately by injection of 4%

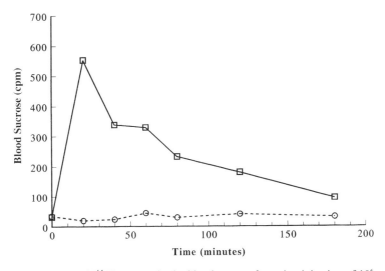

Figure 23-2. Appearance of [^{14}C]-sucrose in the bloodstream after microinjection of 10^6 cpm into the lumen of the mammary gland in pregnant and lactating mice. After injection, the [^{14}C]sucrose level in the bloodstream rapidly increased then declined in the pregnant mouse as the isotope was cleared by the kidney (open squares). The level of [^{14}C]-sucrose remained at background in the lactating mouse (open circles).

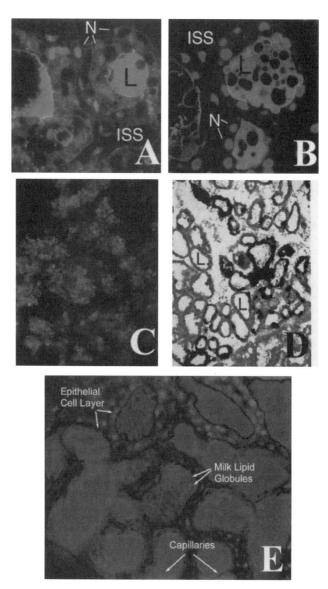

Figure 23-3. Views of injected mammary gland. (A) Distribution of FITC–albumin in the mammary glands of a pregnant mouse. Several alveoli with green fluorescence from the FITC–albumin in the lumina are shown. Nuclei (N) are stained with DAPI (blue). Note the leakage of the FITC–albumin from the lumen into the basolateral and interstitial space (ISS) of the mammary alveoli. (B) Distribution of FITC–albumin in sections of mammary glands of a lactating mouse. The FITC–albumin is confined to the lumen. 400×. (C) Adenovirus transduction of mammary epithelium. Low-power view (40×) on the FITC channel of GFP transduction of fourth mammary gland visualized in an anesthetized mouse prepared as described in text. (D) Section of mammary gland transduced with virus containing gene for *LacZ*. Section stained with Bluo-gal (Sigma) as described by Sanes *et al.* (7). (E) Visualization of the mammary lumen and nuclei of mammary alveoli in the live mouse. The fourth mammary gland of a 10-day lactating mouse was injected with Cy3-labeled IgG and the vital dye DAPI. The nuclei of the alveolar cells are shown in blue. Dark lines crossing the alveoli are capillaries. Blood cells can be seen to move in these vessels under transmitted light (not shown). (For a color representation of this, see figure facing page 268.)

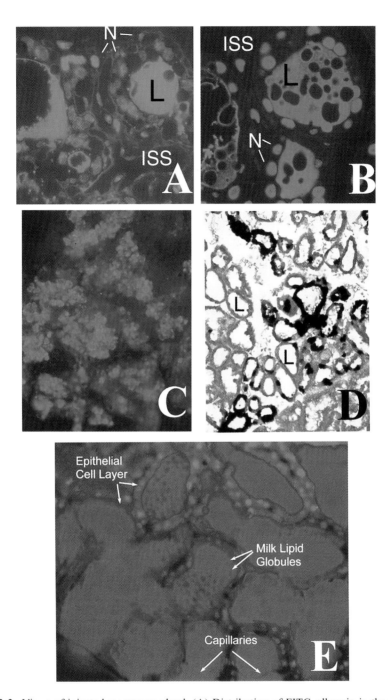

Figure 23-3. Views of injected mammary gland. (A) Distribution of FITC–albumin in the mammary glands of a pregnant mouse. Several alveoli with green fluorescence from the FITC–albumin in the lumina are shown. Nuclei (N) are stained with DAPI (blue). Note the leakage of the FITC–albumin from the lumen into the basolateral and interstitial space (ISS) of the mammary alveoli. (B) Distribution of FITC–albumin in sections of mammary glands of a lactating mouse. The FITC–albumin is confined to the lumen. 400×. (C) Adenovirus transduction of mammary epithelium. Low-power view (40×) on the FITC channel of GFP transduction of fourth mammary gland visualized in an anesthetized mouse prepared as described in text. (D) Section of mammary gland transduced with virus containing gene for *LacZ*. Section stained with Bluo-gal (Sigma) as described by Sanes *et al.* (7). (E) Visualization of the mammary lumen and nuclei of mammary alveoli in the live mouse. The fourth mammary gland of a 10-day lactating mouse was injected with Cy3-labeled IgG and the vital dye DAPI. The nuclei of the alveolar cells are shown in blue. Dark lines crossing the alveoli are capillaries. Blood cells can be seen to move in these vessels under transmitted light (not shown).

paraformaldehyde in PBS up-the-teat to fix the tissue. After dissection the gland was embedded in polymethacrylate embedding medium (JB4), sectioned, and viewed with the digital confocal microscope. Subsequent fluorescent microscopy showed that during lactation, the FITC–BSA was present exclusively within the lumen (Figure 23-3B), while during pregnancy the FITC–BSA was found throughout interstitial space of the mammary gland as well as in the lumen (Figure 23-3A). Although data obtained using protein probes are less quantitative than those using radiolabeled tracer, such probes do allow the leakage path of the tracer to be followed morphologically. In this case the tracer allowed us to ascertain that the probe leaked around the cells rather than being transcytosed, since the injected FITC–BSA was seen in the paracellular space but was not detectable within the mammary epithelial cells.

Adenoviral Transduction of Luminal Epithelium

Figure 23-3C shows a low-power view of a mammary gland from a 3-day lactating mouse transduced with adenovirus containing the GFP gene on day 19 of pregnancy. At this magnification, which does not distinguish individual cells, a large proportion of the gland appears to be transduced. In order to better estimate the proportion of cells transduced, a mouse was similarly injected with a virus containing the *lacZ* gene. The gland was dissected, reacted with the *lacZ* chromagen Bluo-gal (Sigma) to obtain the characteristic blue color and processed for frozen-section microscopy. A representative section is shown in Figure 23-3D. Many cells in the section stain a very dark blue, indicating a high degree of expression. In some alveoli all the cells appear to be stained. These alveoli are expanded and contain evidence of milk in the lumen, suggesting that neither the adenovirus transduction nor the presence of the foreign gene, *lacZ*, interferes with the normal function of the gland. However, the proportion of cells transduced is small. This degree of transduction needs to be kept in mind when experiments are planned, particularly if morphological assays are not to be used. If the criteria for the effect of a particular gene substitution are morphological, then the presence of adjacent transduced and untransduced cells and alveoli provides a control for the effect of the transgene.

Visualization of the Mammary Lumen and Epithelium *In Vivo*

We have found that the lumen of the mammary gland can be visualized with injection up the teat of fluorescent dyes. Figure 23-3E shows a digitally deconvolved view of the mammary gland of a living mouse that had received an injection of 150 µl of Cy3-labeled IgG (0.375 mg/ml) with 40 µg/ml DAPI, to visualize the nuclei. The milk fat globules are clearly visible in the lumen of many of the alveoli, and the DAPI has indeed rendered the nuclei visible. We hope to use this technique, perhaps in conjunction with lipophilic dyes, to visualize milk fat globule secretion. The possibility that calcium binding dyes can be used to quantitate the level of intracellular calcium in various stages of lactation is intriguing. We have just begun to explore this area and are still working out the possibilities and limitations of the technique.

REFERENCES

1. J. L. Linzell and M. Peaker (1971). The permeability of mammary ducts. *J. Physiol.* **216:**701–716.
2. J. L. Linzell and M. Peaker (1974). Changes in colostrum composition and in the permeability of the mammary epithelium at about the time of parturition in the goat. *J. Physiol.* **243:**129–151.

3. M. C. Neville and M. Peaker (1979). The secretion of calcium and phosphorus into milk. *J. Physiol.* **313:** 561–570.

4. J. Yang, T. Tsukamoto, N. Popnikolov, R. C. Guzman, X. Y. Chen, J. H. Yang, and S. Nandi (1995). Adenoviral-mediated gene transfer into primary human and mouse mammary epithelial cells *in vitro* and *in vivo*. *Cancer Lett.* **98:**9–17.

5. M. H. Jeng, C. Kao, L. Sivaraman, S. Krnacik, L. W. K. Chung, D. Medina, O. M. Conneely, and B. W. O'Malley (1998). Reconstitution of an estrogen-dependent transcriptional activation of an adenoviral target gene in select regions of the rat mammary gland. *Endocrinology.* **139:**2916–2925.

6. G. Chinnadurai, S. Chinnadurai, and J. Brusca (1979). Physical mapping of a large-plaque mutation of adenovirus type 2. *J. Virol.* **32:**623–628.

7. J. R. Sanes, J. L. Rubenstein, and J. F. Nicolas (1986). Use of a recombinant retrovirus to study postimplantation cell lineage in mouse embryos. *EMBO J.* **5:**3133–3142.

Chapter 24

Adenoviral and Transgenic Approaches for the Conditional Deletion of Genes from Mammary Tissue

Kay-Uwe Wagner, Edmund B. Rucker III, and Lothar Hennighausen

Abstract. Over the past decade the tools of gene targeting have permitted an unparalleled insight into genetic pathways that control mammary development and tumorigenesis in the mouse. However, the role of many genes in development and disease remains elusive, since their deletion from the mouse genome is either lethal for the mouse or does not mimic human disease progression. Thus, targeting gene deletions or modifications precisely to mammary epithelial cells during distinct time windows is a promising approach to establish high-fidelity mouse models for the study of development and disease.

Abbreviations. adenoviral (Ad); β-lactoglobulin (BLG); cytomegalovirus (CMV); embryonic stem (ES); gene of interest (GOI); long terminal repeat (LTR); mouse mammary tumor virus (MMTV); whey acidic protein (WAP).

INTRODUCTION

For more than a decade, gene targeting and the generation of knockout mice have been powerful genetic tools to evaluate gene functions in the context of the living organism. This approach has provided mechanistic insight into genetic pathways guiding mammary development and function (1). In many cases, however, the deletion of a gene results in embryonic lethality, and more sophisticated approaches have to be employed to study development of the mammary epithelium. If the fetus dies after day E13.5, transplantation of a mutant mammary gland anlagen into the cleared fat pad of a wild-type recipient can be used to study epithelial development (2). However, in those cases in which the fetus dies prior to E13.5 (e.g., deletion of *Brca1*, *Brca2*, *Rad51*, or *Bcl-x*), mammary anlagen cannot be rescued by transplantation. Furthermore, a phenotype observed in the mammary epithelium of viable gene deletion mice may not be the result of cell autonomous mechanisms. The deletion of

Kay-Uwe Wagner, Edmund B. Rucker III, and Lothar Hennighausen Laboratory of Genetics and Physiology, National Institute of Diabetes, Digestive, and Kidney Diseases, National Institutes of Health, Bethesda, Maryland 20892. *Current address for Kay-Uwe Wayner*: Eppley Institute for Research in Cancer and Allied Diseases, University of Nebraska Medical Center Omaha, Nebraske 68198-6805.

Methods in Mammary Gland Biology and Breast Cancer Research, edited by Ip and Asch. Kluwer Academic/Plenum Publishers, New York, 2000.

some genes results in the altered synthesis or release of systemic factors, which in turn causes secondary effects on the mammary epithelium (3, 4). To more accurately examine molecular pathways that lead to distinct alterations in the mammary epithelium of certain mouse models, it is necessary to separate primary functions of a protein in the developing tissue from secondary effects. An understanding of the mechanisms becomes even more complex when other exogenous factors, such as aberrant nursing behavior, become modulating factors (5). Furthermore, it has been reported that the genetic background can modulate the penetrance of phenotypes (6, 7). To minimize these limitations new technologies are required that allow for the specific alteration of genes in defined cell types. Not only are developmental biologists in need of such tools, but cancer researchers would also benefit from an improved knock-out technology. Some mutations of tumor suppressor genes introduced into the germ line of mice result in different types of tumors than expected from the human situation. For example, mutations in the *Rb* gene cause retinoblastomas in humans, whereas mice lacking *Rb* develop pituitary tumors (8). Besides germ-line mutations, most human cancers are the result of sporadic acquired mutations in a limited number of cells that are surrounded by normal tissues. Such defined mutations can now be modeled in a temporal and spatial fashion with a new technology called *conditional or tissue-specific gene targeting*.

THE Cre-loxP RECOMBINATION SYSTEM IS A TOOL FOR CONDITIONAL GENE TARGETING

Cre-loxP and Flp-frt are two recombination systems that were adopted from their original hosts (bacteriophage P1 and *Saccharomyces cerevisiae*, respectively) to generate site-specific DNA modifications in tissue culture cells (9) or in transgenic mice (10–12). They are both binary systems, in which the recombinase (Cre or Flp) recognizes its specific target sequence (loxP or frt) and catalyzes the deletion, insertion, or inversion of the DNA sequence located between the target sites. Initially, the Cre-loxP system was shown to be more efficient than the Flp-frt system in embryonic stem (ES) cells or transgenic mice. Despite recent improvements of the Flp-frt system (13), the Cre-loxP recombination system is already more widely used, and a large number of mutant mice exists with either a Cre transgene (for a list of mice see http://www.mshri.on.ca/nagy/cre.htm) or a targeted endogenous gene with inserted loxP sites ("floxed" genes). After legal issues regarding the unrestricted use of the Cre-loxP system in basic research have been settled (14), this system will probably remain the leading technology for conditional gene modifications in the future.

The mechanism underlying the Cre-loxP system is illustrated in Figure 24-1. Briefly, a loxP (locus-of-crossing-over) site is a 34 bp DNA sequence (Figure 24-1A) consisting of two inverted repeats and a nonpalindromic spacer region that determines its orientation. Several monomers of Cre recombinase bind to each of the loxP recognition sites and excise the DNA fragment between two directly orientated loxP sites as a circular segment, leaving one loxP site in the chromosome (Figure 24-1B). To a lesser extent, this recombination event is reversible (integration). Two other excellent features of the Cre-loxP recombination system have been revealed recently: First, the distance between two loxP sites does not seem to be a limiting factor because several cM of intervening sequences between loxP sites have been successfully deleted (15). Second, recombination events between homologous and even non-homologous chromosomes can be achieved (16). The Cre-loxP system will not only be used to delete important parts of a particular gene in an organ of interest, for example the mammary gland, but also to induce cytogenetic modifications, such as chromosomal loss or rearrangements on mouse chromosomes, in a tissue-specific fashion.

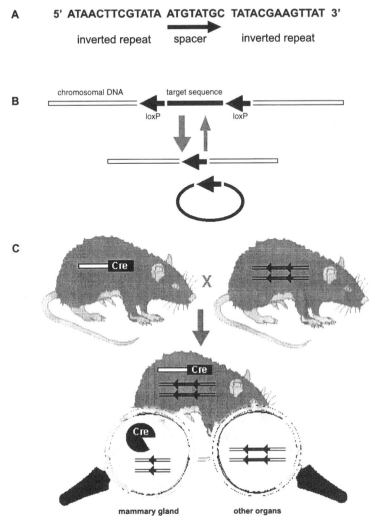

A 5' ATAACTTCGTATA ATGTATGC TATACGAAGTTAT 3'

inverted repeat spacer inverted repeat

B chromosomal DNA target sequence

loxP loxP

C Cre

X

Cre

Cre

mammary gland other organs

Figure 24-1. Characteristics of the Cre-loxP recombination system. (A) Sequence of a loxP (locus-of-crossing-over) recognition site. (B) Cre-mediated excision of a target sequence flanked by two directly orientated loxP sites. (C) Simplified breeding strategy for a tissue-specific gene deletion in transgenic mice.

Taken together, the alteration of loci that are syntenic to the human genome and that are involved in mammary tumorigenesis will permit the design of high-fidelity mouse models for breast cancer. The first and most important step for mammary gland biologists toward this long-term goal is the development of methods to target the expression of Cre recombinase to specific cell types in the mammary tissue. Once these tools have been established, they can be combined with mouse models that contain one or more floxed loci. In this chapter we describe techniques used to express Cre specifically in the mammary epithelium. Furthermore, we discuss common strategies to insert loxP recognition sites into defined genes by gene targeting.

TECHNIQUES TO EXPRESS Cre RECOMBINASE SPECIFICALLY IN THE MAMMARY GLAND

Transgenic Approach

The transgenic approach requires the generation of transgenic mice that express Cre recombinase specifically in mammary tissue. Upon crossing these mice into strains that contain a floxed gene (gene flanked by loxP sites), the mammary-specific deletion of this gene can be achieved (Figure 24-1C). Depending on the spatial and temporal expression of the Cre transgene, excision of the floxed target gene occurs only in those cells that expressed active recombinase at any time during its ontogeny. The floxed target gene remains unrecombined in all those cells that lacked Cre expression. Since a complete inactivation requires the Cre-mediated deletion of both alleles, it is an advantage to introduce a conventional knockout allele. In progeny that carry the Cre transgene, along with a floxed and a knockout allele, deletion of the floxed gene can be achieved more easily.

Several genetic regulatory elements have been used successfully to target distinct cell types in mammary tissue. The LTR of the mouse mammary tumor virus (MMTV) and promoters of milk protein genes, such as the mouse whey acidic protein gene (WAP) and the ovine β-lactoglobulin gene (BLG), have been used to target growth factors and foreign proteins to various compartments of the mammary epithelium. Other promoters can be utilized for a targeted expression of transgenes in the myoepithelium (keratin 14 promoter) or the adipose stroma (aP2 promoter). Some of these promoters have also been applied to target Cre recombinase to mammary tissue. Formerly, MMTV-Cre, WAP-Cre (17), and BLG-Cre (18) transgenic mice have been reported that express Cre in the ductal and lobuloalveolar epithelium. The aP2-Cre mice can be used to delete genes in adipocytes (19). Transgenic lines with a targeted expression of Cre in the fibrous stroma or myoepithelium have not yet been published. However, no promoters are available to date that permit the expression of Cre exclusively in connective tissues of the mammary gland.

MMTV-Cre Transgenic Lines

The value of a Cre transgenic line for tissue-specific gene deletion is determined by at least two parameters: First, the amount of background recombination in other organs due to a "leakiness" of the regulatory elements in the transgene or the site of integration. Second, the extent of recombination within defined cell types as the result of a mosaic expression pattern of the Cre transgene. Although "tissue-specific" promoters have been used successfully to target growth factors to various cell types, many may not be adequate to regulate Cre recombinase expression tightly (20). Transient activation of the transgene during earlier developmental stages leads to low levels of Cre expression, which in turn can result in significant background recombination. For example, the MMTV–LTR is highly expressed in only a few tissues of adult mice, but MMTV-Cre-mediated recombination was detected in most organs, indicating that the LTR was active at earlier developmental stages or at constant low levels (17). This expression pattern is not dependent on the integration site of the transgene since it was observed in four independent lines. Some MMTV-Cre strains even exhibit extensive recombination in the female germ line, which seems to be integration-site dependent. The germ-line recombination was verified by crossing wild-type males with females that had the MMTV-Cre transgene and one floxed allele of an endogenous locus. The transmission of the floxed allele was analyzed in mice of the subsequent generation that had inherited the loxP locus but not the Cre transgene (segregated loxP allele). The MMTV-Cre line A shows a 100% recombination efficiency in oocytes, whereas the line D does not show any recombination in germ cells (Wagner, unpublished). Because of this feature, the MMTV-Cre line A was used successfully in several experiments to create complete knockout alleles from floxed loci (Rucker and Wagner, unpublished).

Despite the fact that MMTV-Cre mice exhibit background recombination in a variety of organs, these strains are still valuable for mammary-specific gene deletion experiments. In contrast to conventional belief, a mosaic deletion of genes that are essential for early embryonic development did not result in prenatal lethality (21; Wagner and Rucker, unpublished). MMTV-Cre transgenic mice can be used to delete genes in the ductal epithelium of virgin females without administration of exogenous hormones (17). This feature is important not only for studying gene function during ductal development but also for modeling specific types of cancer, such as ductal carcinoma *in situ* (21), and for experiments that require treatment of mice with mutagens such as DMBA or radiation. Nevertheless, the amount and timing of MMTV-Cre-mediated recombination in the ductal epithelium of various lines remains to be determined when suitable reporter mice become available.

If MMTV-Cre mice are to be used in mammary-specific gene deletion experiments one needs to be aware of several important limitation. All lines, regardless of their ability to recombine floxed loci in the germ line, exhibit Cre-mediated recombination in many tissues, including the tail. If a PCR assay on DNA of a tail biopsy is used to verify the genotype of a given mouse that has inherited the MMTV-Cre transgene from one parent and a loxP allele from the other parent, it is also possible to identify a recombined locus. Therefore, it is not a PCR artifact if three alleles (wild type, floxed, recombined–null) are detected in these transgenic mice. In fact, the PCR assay for the recombined allele can be used to verify the presence of MMTV-Cre in intercrosses (F1 generation). However, it is practically impossible to determine exactly the genotype by PCR in the subsequent (F2) generation when a recombined–null allele is used in combination with a floxed locus and a MMTV-Cre transgene. The null–recombined allele can be detected in mice that have inherited the MMTV-Cre transgene and either two floxed alleles or one floxed and one null–recombined allele. This problem can be bypassed by using Southern blotting or a null allele from a conventional knockout that can be detected independently from the floxed or recombined locus in a separate PCR assay. Another option to avoid this obstacle is a specific mating strategy. There are no limitations in breeding schemes if one utilizes exclusively floxed alleles in combination with MMTV-Cre lines that do not show any expression of Cre in the germ line, for instance mice of the MMTV-Cre line D. Alternatively, the following mating scheme can be applied if one uses a null–recombined allele of a gene of interest (GOI) to increase the recombination efficiency:

$$\text{Female or male} \qquad \text{Male or female}$$
$$\text{MMTV-Cre(D) GOI}^{\text{null/wild type}} \times \text{MMTV-Cre(D) GOI}^{\text{lox/lox}}$$

Homozygous knockout (null) mice could be used to simplify the breeding strategy if this genotype does not lead to early lethality or reproductive problems. The breeding scheme has to be modified if a strain is used that expresses Cre in the female germ line, such as MMTV-Cre line A. For maintaining a nonrecombined loxP allele of the GOI one needs to follow this breeding strategy:

$$\text{Female} \qquad \text{Male}$$
$$\text{GOI}^{\text{lox/lox}} \times \text{MMTV-Cre(A) GOI}^{\text{lox/lox}}$$

A breeding strategy with a null allele via Cre-mediated recombination in the female germ line is very simple and can be performed efficiently with this mating scheme:

Female   Male

MMTV-Cre(A) GOI$^{lox/lox}$ × MMTV-Cre(A) GOI$^{lox/lox}$

Since all floxed loci will be recombined in the oocyte, all littermates will inherit uniformly a null–recombined allele from the mother and a floxed locus from the father. This efficient breeding strategy is only suitable when the GOI is not essential for oocyte development. It might be problematic if a deletion of the gene affects the survival of the pups due to the inability of the female to lactate. In that case the pups can be fostered, or the matings have to be performed in a less efficient way by using MMTV-Cre(A) GOI$^{lox/wild\ type}$ or GOI$^{null/wild\ type}$ females.

Cre Expression under Regulatory Elements of Milk Protein Genes

WAP-Cre (17) and BLG-Cre (18) transgenic mice are valuable tools to delete genes specifically from the mammary epithelium. Since WAP and BLG are milk protein genes, it is not surprising that Cre-mediated recombination increased during pregnancy and peaked at lactation. Between 50% and 80% of the epithelium underwent recombination (18, 22), and both strains exhibited very little recombination in other tissues. We have evidence to suggest that these low levels of recombination are of no physiological consequences. For instance, the deletion of the *Bcl-x* gene from the mouse genome results in massive neuronal cell death (23), but the low-level recombination in the brain of WAP-Cre/*Bcl-x*$^{loxP/null}$ mice is without apparent physiological consequences (Rucker, unpublished). Since Cre expression in the WAP-Cre and BLG-Cre transgenic mice is highest during pregnancy and lactation, they can be used to delete genes in these stages of mammogenesis. In contrast, the recombination efficiency is significantly lower in virgin mice. Although the secretory epithelium undergoes programmed cell death after the pups are weaned, some recombined cells remain in the gland of WAP-Cre transgenics (17). During subsequent pregnancies those cells probably give rise to a new population of epithelium with pre-recombined alleles, thus explaining the higher recombination efficiency in subsequent pregnancies.

WAP-Cre mice have been used to delete the *Brca1* gene specifically from the mammary epithelium (21). The loss of BRCA1 resulted in abnormal ductal outgrowth and the formation of mammary tumors after a long latency. BRCA1 deficiency led to genetic instability and increased apoptosis. In subsequent pregnancies, WAP-Cre expression initiated numerous recombination events. This was essential for the onset of tumorigenesis in this disease model and is important from a technical perspective. For example, a single recombination event initiated by transient expression of Cre via adenoviral vectors (AdCre) during the first pregnancy did not result in the induction of tumors despite a reasonably large number of recombined cells. Those manipulated cells could be detected by PCR also after several pregnancies, but no tumors originated in AdCre-treated *Brca1*$^{fl/null}$ females during a period of 20 months (Wagner and Xu, unpublished). Therefore, we hypothesize that WAP-Cre expression is necessary to generate an increasing number of BRCA1-deficient cells during every pregnancy period. These cells are susceptible to alterations of the DNA since they are rapidly dividing and, coincidentally, lack BRCA1. The BRCA1 protein is a caretaker, not a gatekeeper. Among other functions, BRCA1 has been suggested to act in a complex with proteins (e.g., Rad51) that are essential for DNA repair. In the mammary gland, the expression of BRCA1 is elevated in dividing epithelial cells especially during pregnancy (for a review see Ref. 24).

Hence, WAP-Cre-mediated *Brca1* gene deletion during pregnancy predisposes a large pool of cells to acquire additional mutations. We do not know whether these mutations follow a common pattern. However, some mutations frequently affect gatekeeper genes such as *Trp53* (21).

Improved Cre Transgenic Strains for Mammary-Specific Gene Deletion

Because of the inherent limitations encountered in the MMTV-Cre, WAP-Cre, and BLG-Cre mice, it may be necessary to introduce additional levels of control. First, an inducible Cre recombinase can be utilized either through dual systems, such as the tetracycline inducible system (25), or the fusion of Cre to other regulatory proteins, such as estrogen receptor (26), progesterone receptor (27), or glucocorticoid receptor binding domains (28). Second, the inducible Cre recombinase needs to be targeted to the mammary gland in such a way that the window of Cre expression is expanded and the mosaic expression of the transgene is minimized. Unfortunately, both criteria cannot be fully accomplished with the genetic tools available today. For instance, the efficiency of recombination in binary inducible systems is unsatisfactory (25), and the utilization of hormone binding domains in Cre fusion constructs has limitations since all ligands (estrogen, tamoxifen, dexamethasone, etc.) are also biologically active in the gland. The mosaic expression of a Cre transgene in the mammary epithelial compartment may be eliminated through a knock-in approach, i.e., the insertion of the Cre coding sequence into an endogenous locus that is expressed in the mammary gland. An earlier expression of this locus in other organs is not a limiting factor when it is combined with one of the Cre inducible systems mentioned.

Cre Expression in the Mammary Gland through Adenovirus-Mediated Gene Transfer

Adenovirus-mediated gene transfer is a suitable approach for the temporal expression of Cre. Recombinant adenoviral (Ad) vectors are able to infect nondividing cells without integrating into the genome of the host. Therefore, they are perfect tools to shuttle foreign genes into a variety of tissues. Cre has been targeted successfully with Ad vectors to various cell types *in vitro* (29) and *in vivo* (30, 31). To examine the possible utilization of those vectors for a mammary gland-specific gene deletion, we have delivered an AdCre vector to mammary tissue by surgical injection. Furthermore, we have infected primary mammary epithelial cells with AdCre in an attempt to combine an *in vitro* gene deletion technology with the mammary transplantation method (22).

Direct Injection of AdCre into the Mammary Gland

MATERIALS AND INSTRUMENTATION.   Although recombinant adenoviral vectors are replication deficient, special care should be taken to avoid contamination or self-infection. The production and purification of adenovirus require a P2 cell culture facility, and we recommend performing the transfer of the vectors into the mouse in a biosafety hood. Infected instruments should be sterilized, and all nonrecyclable materials should be treated as biological waste. The following instruments and materials should be available: dissecting microscope (e.g., Zeiss Stemi SV11), 50- or 100-μl Hamilton syringe with a 25-gauge ($\frac{5}{8}$ inch) needle (purchased from Thomas Scientific), cotton swab, cork board, wound clips, and other instruments to perform a surgery as described by Robinson *et al.* in Chapter 26 this volume (2).

REAGENTS AND REAGENT PREPARATION

1. A recombinant adenovirus vector containing a CAG-Cre transgene (AxCANCre) was described earlier (29). CAG is a ubiquitously expressed regulatory element containing the cytomegalovirus (CMV) immediate early enhancer and regulatory elements of chicken β-actin promoter.

2. The adenovirus was propagated in 293 cells (Quantum Biotechnology, Canada) and purified according to a procedure described in detail by Li *et al.* in Chapter 21, this volume (32). The purified virus was stored in 20- to 50-μl aliquots (2.8×10^9 pfu) at −70°C. The viral stock was thawed on wet ice, diluted 1 : 10 with chilled 1 × PBS (Gibco BRL), and used instantly for injection. The dilution step is important to adjust the final virus concentration and to lower the glycerol concentration to ensure maximum infectivity.

DETAILED PROCEDURES. The mice were anesthetized and placed under a dissecting microscope. Initially we tried to inject the viral solution through the nipple by using a fine glass needle. However, we were not able to inject enough solution to penetrate the gland. Instead, we delivered the virus by surgical injection into one inguinal gland (no. 4) as shown in Figure 24-2. For the surgical procedure refer to Chapter 26 in this volume (2). The skin was dissected from the body wall and the gland was exposed by pinning the skin flap to a cork board. A 100-μl Hamilton syringe with a 25-gauge needle was used to administer the viral solution. The preferred injection site was close to the nipple at the base of the ductal tree. The viral

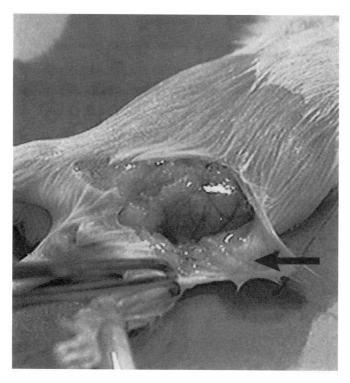

Figure 24-2. Exposure of the left gland no. 4 prior to injection with recombinant adenovirus by surgical means. The arrow indicates the injection site near the ductal base.

solution (10 to 30 μl) was injected very slowly into the gland. This procedure leads quite often to an accumulation of fluids in the form of a small cyst. Most of the viral solution stayed in place after the needle was cautiously withdrawn from the injection site. Occasionally, very small amounts of liquid appeared after retraction, and cotton swabs were used to remove them immediately. After injection, the surgical site was closed with wound clips. All materials used during the procedure were disinfected immediately, autoclaved, and disposed according to safety guidelines for hazardous materials.

IMPORTANT NOTES.   A single injection is sufficient to infect a large portion of the mammary gland no. 4 as determined by co-injection of a Cre vector and a loxP reporter virus (22). Since the Cre construct contains the CAG promoter, it expresses transiently in all cell types (epithelium or stroma) that are susceptible to adenoviral infection. We conclude from our co-injection experiment that adenoviral vectors infect predominantly the epithelial compartment and to a lesser degree adipocytes. The virus is able to migrate a considerable distance from the basis of the ductal tree (injection site) through smaller ducts into the alveolar compartment. This suggests that most of the viral solution spreads through the ductal system and less of the suspension migrates through the fat pad. However, we also observed a massive invasion of lymphocytes into all regions of the gland.

Once injected, AdCre can efficiently mediate the recombination between loxP sites on chromosomes *in vivo*. Three days after the viral transfer, the recombination was examined by PCR on a reporter construct (22) and the floxed *Brca1* locus (Wagner and Xu, unpublished). Mammary-specific recombination was achieved in virgin, pregnant, and lactating glands. Among all other organs that were analyzed for background recombination, only the liver showed detectable amounts of Cre-mediated gene deletion. The liver-specific Cre activation was found repeatedly, and we assume that viral particles migrated from the mammary gland via the circulation to that organ. The passage of viral particles into the capillary system of the bloodstream could have been caused by the surgical injection method. As shown previously, the liver is extremely susceptible to adenovirus infection when viral particles were injected intravenously (31).

Furthermore, we could demonstrate that mammary gland remodeling during involution influences the amount of recombination (22). AdCre injection during the first pregnancy resulted in satisfactory recombination efficiencies. However, when analyzed during the second pregnancy cycle, 6 to 8 weeks after virus administration, only a few recombined cells remained in the mammary gland and the recombination efficiency decreased significantly. These observations suggest that mammary gland remodeling during the reproductive phase has a significant influence on the recombination efficiency. This may distinguish the mammary gland from other organs that do not undergo cyclic renewal of various cell types. These data are of particular interest when this technology is applied for studies in the mammary gland that require a high amount of recombination over a long period of time in order to determine a measurable effect of the deleted gene on the physiology of the gland. Under experimental conditions using an inactive floxed transgene, there was also no selective pressure on either the recombined or unrecombined allele. However, the loss of BRCA1 due to Cre-mediated excision leads to programmed cell death because of genomic instability and the subsequent activation of apoptotic pathways. Taken together, there are several intracellular and extracellular mechanisms that can have a profound influence on the efficiency of gene deletion by using AdCre: (1) loss of cells due to immune response against viral proteins in infected tissues; (2) loss of cells due to apoptosis at the end of each consecutive reproductive cycle; (3) loss of cells triggered by apoptotic pathways due to the Cre-mediated excision of the targeted gene. Nevertheless, a reduced level of recombination in subsequent pregnancies may not be a limiting factor for a mammary-specific knockout of a tumor suppressor gene that is a gatekeeper rather than a caretaker. In that case, the recombination event could lead to a selective amplification of the remaining recombined cells (i.e., tumor formation).

A POTENTIAL COMBINATION OF MAMMARY TRANSPLANTATION AND AdCre-MEDIATED GENE DELETION

The property of mammary epithelium to undergo extensive remodeling after weaning raised experimental problems in utilizing the adenoviral approach to delete genes in the gland. However, this characteristic might serve as the basis for other emerging Cre-loxP technologies. The presence of stem cells in the gland, which give rise to differentiated cell types of the mammary epithelium (ducts, alveoli), allows an *ex vivo* manipulation and subsequent transplantation of modified epithelial cells. A combination of AdCre with cell transplantation (Figure 24-3) could greatly enhance the recombination efficiency. This approach will require isolation of epithelial cells from a donor with a floxed gene, infection with AdCre, and transplantation of the recombined cells into a recipient with a cleared fat pad. These knockout cells will then contribute to the reconstitution of the ductal tree. In initial studies, we were able to show that HC11 cells (22) and primary epithelial cells (32) can be infected very efficiently with adenovirus and that Cre-mediated recombination can be achieved in culture (22). Primary cells from both virgin and lactating animals showed a considerable amount of excision. Potentially, these cells could be transplanted into a cleared fat pad by using a technique similar to that described by Robinson and co-workers in this volume (2). The success of this

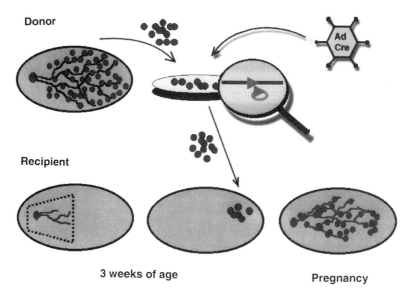

Figure 24-3. Combination of mammary transplantation and AdCre-mediated gene deletion. This approach requires the isolation of epithelial cells from a donor with floxed alleles of a target gene, the infection with AdCre *in vitro*, and the transplantation of the recombined cells into a wild-type recipient. These knockout cells contribute to the reconstitution of the ductal tree if no selection against stem cells with recombined alleles occurs.

technique depends largely on selective mechanisms against recombined stem cells versus unrecombined cells during ductal outgrowth. Nevertheless, when this technology is markedly improved, it will serve as a new tool to study the loss of function of specific genes in the mammary gland.

TRANSGENIC VERSUS ADENOVIRAL APPROACH

An accurate comparison of different techniques for the deletion of genes from mammary tissue is difficult. Generally, it is almost impossible to compare published data about deletion efficiencies between various floxed loci or a particular locus in different organs and simply project these results to the tools used in these specific approaches. The position of the floxed locus and the distance between the loxP sites can greatly influence the recombination efficiency. In addition, selective pressure (positive or negative) on the growth of recombined alleles in different organs may not adequately represent the true extent of recombination. For example, a conditional knockout of *Brca1* in the mammary gland leads to genomic instability and increased apoptosis (21). Therefore, one should expect a different scenario from gene deletions that act in pro-apoptotic pathways. The experimental design will determine whether a transgenic or adenoviral approach should be used. The transgenic approach is clearly the method of choice when high levels of recombination over a longer period of time (e.g., several lactation periods) are required to evaluate physiological effects. For short-term experiments or certain tumorigenicity studies, the adenoviral approach is of particular interest because this method requires less mouse breeding and the recombination event can be achieved at a specific developmental stage (time point of AdCre injection). However, several properties of the AdCre technology need to be improved. First, the immune response against the adenovirus needs to be minimized. The invasion of immune cells into the mammary gland could be significantly lowered through the use of Ad vectors that do not contain viral genes (33) or through the use of lenti viruses. Second, the tissue specificity of Cre expression needs to be improved. AdCre can infect different cell types in the mammary gland. Subsequently, the recombinase excises the floxed gene in all of these cell types since the Cre transgene is under the control of a ubiquitously expressed promoter (e.g., CAG). Therefore, these promoters need to be replaced with regulatory elements for the epithelial compartment. At present, this could be the MMTV–LTR. The utilization of a tissue-specific promoter will also reduce background recombination in other organs.

INSERTION OF loxP RECOGNITION SITES INTO DEFINED LOCI

Gene targeting is a technique that allows for the intentional alteration of a defined locus within the genome. It can be used to delete, change, or insert additional sequences (e.g., loxP sites) into endogenous genes. The general schematic for gene targeting in ES cells and targeting construct design are based on a positive–negative selection system shown in Figure 24-4. The first step of the system is based on using a positive selectable cassette, the neomycin phosphotransferase gene (*neo*), which is flanked by two regions of homology to the target gene. Therefore, random or homologous integration of this DNA results in the resistance of cells to G418. The second step involves the negative selection cassette, the HSV-thymidine kinase gene (TK), which is placed outside the region of homology in the vector. This TK cassette is integrated into the host chromosome if random integration occurs, but it is

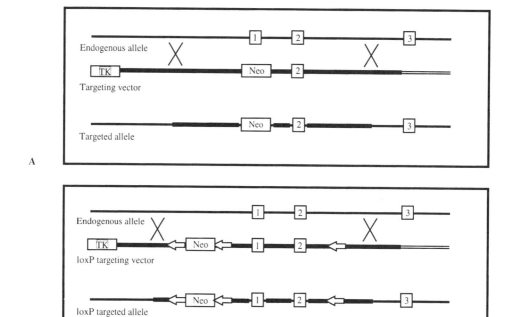

Figure 24-4. Targeting strategy for a conventional gene knockout (A) and the introduction of loxP sites (open arrowhead) for a tissue-specific gene deletion approach (B) based on the positive–negative selection system in embryonic stem cells. (B) The selectable marker, which itself is flanked by loxP sites, is placed in the 5′-upstream region of the gene. The extrinsic loxP site is located 3′ in an intron. Cre-mediated gene deletion can be achieved by recombination between the extrinsic loxP site and either one of the loxP sites of the floxed neomycin cassette. The selectable marker can be removed by partial Cre-mediated recombination between the two loxP sites flanking the neomycin cassette.

removed if homologous recombination takes place. Therefore, adding gancyclovir to the growth medium kills any cells containing the HSV-TK due to random integration.

Figure 24-4A shows a classical gene deletion approach where the promoter and first coding exon of a gene are replaced by a neomycin selectable cassette. In a successful targeting event, crossover occurs between the 5′- and 3′-ends of the homologous DNA sequence and the ES cell genomic DNA. The general targeting strategy is similar in the loxP insertion approach (Figure 24-4B). Here the neomycin selection cassette is placed into a noncoding part of the gene that is also not essential for the regulation of gene expression. The selectable marker is surrounded by loxP sites so that it can be removed by partial recombination if necessary. A third loxP site is inserted on the opposite end of the sequence to be deleted. Excision of the gene is achieved when in the presence of Cre recombinase the outermost loxP site recombines with one of the loxP sites apposed to the selectable marker.

IDENTIFICATION OF TARGETED ES CELLS AND CRE-MEDIATED RECOMBINATION EVENTS *IN VIVO*

In order to distinguish between random integration and homologous recombination in isolated ES cell clones, Southern blot hybridization or PCR is performed. The standard for target verification is Southern blot hybrization with flanking (external sequence not included in the targeting construct) and internal probes at the 5′- and 3′-ends of the targeting event. Southern blots are performed with external probes to verify targeting and with internal probes to determine whether an additional random integration of the targeting vector has occurred in the ES cell clone.

After verifying by Southern blot that the targeted allele has been transmitted through the germ line of chimeric mice, it is faster to screen progeny by PCR for the presence of the floxed allele. For this purpose, PCR primers can be designed that flank the third loxP site, and amplification will reveal an endogenous and a targeted allele in heterozygous mice (Figure 24-5, primers 4 and 5). After crossing the Cre transgene into the homozygous floxed background it is necessary to analyze the different products expected from the Cre-mediated recombination event. These include the endogenous, floxed, floxed markerless (Figure 24-5, type I deletion), and complete deletion alleles (Figure 24-5, type III deletion). Quantitative PCR or Southern blot can be performed to estimate the extent of recombination (floxed allele versus complete deletion) in the mammary gland in comparison to other organs. The functional down-regulation of the target gene in the mammary gland is verified by a decreased amount of transcript or protein (Northern or Western blot, *in situ* hybridization, immunocytochemistry, etc.).

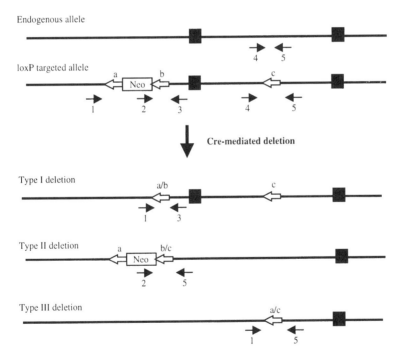

Figure 24-5. Generation of a series of alleles by Cre-mediated recombination following a single targeting event. The introduction of the neomycin selectable marker into various sites of a gene (promoter or intron) can cause hypomorphic or hypermorphic phenotypes. A partial deletion can excise only the selectable marker (type I deletion) or the intervening sequence between marker and exterior loxP site (type II deletion). A complete deletion results in a null allele with only one remaining loxP site in the targeted locus (type III deletion). Solid arrows indicate various PCR primers that can be used in combination to detect the type of Cre-mediated deletion or the presence of a wild type and a floxed allele (primers 4 and 5) for the analysis of the genotype.

In cases when the neomycin selection marker interferes with normal transcription of the gene, the marker should be removed by Cre-mediated recombination either in the ES cells or in the germ line of transgenic mice. Whereas subsequent manipulations on ES cells take the risk that modified ES cells are no longer transmitted through the germ line of chimeric mice, a transgenic approach using EIIa-Cre mice (34) can be employed to excise the floxed neomycin marker *in vivo* (Figure 24-5, type I deletion). The EIIa-Cre transgene exhibits a weak expression in embryonic progenitor cells that contribute to the germ line. This weak Cre expression leads to a partial recombination of the floxed allele, i.e., the elimination of the neomycin cassette. Mice that are heterozygous for the floxed allele and contain the EIIa-Cre transgene should be crossed with wild-type mice for two reasons: first, to verify that recombination has occurred in the germ line and is transmissible; second, to eliminate the Cre transgene that would otherwise cause further gene deletions in subsequent generations. A conditional approach requires breeding to homozygosity of the floxed allele combined with introduction of the Cre transgene. To maximize the extent of recombination it may be necessary to generate mice that carry a null allele (Figure 24-5, type III deletion) and a floxed allele in addition to the Cre transgene. As shown earlier, a null allele can be easily generated by transmitting the floxed allele through the female germline of MMTV-Cre (A) transgenic mice (17).

Although the time and effort are considerable in pursuing the conditional approach, the wealth of information from generating a series of different alleles might outweigh this concern. The altered alleles might display different expression profiles, which then could lead to various phenotypes. For instance, several *N-myc* alleles were generated that gave rise to distinct developmental defects (35). The *Fgf-8* gene, flanked by loxP and frt sites (36), was modified through expression of Cre or Flp recombinase to generate a series of alleles that demonstrated the importance of this gene in gastrulation, cardiac, and brain development. Therefore, a single targeting event can be used to examine a combination of subtle and complex phenotypes in the mouse.

OUTLOOK

A major advantage of the Cre-loxP technology is the interchangeability of its components. Mammary gland researchers will benefit greatly from the numerous mouse lines containing floxed genes previously developed for tissue-specific knockouts in other organs. By simply crossing these floxed alleles into mammary-specific Cre transgenics that are already available, entirely new experimental models can be developed. Nevertheless, the variety of tools for mammary-specific gene deletion needs to be extended, for instance, by combining Cre recombinase with other inducible systems and by using adenoviral Cre vectors in conjunction with epithelial transplantation techniques. It may also be beneficial to generate transgenic lines by targeted insertion of the Cre coding sequence into a milk protein locus to eliminate the mosaic expression of a Cre transgene in the mammary epithelial compartment. However, since milk protein genes and other important loci for mammary gland development and breast cancer are confined to the same chromosome (for example, *Wap*, *Brca1*, and *Trp53* are linked on chromosome 11, and the *Casein* genes and *Brca2* are coupled on chromosome 5), it is in certain cases difficult to achieve the final combination of a Cre transgene, a floxed allele, and a knockout allele by simple mating schemes. Therefore, it is important that different Cre expressing lines including conventional transgenics are accessible to the scientific community.

Cre transgenic mouse strains are useful not only for tissue-specific gene deletions, but also for a tissue-specific activation of transgenes by using a floxed transcriptional stop sequence between a ubiquitously expressed promoter and the protein coding sequence. Such conditionally activated transgenes can be delivered by standard pronuclear injection into zygotes, gene targeting in ES cells, or viral vectors. To date, the latter approach has only been used in reporter constructs to monitor the recombination event (17), but it could also be utilized to express other biologically relevant molecules. Furthermore, it is of great importance to develop a reporter strain that is highly expressed throughout mammary gland development and that allows for the detection of the Cre-mediated recombination within individual cells. A potentially useful reporter line with a targeted *Rosa26* gene was published recently (37) and should be tested specifically for this purpose. A variety of transgenic reporter strains with other ubiquitously expressed promoters have been published, but so far none of them has been utilized successfully in mammary-specific gene deletion experiments.

Although further refinements are necessary, initial technical hurdles to target the Cre specifically to the mammary gland have been conquered. Mammary-specific tools for gene deletion are currently being tested for their efficacy *in vivo* by deleting floxed genes that are suggested to be essential for mammary epithelial development. The WAP-Cre and MMTV-Cre transgenic lines have recently passed this litmus test, since they were utilized to generate the first mouse model for breast cancer by mammary-specific gene targeting (21). These transgenic tools, now distributed by the Jackson Laboratory, will facilitate new insights into the function of genes during mammary development and tumorigenesis.

ACKNOWLEDGMENTS. The authors would like to thank Dr. Izumu Saito for providing us with the adenoviral vectors and Dr. Gertraud W. Robinson and Dr. Daniel Schoeffner for critically reading the manuscript. KUW was supported by a grant from the DFG (Wa-1119/1-1).

NOTE ADDED IN PROOF

WAP-Cre, MMTV-Cre (A), and MMTV-Cre (D) transgenic mice are now available from the Jackson Laboratory under the following strain codes: B6129-TgN(WapCre)11738 Mam, B6129-Tgn(MMTV-Cre)1 Mam, and B6129-Tgn(MMTV-Cre)4 Mam. Recently, BLG-Cre mice have also been used to delete the Stat3 gene in the lactating mammary gland (Chapman *et al. Genes Dev* 1999 13(19):2604–2616), and the first successful attempt to combine the Cre-lox technique with the tetracycline inducible system in the mammary gland has been reported (Utomo *et al. Nat. Biotechnol.* 1999(11):1091–1096).

REFERENCES

1. L. Hennighausen and G. W. Robinson (1998). Think globally, act locally: the making of a mouse mammary gland. *Genes Dev.* **12**(4):449–455.
2. G. W. Robinson, D. Accili, and L. Hennighausen (2000). Rescue of mammary epithelium of early lethal phenotypes by embryonic mammary gland transplantation as exemplified with insulin receptor null mice, Chapter 26 this volume.
3. N. D. Horseman, W. Zhao, E. Montecino-Rodriguez, M. Tanaka, K. Nakashima, S. J. Engle, F. Smith, E. Markoff, and K. Dorshkind (1997). Defective mammopoiesis, but normal hematopoiesis, in mice with a targeted disruption of the prolactin gene. *EMBO J.* **16**:6926–6935.
4. K. U. Wagner, W. S. Young, X. Liu, E. I. Ginns, M. Li, P. A. Furth, and L. Hennighausen (1997). Oxytocin and milk removal are required for post-partum mammary-gland development. *Genes and Function* **1**(4):233–244.
5. J. R. Brown, H. Ye, R. T. Bronson, P. Dikkes, and M. E. Greenberg (1996). A defect in nurturing in mice lacking the immediate early gene fosB. *Cell* **86**:297–309.

6. L. A. Donehower, M. Harvey, H. Vogel, M. J. McArthur, C. A. J. Montgomery, S. H. Park, T. Thompson, R. J. Ford, and A. Bradley (1996). Effects of genetic background on tumorigenesis in p53-deficient mice. *Mol. Carcinog.* **14**:16–22.

7. D. W. Threadgill, A. A. Dlugosz, L. A. Hansen, T. Tennenbaum, U. Lichti, D. Yee, C. LaMantia, T. Mourton, K. Herrup, and R. C. Harris (1995). Targeted disruption of mouse EGF receptor: effect of genetic background on mutant phenotype. *Science* **269**:230–234.

8. T. Jacks, A. Fazeli, E. M. Schmitt, R. T. Bronson, M. A. Goodell, and R. A. Weinberg (1992). Effects of an Rb mutation in the mouse. *Nature* **359**:295–300.

9. B. Sauer and N. Henderson (1988). Site-specific DNA recombination in mammalian cells by the Cre recombinase of bacteriophage P1. *Proc. Natl. Acad. Sci. U.S.A.* **85**:5166–5170.

10. P. C. Orban, D. Chui, and J. D. Marth (1992). Tissue- and site-specific DNA recombination in transgenic mice. *Proc. Natl. Acad. Sci. U.S.A.* **89**:6861–6865.

11. M. Lakso, B. Sauer, B. J. Mosinger, E. J. Lee, R. W. Manning, S. H. Yu, K. L. Mulder, and H. Westphal (1992). Targeted oncogene activation by site-specific recombination in transgenic mice. *Proc. Natl. Acad. Sci. U.S.A.* **89**:6232–6236.

12. H. Gu, J. D. Marth, P. C. Orban, H. Mossmann, and K. Rajewsky (1994). Deletion of a DNA polymerase beta gene segment in T cells using cell type-specific gene targeting. *Science* **265**:103–106.

13. F. Buchholz, P. O. Angrand, and A. F. Stewart (1998). Improved properties of FLP recombinase evolved by cycling mutagenesis. *Nat. Biotechnol.* **16**:657–662.

14. E. Marshall (1998). NIH, DuPont declare truce in mouse war. *Science* **281**:1261–1262.

15. R. Ramirez-Solis, P. Liu, and A. Bradley (1995). Chromosome engineering in mice. *Nature* **378**:720–724.

16. J. Van Deursen, M. Fornerod, B. Van Rees, and G. Grosveld (1995). Cre-mediated site-specific translocation between nonhomologous mouse chromosomes. *Proc. Natl. Acad. Sci. U.S.A.* **92**:7376–7380.

17. K. U. Wagner, R. J. Wall, L. St.-Onge, P. Gruss, A. Wynshaw-Boris, L. Garrett, M. Li, P. A. Furth, and L. Hennighausen (1997). Cre-mediated gene deletion in the mammary gland. *Nucleic Acids Res.* **25**(21):4323–4330.

18. S. Selbert, D. J. Bentley, D. W. Melton, D. Rannie, P. Lourenco, C. J. Watson, and A. R. Clarke (1998). Efficient BLG-Cre mediated gene deletion in the mammary gland. *Transgenic Res.* **7**:387–396.

19. C. Barlow, M. Schroeder, J. Lekstrom-Himes, H. Kylefjord, C. X. Deng, A. Wynshaw-Boris, B. M. Spiegelman, and K. G. Xanthopoulos (1997). Targeted expression of Cre recombinase to adipose tissue of transgenic mice directs adipose-specific excision of loxP-flanked gene segments [published erratum appears in *Nucleic Acids Res.* **25**(21):4429 (1997)]. *Nucleic Acids Res.* **25**:2543–2545.

20. U. A. Betz, C. A. Vosshenrich, K. Rajewsky, and W. Muller (1996). Bypass of lethality with mosaic mice generated by Cre-loxP-mediated recombination. *Curr. Biol.* **6**:1307–1316.

21. X. Xu, K. U. Wagner, D. Larson, Z. Weaver, C. Li, T. Ried, L. Hennighausen, A. Wynshaw-Boris, and C. X. Deng (1999). Conditional mutation of Brca1 in mammary epithelial cells results in blunted ductal morphogenesis and tumour formation. *Nat. Genet.* **22**:37–43.

22. K. U. Wagner (1998). Adenoviral and transgenic approaches to delete genes from mammary tissue via Cre-lox recombination. Workshop on Conditional Genetic Technologies in the Mouse, Cold Spring Harbor Laboratory, August 31–September 2, 1998. The multimedia online lecture (audio and slide presentation) is accessible at http://www.leadingstrand.org.

23. N. Motoyama, F. Wang, K. A. Roth, H. Sawa, K. Nakayama, I. Negishi, S. Senju, Q. Zhang, and S. Fujii (1995). Massive cell death of immature hematopoietic cells and neurons in Bcl-x-deficient mice. *Science* **267**:1506–1510.

24. L. A. Chodosh (1998). Expression of BRCA1 and BRCA2 in normal and neoplastic cells. *J. Mammary Gland Biol.* **3**(4):389–402.

25. L. St.-Onge, P. A. Furth, and P. Gruss (1996). Temporal control of the Cre recombinase in transgenic mice by a tetracycline responsive promoter. *Nucleic Acids Res.* **24**:3875–3877.

26. Y. Zhang, C. Riesterer, A. M. Ayrall, F. Sablitzky, T. D. Littlewood, and M. Reth (1996). Inducible site-directed recombination in mouse embryonic stem cells. *Nucleic Acids Res.* **24**:543–548.

27. C. Kellendonk, F. Tronche, A. P. Monaghan, P. O. Angrand, F. Stewart, and G. Schutz (1996). Regulation of Cre recombinase activity by the synthetic steroid RU 486. *Nucleic Acids Res.* **24**:1404–1411.

28. J. Brocard, R. Feil, P. Chambon, and D. Metzger (1998). A chimeric Cre recombinase inducible by synthetic, but not by natural ligands of the glucocorticoid receptor. *Nucleic Acids Res.* **26**:4086–4090.

29. Y. Kanegae, G. Lee, Y. Sato, M. Tanaka, M. Nakai, T. Sakaki, S. Sugano, and I. Saito (1995). Efficient gene activation in mammalian cells by using recombinant adenovirus expressing site-specific Cre recombinase. *Nucleic Acids Res.* **23**:3816–3821.

30. Y. Wang, L. A. Krushel, and G. M. Edelman (1996). Targeted DNA recombination in vivo using an aden-ovirus carrying the cre recombinase gene. *Proc. Natl. Acad. Sci. U.S.A.* **93**:3932–3936.

31. Y. H. Lee, B. Sauer, P. F. Johnson, and F. J. Gonzalez (1997). Disruption of the c/ebp alpha gene in adult mouse liver. *Mol. Cell Biol.* **17**:6014–6022.

32. M. Li, K. U. Wagner, and P. A. Furth (1999). Transfection of primary mammary epithelial cells by viral and nonviral methods, Chapter 21 this volume.

33. R. J. Parks, L. Chen, M. Anton, U. Sankar, M. A. Rudnicki, and F. L. Graham (1996). A helper-dependent adenovirus vector system: removal of helper virus by Cre-mediated excision of the viral packaging signal. *Proc. Natl. Acad. Sci. U.S.A.* **93**:13565–13570.

34. M. Lakso, J. G. Pichel, J. R. Gorman, B. Sauer, Y. Okamoto, E. Lee, F. W. Alt, and H. Westphal (1996). Effi-cient *in vivo* manipulation of mouse genomic sequences at the zygote stage. *Proc. Natl. Acad. Sci. U.S.A.* **93**:5860–5865.

35. A. Nagy, C. Moens, E. Ivanyi, J. Pawling, M. Gertsenstein, A. K. Hadjantonakis, M. Pirity, and J. Rossant (1998). Dissecting the role of N-myc in development using a single targeting vector to generate a series of alleles. *Curr. Biol.* **8**:661–664.

36. E. N. Meyers, M. Lewandoski, and G. R. Martin (1998). An Fgf8 mutant allelic series generated by Cre- and Flp-mediated recombination. *Nat. Genet.* **18**:136–141.

37. P. Soriano (1999). Generalized lacZ expression with the ROSA26 Cre reporter strain. *Nat. Genet.* **21**:70–71.

Chapter 25

Transplantation and Tissue Recombination Techniques to Study Mammary Gland Biology

Gerald R. Cunha, Yun Kit Hom, Peter Young, and Joel Brody

Abstract.   Because certain mutant transgenic mice die prematurely or are infertile, the study of the mammary gland is hampered. To circumvent this problem, mammary transplantation techniques can be used to "rescue" mammary glands from embryonic or neonatal lethal mutants. Similarly, for infertile mutants transplantation techniques can be used to grow mammary glands under all types of hormonal conditions. This chapter gives detailed technical protocols for transplantation techniques and methods for preparing tissue recombinants composed of embryonic mammary mesenchyme and epithelium or mammary fat pad and epithelium. These procedures greatly extend the utility of many of the transgenic and gene knockout mice that are available.

Abbreviations. α-estrogen receptor knockout (α-ERKO); β-estrogen receptor knockout (β-ERKO); progesterone receptor knockout (PRKO); prolactin receptor knockout (PrlR-KO).

INTRODUCTION

The availability of numerous types of transgenic and gene knockout mice has allowed the *in vivo* analysis of the molecular pathways that regulate growth, development, and carcinogenesis of the mammary gland. For those mutant mouse strains that are fully viable, the mammary gland is available for investigation at all developmental stages (embryonic to senescent stages). However, for certain mutant mice the study of the mammary gland is hampered because the mutants die prematurely during embryonic, neonatal, or early adult stages. Alternatively, certain mutant mice may not be fertile, and therefore they are not capable of becoming pregnant. This hampers analysis of the mammary gland during pregnancy and lactation. In this chapter, methods are described to overcome these limitations through the use of tissue transplantation and epithelial–mesenchymal tissue recombination technology.

Gerald R. Cunha, Yun Kit Hom, Peter Young, and Joel Brody   **Department of Anatomy, University of California, San Francisco, California 94143.**

Methods in Mammary Gland Biology and Breast Cancer Research, edited by Ip and Asch. Kluwer Academic/Plenum Publishers, New York, 2000.

RESCUE OF DEVELOPING MAMMARY GLANDS: GENERAL CONSIDERATIONS

Many of the techniques described in this chapter utilize the dissection of tissues from donor animals (embryos, neonates, or adults) as well as surgical transplantation techniques. For both purposes standard dissecting instruments will be required along with certain more specialized items. The following materials and equipment are needed:

- Dissecting microscope with illumination capabilities above and below the specimen stage
- Dissecting instruments (scissors of various sizes, forceps of various sizes, including no. 5 Dumont forceps (Cat. No. 11251-20, Fine Science Tools, Foster City, CA)
- Graefe microdissecting knife (Cat. No. 10071-12, Fine Science Tools)
- Spring-loaded Vannas scissors (Cat. No. 15100-09, Fine Science Tools)
- Pasteur pipettes
- Hank's salt solution
- Maximov depression slides (Fisher, Pittsburgh, PA)
- 1-ml tuberculin syringes, wound clips, and applicator (Fisher)
- Avertin (see the sequel) or Nembutal (Abbot Laboratories, North Chicago, IL)

The basic method involves the grafting of microdissected mammary tissue obtained from the donor at least 1 day prior to its expected demise. The microdissected mammary rudiment can be grafted into a mammary fat pad devoid of epithelium (cleared fat pad) or to other sites, such as beneath the renal capsule. The hormonal status of the host can be manipulated experimentally according to the goal of the experiment. Important considerations include selection of the graft site, age of the mutant mouse donor, type of mutant, and endocrine parameters.

SELECTION OF THE GRAFT SITE

Choice of the graft site is influenced by the goal of the experiment and, especially, whether the mutation affects the mammary epithelium, stroma, or both. In cases in which the gene in question is expressed in both epithelium and stroma–fat pad, gene knockout eliminates the gene simultaneously from both tissues. For example, in the epidermal growth factor receptor knockout (EGFR-KO) mouse epithelial and stromal cells are devoid of the EGF receptor. If EGFR-KO epithelium is grafted into a cleared mammary fat pad of a nude mouse, it should be recognized that the fat pad of the nude mouse is wild type with respect to the EGFR. For this reason, transplantation of EGFR-KO mammary epithelium into a wild-type nude mouse fat pad creates a chimeric mammary gland with wild-type stroma and EGFR-KO epithelium. Such a construct is different from an EGFR-KO mammary gland in which EGFR signaling is simultaneously absent in the mammary epithelium and in the fat pad. Since EGFR-KO mice usually die in the neonatal period, the only method of determining the mammary phenotype in EGFR-KO mice is through whole mammary gland transplantation. Such "rescued" EGFR-KO mammary glands exhibited severely impaired ductal growth (1). Thus, when the genetic manipulation affects epithelium and stroma simultaneously, the phenotype of mutant mammary rudiments must be assessed by grafting the entire mammary rudiment (fat pad and ducts) to a "neutral" graft site. For this purpose complete mammary gland rudiments can be isolated from mutant embryos or neonates and grafted under the renal capsule or to subcutaneous sites of syngeneic or athymic nude mouse hosts. In these graft sites mammary gland development will usually not be influenced by host wild-type cells of the graft site.

Renal Capsule Graft Site

Immunologic parameters must be considered so that the graft will not be rejected. If the donor tissue is from an inbred strain of mouse (or rat), the recipient host should be from the same strain. If the donor is an outbred mouse or a mouse of mixed genetic background, an immuno-incompetent host should be used. For almost all experiments the athymic nude mouse is the host of choice because of its relatively low cost. The outbred CD-1 athymic nude mouse is an excellent inexpensive recipient host. The athymic nude mouse has a low level of residual immunologic function and, in some cases, has been known to reject grafts (2). If grafts are rejected or if severe lymphocytic infiltration is observed in histological sections of the grafts, it is advisable to use a completely immuno-incompetent recipient host, such as the SCID mouse.

The process of renal capsule grafting is described and illustrated in detail in the following website: http://mammary.nih.gov/tools/mousework/Cunha001/index.html. The first step is anesthetizing the recipient host with Avertin or Nembutal. Avertin is prepared with 2,2,2-tribromoethanol and *tert*-amyl alcohol (Aldrich, Milwaukee, WI). To make the Avertin stock solution, 25 g of tribromoethanol is dissolved in 1.5 ml of *tert*-amyl alcohol heated to 40–50°C. When completely dissolved wrap the bottle in aluminum foil and store at 4°C. The working solution is made by mixing 19.75 ml Hank's salt solution with 0.25 ml of the Avertin stock. The mixture is warmed and stirred to dissolve the stock. The dosage is 0.02 ml/g body weight (e.g., 25-g mouse receives 0.5 ml) by intraperitoneal injection. Alternatively, Nembutal (Abbot Laboratories) can be used. Nembutal comes as a 50 mg/ml stock solution. This concentrated stock solution is diluted to 6 mg/ml with a diluent of ethanol, propylene glycol, and distilled water (1 : 2 : 7). The final dose given is 0.01 ml/g body weight by intraperitoneal injection.

The surgical method for renal capsule grafting is as follows. Animals are weighed and anesthetized by Avertin (125 mg/kg) or Nembutal (50–90 mg/kg) or as recommended by your local Animal Care Committee. The back skin is lifted with a pair of blunt forceps. A midline incision is made in the skin with scissors approximately an inch in length. The skin is separated by blunt dissection from the underlying body wall on both sides of the skin incision for bilateral grafting or on one side only. The animal is placed on its side, and the location of the kidney is identified by viewing it through the relatively transparent body wall. An incision is made in the body wall approximately the length of the long axis of the kidney. The kidney is "popped out" of the incision in the body wall by applying pressure on either side of the kidney using the forefinger and thumb. The exteriorized kidney is allowed to rest externally on the body wall. In female hosts, extrusion of the kidney from the body cavity can be facilitated by pulling on the ovarian fat pad (at the lower pole of the kidney) with a pair of blunt forceps and gently guiding the kidney through the opening in the body wall. A pair of no. 5 forceps is used to gently pinch and lift the delicate renal capsule from the parenchyma of the kidney so that a 2- to 4-mm incision can be made in the capsule with fine spring-loaded scissors. The size of the incision in the capsule is determined by the size of the graft. A glass Pasteur pipette, which has been drawn thin and fire-polished with a rounded closed end, is manipulated under the capsule tangential to the surface of the kidney. By blunt dissection a pocket is created between the renal capsule and the parenchyma. Great care should be taken not to damage the renal parenchyma to minimize bleeding. Grafts are transferred to the surface of the kidney by using a blunt scalpel. The cut edge of the kidney capsule is lifted with a pair of fine forceps, and the graft is pushed into the pocket under the capsule by using the

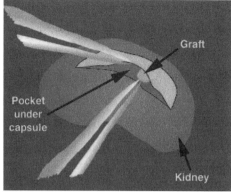

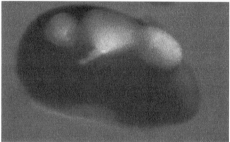

Figure 25-1. (Upper) With no. 5 forceps the renal capsule is pinched and lifted from the underlying renal parenchyma so that a 2- to 4-mm incision can be made in the capsule with fine spring-loaded scissors. A finely drawn fire-polished glass Pasteur pipette is manipulated under the capsule to create a pocket between the renal capsule and the parenchyma. Grafts are transferred to the surface of the kidney by using a blunt scalpel. The cut edge of the kidney capsule is lifted with a pair of fine forceps, and the graft is pushed into the pocket under the capsule by the polished glass pipette or forceps. (Lower) Grafts of neonatal mouse mammary glands grown under the renal capsule after 1 month of growth.

polished glass pipette or forceps (Figure 25-1a). Figure 25-1b shows a renal graft of a neonatal mouse mammary gland after 1 month of growth.

Graft size is an important issue. Although the grafts can be large (covering up to half of the surface of the kidney), graft thickness should not exceed 2 mm. Implantation of grafts thicker than 2 mm will result in central necrosis of the graft prior to establishment of vascularization. Several small grafts can be placed under the kidney capsule with no apparent ill effect to the host. If, during the course of grafting, the capsule becomes dehydrated, it should be moistened with physiologic saline. When grafting is complete, the kidney is gently eased back into the body cavity with forceps. The operation can be repeated with the contralateral kidney. When grafting is finished, the body wall is sutured, and the edges of the back skin are aligned and closed with wound clips. The animal is allowed to recover in the absence of nonanesthetized animals.

Subcutaneous Graft Site

The goal of a subcutaneous graft site is to insert the graft into a subcutaneous pocket between the skin and the muscular body wall positioned between mammary glands 3 and 4 in such a manner that the grafted mammary tissue does not contact the adjacent mammary glands. For this procedure it is essential to know the exact positions of the no. 3 and no. 4 mammary glands. Thus, prior examination of the spatial distribution of the mammary glands should be ascertained by reflecting the ventral skin laterally from the midline on "practice animals." Once the positions of no. 3 and no. 4 mammary glands are known, a 1-cm incision is made through the skin mid-ventrally with scissors in anesthetized mouse or rat hosts midway between the positions of mammary glands 3 and 4. By blunt dissection pockets are created on both sides between the skin and the muscular body wall, extending about 1.5 cm laterally. A mammary gland graft is inserted into the subcutaneous pocket. This procedure can be repeated on the contralateral side. Finally, the skin incision is closed with wound clips, and the animal is allowed to recover. Take rate is usually lower in subcutaneous versus renal grafts sites because the renal site is more vascular than the subcutaneous site.

Cleared Mammary Fat Pad Graft Site

Supplies for preparing cleared mammary fat pad are similar to those required for rescue of mammary rudiments. A cautery device (Arista, New York, NY) is a useful addition. The cleared mammary fat pad is the graft site of choice when the mutation (transgene or null gene) only affects the epithelium. The technique of grafting mammary epithelial tissue into the cleared mammary fat pad was developed decades ago by De Ome's group at UC Berkeley (3). This technique is fully illustrated in an NIH website (http://mammary.nih.gov/tools/mouse-work/index.html) and is described in this volume by Young (Chapter 6). This technique takes advantage of the fact that at 3 weeks, postnatal mammary ducts are near the nipple. At 3 weeks of age, the female mouse is anesthetized and taped on its back to a cork board by its arms and legs. A longitudinal mid-ventral incision is made through the skin from the lower thoracic region to a point about 0.25 cm from the external genitalia. From the caudal end of the first skin incision bilateral incisions are extended to the proximal aspect of the legs. Both skin flaps are reflected laterally from the body wall and pinned, thus exposing the deep surface of the skin and exposing the abdominal (no. 4) and inguinal (no. 5) pairs of mammary glands. The no. 4 abdominal pair of glands are the ones to be used for clearing and transplantation since these are the largest mammary glands in the female mouse and are the easiest to manipulate. The nipple of the no. 4 mammary gland should be located with the aid of a dissecting microscope. Clearing begins when the nipple and main ducts are cauterized or surgically excised. This procedure is followed by removal of the medial portion of the mammary fat pad, which may contain mammary ducts. Finally, the mammary fat "bridge" between the abdominal and inguinal (no. 5) gland is cauterized as described by Young (Chapter 6). The result is a fat pad devoid of ductal tissue.

Actual transplantation into the cleared mammary fat pad is performed by any of the following methods, depending on the physical state of the transplant (cells suspension versus intact tissue fragments). For transplantation of mammary tissue into the cleared mammary fat pad, it is advisable to clear the fat pad and transplant at the same time so that the host is subjected to only one operation. If the mammary epithelial cells are in the form of a cell suspension, they can be injected by Hamilton microsyringe (Hamilton, Reno, NE) into the previously cleared fat pad. For this purpose a bolus of about 1×10^6 epithelial cells suspended in nutrient medium, in liquid collagen, or in liquid Matrigel is injected in a 20 µl volume. If the mammary epithelial cells are in the form of tissue fragments ≤1 mm³, a small pocket is created in the exposed cleared fat pad by blunt dissection with no. 5 Dumont forceps. Under observation with the dissecting microscope the tissue graft is inserted into the pocket with forceps or a finely drawn holding pipette. The holding pipette is prepared by manually pulling a Pasteur pipette after heating over a small flame. The finely drawn pipette should be scored with a 1-inch-diameter Dremel tool carborundum disk (available at a hardware store) or a diamond pen (VWR, San Francisco, CA) so that it breaks cleanly at the correct diameter. Drawn pipettes with jagged tips should be discarded. By either technique the graft is deposited into the pocket created in the fat pad under examination with a dissecting microscope. During implantation of the graft, it can be difficult to verify that the graft has been retained within the pocket in the fat pad. If the graft is first coated with sterile dry charcoal particles (Norit A, Sigma, St. Louis), the operator can be sure that the graft has been successfully inserted into the graft site. After the right and left no. 4 fat pads are grafted, the skin is closed with wound clips.

SELECTION OF THE DONOR TISSUE

Rescue of mammary rudiments is dictated when the mutant mice die during embryonic or neonatal periods. Thus, the nature of the donor tissue for transplantation is determined by the age of the donor, which will dictate the morphological pattern and developmental stage of the mammary rudiment to be grafted. For this reason knowledge of mammary development is essential.

Mouse mammary epithelial rudiments appear at 12 days of gestation (4, 5) as solid spherical epithelial buds. These buds can be easily recognized through a dissecting microscope illuminated from below (Figure 25-2a). The embryonic mammary rudiments of female and male mouse embryos are initially spherical epithelial buds connected by a stalk to the epidermis (Figure 25-2b). In many strains of mice the male mammary rudiments normally regress in response to endogenous testosterone during days 13 to 16 of gestation (6). In female embryos the elongation of the epithelial bud generates the primary duct, which begins to undergo ductal branching morphogenesis on about day 17 of gestation (5–7). By 18 days of

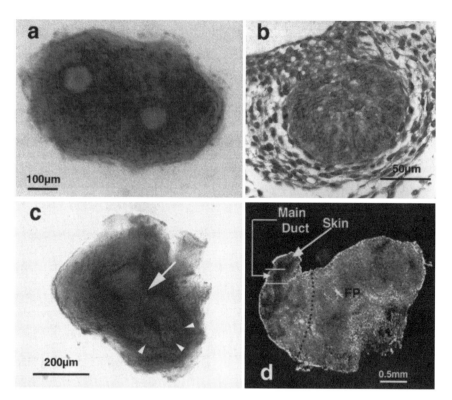

Figure 25-2. (a) With transmitted light from below, 13-day embryonic mammary rudiments are easily observed in dissected fragments of ventral skin. For the purposes of grafting or for the separation of the embryonic mammary rudiment into epithelium and mesenchyme, the specimen should be trimmed, as indicated by the boxed area. (b) Histological section of a 13-day embryonic mammary gland showing its connection to the overlying epidermis. (c) Whole mount of an unfixed, unstained 18-day embryonic mammary gland. Note the primary mammary duct (arrow) and its branches (arrowheads). (d) A fixed and stained whole mount of a mammary gland of a newborn mouse. At birth 6 to 10 ductal branches are just beginning to invade the edge of the fat pad.

gestation the primary mammary duct has given rise to 2 or 3 branches (Figure 25-2c), and by birth about 6 to 10 ductal branches are present that are just beginning to invade the edge of the mammary fat pad (Figure 25-2d). From birth to about 30 days postnatal the mammary ductal tree undergoes little growth or ductal branching. Beginning at about 30 days, postnatal mammary end buds reappear when ductal growth and branching morphogenesis of the mammary gland are stimulated by estrogens.

Although the age of the donor can vary considerably, there are basically three scenarios for rescue of mammary rudiments from donors: derivation of the mammary rudiments from (a) embryonic, (b) perinatal, and (c) weanling donors. In the case of the embryonic mammary gland (12 to about 16 days of gestation), the fat pad has not yet differentiated. The mammary epithelial rudiment is attached to the deep surface of the epidermis and is spherical or elongated, unbranched, and surrounded by mesenchyme. To isolate the embryonic mammary rudiment from 12- to 17-day embryos, strips of body wall or skin are dissected from the ventral body surface in the region of the groin to the axilla. Five mammary rudiments are present on each side in mice even though it is rare that all 10 mammary rudiments will be found. Dumont no. 5 forceps (Cat. No. 11251-20, Fine Science Tools, Foster City, CA) and spring-loaded student Vannas scissors (Cat. No. 15100-09, Fine Science Tools) are the instruments of choice to isolate strips of ventral body wall and skin containing the mammary rudiments. To accomplish this, embryos should be transferred to small dishes containing a physiological salt solution such as phosphate buffered saline (PBS) or culture medium. The depth of the medium in the dish should be sufficient to completely cover the embryos so that surface tension does not interfere with manipulation of the embryos. If insufficient medium is present, it will be difficult to turn the embryos from side to side. At 14 days of gestation (day 0 = day of detection of the vaginal plug), a fascial plane allows easy separation of the skin from the underlying muscular body wall. Once ventral strips of body wall or skin are isolated through use of a dissecting microscope, they should be transferred to a dish of fresh medium. Blood should be aspirated so that a clear view of the tissues is obtained.

Dissection of embryonic rudiments requires use of a dissecting microscope employing transillumination from below the stage. In embryos at 12 to about 14 to 15 days of gestation, the spherical mammary rudiments are seen as bright translucent spheres surrounded by the slightly darker mesenchyme (Figure 25-2a). The surrounding skin and body wall should be trimmed away from the mammary rudiments without damaging the epithelial rudiment.

Trimming a large segment of skin and body wall to isolate embryonic mammary rudiments can be accomplished in many ways, but it definitely requires steady hands, a dissecting microscope with transillumination, and some type of cutting tool. We have found the following method to be ideal. Use of a Maximov depression slide facilitates the procedure. Number 5 Dumont forceps are used to manipulate the dissected skin into position. A Graefe microdissecting knife (Cat. No. 10071-12, Fine Science Tools) is brought down onto the sheet of skin and body wall near the epithelial rudiment and compresses it (epidermis side down) solidly to the bottom of the dish. The upward slope of the Maximov depression slide (Fisher, Pittsburgh, PA) provides a surface with the correct angle so that the cutting edge of the knife and the surface of the dish are roughly parallel. (With a standard flat culture dish the compression of the tissue to the bottom of the dish will not be as effective because the cutting edge of the knife and the surface of the dish will not be parallel.) Once the tissue is firmly compressed by the scalpel to the bottom of the dish, the forceps are drawn along the bottom of the dish in contact with the scalpel. It is by this method that the actual cutting of embryonic tissue is best accomplished. Other methods are possible (Vannas spring scissors), but we have found that extremely accurate microdissection is better achieved by the method described. After the mammary rudiment is closely trimmed, it can be turned edgewise so that the stalk connected to the epidermis can be severed, thus isolating the mammary rudiment from the overlying skin.

Although 12- to 14-day embryonic mammary rudiments are easily visualized by tran-sillumination, embryonic mammary rudiments at later developmental stages (embryos ≥15 or 16 days of gestation) are difficult to see by transillumination of skin, due to the skin thickness and texture. Embryonic nipples are not easily recognizable externally, and even the most experienced operator will have difficulty finding the mammary rudiments of these older embryos, even though several can usually be found.

Perinatal mammary glands (18 days of gestation, day of birth and up to 7 days post-natal) are isolated from ventral skin stripped from the underlying body wall. At these stages the fat pads are well differentiated. For this reason observation of the deep surface of the ventral skin will reveal the mammary glands. Under transmitted light, the attachment of the main duct to the skin can be identified and severed. The fat pad and the entire branched duct can then be teased from the undersurface of the skin with a pair of forceps or severed with spring-loaded Vannas scissors to yield the entire perinatal mammary gland (ducts plus fat pad) (Figure 25-3a).

For mammary glands of weanlings (3 weeks postnatal) the mammary ducts are located in the fat pad in the region of the nipple. Thus, after the nipple is located the main duct can be identified and severed, and the mammary fat pad with ducts can be detached from the deep surface of the skin.

Isolation of Mammary Epithelium

Supplies

- Culture dishes and tubes (Becton–Dickinson, Franklin Lake, NJ)
- Pipettes
- Bacto-trypsin (1/250, Difco, Detroit, MI)
- Calcium-magnesium-free Hank's salt solution
- Fetal calf serum
- Dulbecco's modified Eagle's medium (DMEM)
- Type III collagenase (Worthington, Lakewood, NJ)
- Hyaluronidase (Sigma)
- Dissecting microscope

Once the mammary rudiments are isolated from embryos, neonates, or weanling donors, the entire mammary rudiment (mesenchyme plus epithelium or fat pad plus ducts) can be grafted directly. Alternatively, the design of the experiment may require grafting the epithelium. Epithelial grafts may be partially cleaned of adherent mesenchymal or stromal tissue with fine forceps, in which case some of the stromal or mesenchymal tissue may be left in place. Alternatively the mammary epithelial rudiments can be subjected to enzymatic treatment so that all stromal tissue is removed before grafting. Embryonic mammary epithelial buds can be freed of mesenchymal tissue following incubation for about 1.5 h in 1% Bacto-trypsin (1/250, Difco) in calcium-magnesium-free Hank's salt solution at 4°C. Following neutralization of the enzyme with 10% fetal bovine serum in medium, the epithelium and mesenchyme are teased apart with fine forceps. Separated epithelium should be stored before grafting in 10% fetal calf serum in medium. Once the fat pad has

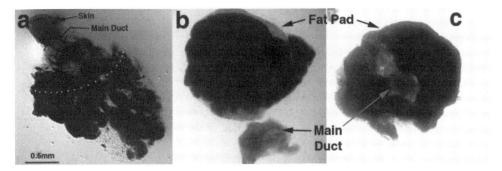

Figure 25-3. (a) An entire neonatal mammary gland dissected from the deep surface of the skin. Note that with transmitted light from below portions of the ductal network are visible. (b) Surgically isolated main duct and fat pad from a neonatal mouse obtained by severing the fat beyond the region containing the ducts (see dotted line in a). (c) Main duct (arrow) inserted into a pocket in the surgically isolated fat pad (FP).

differentiated (late fetal, neonatal, and weanling stages), incubation with collagenase is the method of choice for removing residual stromal tissue from postnatal mammary glands. The method involves digesting mammary tissue with collagenase type III (Worthington, 1 g/L) and hyaluronidase (Sigma, 1 mg/L) for 2–3 h at 37°C in a shaking water bath (8). The stroma and fat pad are thus digested away from the ducts or end buds. Any such residual stromal tissue can be removed with fine forceps under a dissecting microscope. The cleaned ducts or end buds are washed and stored in medium containing 10% fetal bovine serum before use.

Although use of enzymatically cleaned mammary epithelium is the most rigorous approach, the grafting of mammary epithelium with a small amount of residual stroma gives acceptable results when the graft site is the mammary fat pad. The reason is that in grafts containing epithelium plus some residual stroma, the contaminating stroma remains at the graft site, whereas the epithelial ducts grow out and away from its original stroma into the host's fat pad. This was verified in grafts of rat mammary tissue implanted into cleared mammary fat pads of athymic nude mice (9). An advantage of using mammary epithelial rudiments and ducts with residual stroma is that the take rate is vastly higher in comparison to grafts of a comparable amount of enzymatically purified epithelial cells.

INTERPRETATION OF RESULTS OF TRANSPLANTING MAMMARY RUDIMENTS AND TISSUE RECOMBINANTS COMPOSED OF EMBRYONIC OR NEONATAL TISSUES

At the moment of transplantation, mammary rudiments or tissue recombinants composed of embryonic or neonatal tissues are undifferentiated. Over a period of several weeks following transplantation the undifferentiated embryonic or neonatal tissues undergo a process of growth, ductal branching morphogenesis, and differentiation so that after 4 to 8 weeks of growth under the renal capsule, the graft is no longer undifferentiated. Indeed, with sufficient time the grafted embryonic rudiments will express an adult phenotype both morphologically and functionally if the hormonal conditions are appropriate. Thus, even though a tissue recombinant may have been constructed with embryonic tissues, the transplant after 4 to 8 weeks of

Table 25-1. Epithelial Differentiation Expressed by Grafts of Embryonic Mammary Rudiments or Tissue Recombinants Grown *In Vivo*

Epithelial differentiation feature	Reference
Ductal branching morphogenesis	1, 10
Luminal and myoepithelial cells present	10
Milk proteins expressed in response to lactogenic hormones	10, 19
Alveolar structures in response to mammotrophic hormones	10, 19

growth is fully differentiated. For example, when undifferentiated 13-day embryonic skin is combined with embryonic mammary mesenchyme and grown for 4 weeks in a pituitary-grafted female host, the embryonic undifferentiated epidermis differentiates into morphologically recognizable mammary ducts composed of luminal and myoepithelial cells, and the luminal cells express casein and α-lactalbumin (10). The actual developmental process can be studied as it is occurring provided that specimens are harvested at early time points. However, at the end of 4 to 8 weeks of *in vivo* growth, the differentiation status of the "embryonic transplant" is virtually identical to its adult counterpart (the adult host's mammary glands). This observation has been made repeatedly not only for transplants of mammary rudiments or tissue recombinants composed of embryonic or neonatal mammary tissues, but also for comparable transplants of developing female urogenital tract rudiments or tissue recombinants composed of embryonic or neonatal urogenital tissues. Tables 25-1 to 25-3 emphasize the adult-type differentiation expressed by transplants of developing mammary gland and female genital tract tissues grown for 4 or more weeks *in vivo*. Similar observations have been made for transplants of developing male genital tract rudiments and tissue recombinants. The interpretation of this vast amount of data is clear. Transplants of developing organs will differentiate *in vivo*, and once differentiation is complete the transplant is fully mature and comparable to its adult counterpart.

TRANSPLANTATION OF MAMMARY EPITHELIUM

The technique of transplantation of mammary epithelium into the cleared mammary fat pad can be used for many purposes other than that of rescuing mutant mammary epithelium

Table 25-2. Epithelial Features Expressed in Grafts of Embryonic or Neonatal Vaginal Rudiments or Tissue Recombinants Grown *In Vivo*

Feature	Reference
Cornification in response to estrogen	31
Proliferation in response to estrogen	31
Mucification in response to progesterone	Kurita *et al.*, unpublished
Keratin 10 expression in response to estrogen	31
Keratin 14 in basal epithelial cells	Kurita *et al.*, unpublished
Cyclic hormone-dependent change in epithelial differentiation	32
Adult isoforms of syndecan	33

Table 25-3. Differentiation Features Expressed by Grafts of Embryonic or Neonatal Uterine Rudiments of Tissue Recombinants Grown *In Vivo*

Differentiation feature	Reference
Luminal and glandular epithelium	32
Adult isoforms of syndecan in epithelium	33
Estrogen receptor α in epithelium, stroma, and myometrium	Kurita *et al.* (submitted)
Progesterone receptor in epithelium, stroma, and myometrium	Kurita *et al.* (submitted)
Lactoferrin expressed in epithelium	34
Mitogenic response to estradiol by epithelium	30
Anti-mitogenic response to progesterone	35
Differentiation of myometrium	36
Msx-1 expression in epithelium	37

from embryonic or neonatal lethal mice. For aging studies a small fragment of an adult mammary duct can be transplanted into a cleared fat pad to generate a mammary ductal tree that completely fills the fat pad. Once this is achieved in about 8 weeks of growth, mammary ducts can be dissected from the grafted mammary gland and transplanted into the cleared fat pad of a second host. During each transplant generation the small ductal transplant increases dramatically in cell number. This process of mitotic aging can be repeated many times until the mammary epithelial cells senesce and lose their capacity to divide (9). The same fat pad transplantation technique can be used to study carcinogenic progression of hyperplastic alveolar nodules into mammary carcinomas (3, 11). Another use of the fat pad transplantation technique involves the creation of mutant mammary epithelium *in vitro* as a result of infection of mammary epithelial cultures with retroviral vectors. Such infected mammary epithelial cell populations can be injected into cleared fat pads to reconstitute mammary glands with specific genetic alterations in the epithelium (12).

ENDOCRINE PARAMETERS OF MAMMARY DEVELOPMENT

Embryonic mammary development appears to be hormone independent since embryonic mammary glands develop in mice devoid of either functional estrogen receptor-α (α-ERKO) (13), estrogen receptor-β (β-ERKO) (14), progesterone receptor (PRKO) (15), or prolactin receptor (PrlR-KO) (16). In contrast, postnatal ductal growth, which begins during puberty, is estrogen dependent (17) and estrogen receptor-α dependent (13).

Even when mutant mice are viable, renal capsule grafting procedures can be useful for studying the mammary gland under physiologic conditions that are impossible to achieve in the mutant animal *per se*. Mammary gland rudiments transplanted into young virgin (≥30 days old) female hosts are exposed to endogenous hormones (estradiol) sufficient to promote mammary ductal growth when grafted into either the cleared fat pad or under the renal capsule. To achieve ductal side branching and alveolar development within mammary transplants, the hosts can be injected with estradiol and progesterone as described previously (18). To achieve full mammary gland development and milk production, two methods can be used. The mouse host can be mated so that the grafts will be exposed to natural levels of the "hormones of pregnancy" (19). Alternatively, at the time of grafting, an adult pituitary from either a male or a female donor can be implanted under the renal capsule (see Chapter 10 by Medina and Kittrell in this volume). Such pituitary grafts release high levels of prolactin and gonadotrophins (20). In pituitary-grafted mice the host's mammary glands and mammary grafts undergo full functional differentiation and produce milk proteins (21). Thus, depending on the experimental design, grafts of mammary tissue can be subjected to all of the various hormonal conditions to which normal mammary tissue is naturally exposed.

The utility of transplantation techniques to solve endocrine problems is illustrated in the estrogen receptor-α knockout (ERKO) mouse, which is infertile and incapable of pregnancy. We have shown that grafts of ERKO mammary rudiments into nude mouse hosts exhibit comparable impairment of ductal growth as seen *in situ* in ERKO mice. Figure 25-4 shows whole mounts of 60-day ERKO and wild-type mammary glands as well as mammary gland grafts from the newborn grown for 1 month in a female nude mouse host. Note that

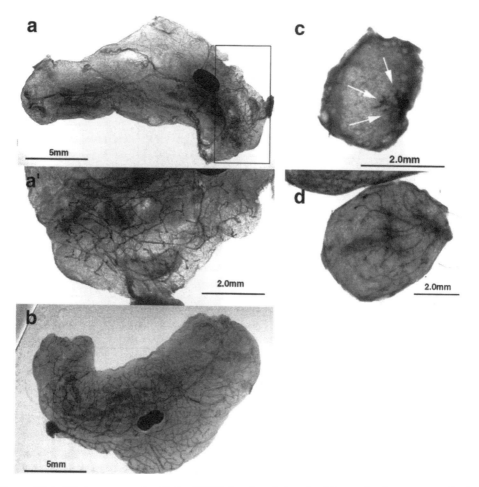

Figure 25-4. Whole mounts of a 60-day ERKO (a, a', and c) and wild-type (b, d) mammary glands. Note that mammary ductal growth is meager in the ERKO mammary gland (a, a') relative to that of a wild-type mammary gland of the same age. (a') Enlargement of the boxed area in (a). (c) Graft of an entire newborn ERKO mammary gland grown for 30 days in a female nude mouse host. Ducts (arrows) have only filled a small portion of the fat pad. (d) Graft of an entire newborn wild-type mammary gland grown for 30 days in a female nude mouse host. Ducts fill over half of the fat pad.

the impaired growth of ERKO mammary ducts *in situ* is also seen in transplants of newborn ERKO mammary glands (Figure 25-4c). This observation is the basis for a grafting experiment, which allows analysis of the effects on the hormones of pregnancy on the ERKO mammary gland. For this purpose intact mammary glands (both mammary ducts and fat pad) from neonatal wild-type and ERKO mice were transplanted to the right and left renal capsules of a female nude mouse host. The host can be mated or grafted with an adult pituitary gland. In either case, the wild-type and ERKO mammary transplants are exposed to mammotrophic hormones, thus allowing analysis of the effects of mammotrophic hormones on mammary glands expressing estrogen receptor-α (ER-α) or devoid of ER-α. By this method it is possible to circumvent the problem of infertility of the ERKO mouse to study the role of ER-α in response of the mammary gland to the hormones of pregnancy.

The availability of α-ERKO, β-ERKO, PRKO, and PrlR-KO mice has led to studies aimed at assessing the respective role of epithelial versus stromal hormone receptors. For this purpose it is possible to graft whole mammary glands, to transplant mutant or wild-type mammary epithelium into cleared fat pads of mutant or wild-type mice, or to graft mammary tissue recombinants composed of mutant or wild-type stroma plus mutant or wild-type epithelium. For such studies it is essential to know whether the hormone receptor is expressed in the epithelium, stroma, or both. Based on current information, ER-α is expressed in both mammary epithelium and stroma (22–24), and ER-β has not been detected in the mammary gland (25). Progesterone receptor (PR) appears to be expressed in mammary epithelium, whereas stromal PR is detected solely in the capsule of the fat pad; therefore, stromal PR is probably not relevant to paracrine stromal–epithelial interactions (26, 27). The prolactin receptor appears to be expressed only in mammary epithelium (28).

TISSUE RECOMBINATION

Appropriate gene knockout mice are particularly useful for defining the cellular mechanisms involved in mammary ductal growth and branching morphogenesis, functional differentiation, hormonal action, growth factor effects, and carcinogenesis. For those mutant mouse lines having informative mammary phenotypes, the knockout mouse can provide compelling validation that a particular signaling pathway is critical for some aspect of mammary biology. However, in many cases examination of the knockout mouse *per se* does not distinguish whether the mammary phenotype is due to an absence of the gene in the epithelium, fat pad, or both. For example, impaired ductal growth in the ERKO mouse could be due to an absence of ER-α in the epithelium, fat pad, or both since both tissues express functional ER-α. To determine whether estrogens elicit ductal growth and branching morphogenesis via epithelial versus the stromal ER-α, tissue recombinants must be constructed between ER-α-positive wild-type (wt) and ER-α-negative ERKO tissues. In this way the tissue separation and recombination technique provides a unique method for experimentally controlling the ER-α status of both stroma and epithelium. Thus, tissue recombinations can be prepared that lack ER-α in stroma (S) and epithelium (E), express ER-α in epithelium or stroma, or do not express ER-α in epithelium and stroma (wt-E+wt-S, ERKO-E+wt-S, wt-E+ ERKO-S, ERKO-E+ ERKO-S). Obviously the basic technique is not restricted to analysis of the respective roles of steroid receptors in mammary epithelium and stroma, but can be used to examine the respective role of any genetic alteration in epithelial versus stromal cells for which a reliable biological endpoint is available. The techniques for preparing such tissue recombinants vary somewhat, depending on the age of the tissues used.

Preparation of Tissue Recombinants with Embryonic Mammary Epithelium and Mesenchyme

Materials

- Finely drawn Pasteur pipettes
- 35- or 60-mm culture dishes (Becton–Dickinson)
- Dumont no. 5 forceps
- Fetal calf serum
- Bacto-Agar (Difco)
- 2 × DMEM H16 medium
- L-Glutamine
- Penicillin
- Streptomycin
- Dissecting microscope equipped for transillumination of the specimen

To make the 1% Bacto-Agar in 1 × DMEM, 50 g of agar are dissolved in 50 ml of distilled water. Cool the dissolved agar to about 50°C and add 50 ml of 2 × DMEM. Mix quickly and aliquot into 25-ml lots. To make the final 0.4% Bacto-Agar plates, liquefy the 1% agar by heating to about 50°C and dilute with 1 × DMEM. Cool to room temperature before using the final agar plates.

Using mammary rudiments from 12- to 16-day-old mice means that the inter-actants will be epithelium and mesenchyme since the fat pad has not yet differentiated. The technique begins with dissection of the embryonic mammary rudiment and attached skin as described previously. Briefly, embryonic mammary rudiments are dissected free of the surrounding body wall from 12- to 16-day rat or mouse embryos. The mammary rudiments are then incubated for 1.5 h in 1% Bacto-trypsin (1/250, Difco) in calcium-magnesium-free Hank's salt solution at 4°C. Following neutralization of the enzyme by transferring the rudiments to 10% fetal bovine serum in medium, the epithelium and mesenchyme are teased apart with fine forceps. Separated mammary epithelium and mesenchyme are stored briefly in 10% fetal calf serum before use. The fragments of mammary mesenchyme are then transferred by pipette to culture dishes containing a solidified agar medium (0.4% Bacto-Agar, Difco) in 1 × DMEM H16 medium supplemented with 2 mM glutamine, 100 IU/ml penicillin, and 100 μg/ml streptomycin. With a drawn-out Pasteur pipette, excess liquid medium is removed from the surface of the agar. The mesenchymes are then pushed into aggregates of four to six mammary mesenchymes. Again, any excess fluid on the surface of the agar is removed by suction by using a drawn-out Pasteur pipette. Tissue recombinants are prepared by transferring two to four mammary epithelial rudiments with an orally controlled holding micropipette to a mesenchymal aggregate previously formed on the agar gel. Following overnight culture at 37°C in a humidified CO_2 incubator, the tissues firmly adhere to each other, and the tissue recombinants can then be transplanted beneath the renal capsule of female syngeneic or athymic nude mouse hosts. Following 1 to 4 weeks of growth, the grafts can be harvested for analysis. Of course, the hormonal status of the host can be controlled as per the experimental design. Using nude mouse hosts it is possible to prepare tissue recombinants with embryonic mesenchyme and epithelium from different genetic backgrounds (gene knockouts) or even from different species (rat–mouse, rat–human, etc.). Such studies are useful to distinguish local versus systemic effects of gene knockout.

Preparation of Tissue Recombinants with Mammary Epithelium and Postnatal Fat Pad

The simplest form of this experiment is the transplantation of small segments of mammary ductal tissue into a cleared mammary fat pad. Taking as an example the use of the epidermal growth factor receptor knockout (EGFR-KO) mouse to determine the respective roles of epithelial versus stromal epidermal growth factor receptors (EGFR) in mammary ductal growth, the four possible tissue recombinants could be prepared by transplanting EGFR-KO mammary epithelium into wild-type or EGFR-KO cleared fat pads and transplanting wild-type mammary epithelium into wild-type or EGFR-KO cleared fat pads. Unfortunately for EGFR-KO mice this simple epithelial transplantation approach is impossible because of the impaired viability of the EGFR-KO mice and immunologic considerations (mixed genetic background). EGFR-KO mice usually die as neonates. Thus, it is not possible to have mature EGFR-KO mice with cleared fat pads. In addition, the EGFR-KO mice are not from genetically inbred stock, which means that transplanted mammary epithelium (MGE) will be rejected. One way around this problem is to breed the mutation of interest onto an athymic background. Although this procedure is certainly possible, animal costs can become prohibitively high. Moreover, this strategy will not solve the problem of neonatal lethality. Using the epithelial transplantation approach, at least half of the possible tissue recombinants can be easily constructed by transplanting wild-type or EGFR-KO mammary epithelium into wild-type (wt) cleared fat pads of nude mice (1). Unfortunately, the reciprocal tissue recombinants (EGFR-KO-FP + wt-MGE and EGFR-KO-FP + EGFR-KO-MGE) are not possible by transplantation of epithelium into cleared fat pads for the reasons stated.

The full range of possible tissue recombinants between wild-type and gene knockout mammary epithelium and fat pad (FP) can be constructed *in vitro* with mammary FP and MGE obtained from neonatal mice. At birth the main mammary duct has branched into 6 to 10 terminal ducts that are just beginning to invade the edge of the fat pad (Figure 25-3a). Once the entire neonatal mammary gland is dissected as described, the main mammary duct is isolated by microdissection, trimmed to length (~100 to 200 μm), and cleaned of extraneous stromal tissue. To prepare the four possible tissue recombinants between wild-type and knockout mammary fat pad and epithelium (E) (wt-FP+wt-E, wt-FP+KO-E, KO-FP+KO-E, KO-FP+wt-E), isolated neonatal mammary rudiments are transilluminated under a dissecting microscope and the fat pad is resected just ahead of the invading epithelial ducts to yield mammary fat pad free of epithelial tissue. Mammary fat pads and cleaned main ducts (Figure 25-3b) of wild type and knockout mice are transferred to nutrient agar plates as described, and a segment of main duct is placed into a pocket created in the fat pad with microforceps (Figure 25-3c). After overnight culture to allow the tissues to adhere, the mammary tissue recombinants are grafted under the renal capsule of female athymic nude mice and allowed to grow for various periods.

This method has been used to assess the respective roles of epithelial versus stromal ER-α in mammary ductal growth. In mammary tissue recombinants constructed with wild-type ER-α-positive fat pad (wt-FP+wt-E and wt-FP+ERKO-E), ductal growth was extensive. Conversely, in mammary tissue recombinants constructed with ERKO ER-α-negative fat pad (KO-FP+KO-E, KO-FP+wt-E), ductal growth was meager (29). These results in the mammary gland and comparable results of ERKO–wt tissue recombinants in the uterus and vagina (30, 31) establish the concept that ductal growth and epithelial proliferation elicited by estrogen in hormone target organs occur via paracrine mechanisms in which ER-α in the stroma and fat pad are the key estrogen target.

Immunologic considerations of potential rejection of grafts are the same for immature (fetal or neonatal) and adult tissue grafts. If it is possible to carry out the entire experiment within an inbred strain, immunologic problems can be averted for the most part. The only exception is the transplantation of male cells into female hosts, because in some strains the HY antigen expressed on male cells may elicit an immunologic reaction.

In summary, renal capsule and cleared fat pad transplantation techniques as well as tissue recombination technology are powerful methods for analysis of the cellular and molecular mechanisms regulating mammary development, growth, ductal branching morphogenesis, function, and carcinogenesis. The rescue by transplantation of mammary rudiments from donor mice from embryonic or neonatal lethal stocks is a useful method for creating experimental models that are otherwise unavailable. In our hands we have rescued mammary tissue from a variety of mutant lines that include Rb-KO, IGF-1-KO, IGF receptor 1-KO, and β4 integrin mutant mice (unpublished observations). It is our impression that this technique is broadly applicable to virtually any mutant mouse line. Tissue recombinant technology has the ability to elucidate the role of a particular gene or signaling pathway in mammary gland biology because it is possible to greatly advance the interpretive power of the transgenic mouse by defining the respective roles of gene expression or gene deficiency in epithelial versus stromal cells. Application of transplantation and tissue recombination technology holds great promise for fine dissection of molecular pathways in the mammary gland.

ACKNOWLEDGMENTS. This work was supported in part by grants CA 58207 and CA44768.

REFERENCES

1. J. F. Wiesen, P. Young, Z. Werb, and G. R. Cunha (1999). Signaling through the stromal epidermal growth factor receptor is necessary for mammary ductal development. *Development* **126**:335–344.
2. L. M. Reid, N. Minato, I. Gresser, J. Holland, A. Kadish, and B. R. Bloom (1981). Influence of anti-mouse interferon serum on the growth and metastasis of tumor cells persistently infected with virus and of human prostatic tumors in athymic nude mice. *Proc. Natl. Acad. Sci. USA* **78**:1171–1175.
3. K. B. De Ome, L. J. Faulkin, Jr., and H. A. Bern (1959). Development of mammary tumors from hyperplastic alveolar nodules transplanted into gland-free mammary fat pads of female C3H mice. *Cancer Res.* **19**:515–520.
4. K. Kratochwil (1975). Experimental analysis of the prenatal development of the mammary gland. *Mod. Probl. Pediat.* **15**:1–15.
5. T. Sakakura (1987). Mammary embryogensis. In C. W. Neville and M. C. Daniel (eds.), *The Mammary Gland: Development, Regulation and Function*, Plenum Press, New York, pp. 37–66.
6. K. Kratochwil (1977). Development and loss of androgen responsiveness in the embryonic rudiment of the mouse mammary gland. *Dev. Biol.* **61**:358–365.
7. G. R. Cunha and Y. H. Hom (1996). Role of mesenchymal-epithelial interactions in mammary gland development. *J. Mammary Gland Biol. Neoplasia* **1**:21–35.
8. J. Richards, R. Guzman, M. Konrad, J. Yang, and S. Nandi (1982). Growth of mouse mammary gland end buds cultured in a collagen gel matrix. *Exp. Cell Res.* **141**:433–443.
9. C. W. Daniel, J. M. Shannon, and G. R. Cunha (1983). Transplanted mammary epithelium grows in association with host stroma: aging of serially transplanted mammary gland is intrinsic to epithelial cells. *Mech. Aging Dev.* **23**:259–264.
10. G. R. Cunha, P. Young, K. Christov, R. Guzman, S. Nandi, F. Talamantes, and G. Thordarson (1995). Mammary phenotypic expression induced in epidermal cells by embryonic mammary mesenchyme. *Acta Anat.* **152**:195–204.

11. S. Miyamoto, R. C. Guzman, R. C. Osborn, and S. Nandi (1988). Neoplastic transformation of mouse mammary epithelial cells by *in vitro* exposure to *N*-methyl-*N*-nitrosourea. *Proc. Natl. Acad. Sci. USA* **85**:477–481.

12. P. A. Edwards, S. E. Hiby, J. Papkoff, and J. M. Bradbury (1992). Hyperplasia of mouse mammary epithelium induced by expression of the Wnt-1 (int-1) oncogene in reconstituted mammary gland. *Oncogene* **7**:2041–2051.

13. K. S. Korach (1994). Insights from the study of animals lacking functional estrogen receptor. *Science* **266**:1524–1527.

14. J. H. Krege, J. B. Hodgin, J. F. Couse, E. Enmark, M. Warner, J. F. Mahler, M. Sar, K. S. Korach, J. Gustafsson, and O. Smithies (1998). Generation and reproductive phenotypes of mice lacking estrogen receptor beta. *Proc. Natl. Acad. Sci. USA* **95**:15677–15682.

15. J. P. Lydon, F. J. DeMayo, C. R. Funk, S. K. Mani, A. R. Hughes, C. A. Montgomery, G. Shyamala, O. M. Conneely, and B. W. O'Malley (1995). Mice lacking progesterone receptor exhibit pleiotropic reproductive abnormalities. *Genes Dev.* **9**:2266–2278.

16. C. J. Ormandy, A. Camus, J. Barra, D. Damotte, B. Lucas, H. Buteau, M. Edery, N. Brousse, C. Babinet, N. Binart, and P. A. Kelly (1997). Null mutation of the prolactin receptor gene produces multiple reproductive defects in the mouse. *Genes Dev.* **11**:167–178.

17. S. Nandi (1958). Endocrine control of mammary gland development and function in the C3H/He Crgl mouse. *J. Natl. Inst.* **21**:1039–1063.

18. R. C. Humphreys, J. Lydon, B. W. O'Malley, and J. M. Rosen (1997). Mammary gland development is mediated by both stromal and epithelial progesterone receptors. *Mol. Endocrinol.* **11**:801–811.

19. T. Sakakura, Y. Nishizuka, and C. J. Dawe (1976). Mesenchyme-dependent morphogenesis and epithelium-specific cytodifferentiation in mouse mammary gland. *Science* **194**:1439–1441.

20. R. A. Adler (1986). The anterior pituitary-grafted rat: a valid model of chronic hyperprolactinemia. *Endocrine Rev.* **7**:302–313.

21. G. R. Cunha, P. Young, S. Hamamoto, R. Guzman, and S. Nandi (1992). Developmental response of adult mammary epithelial cells to various fetal and neonatal mesenchymes. *Epithelial Cell Biol.* **1**:105–118.

22. N. Zeps, J. M. Bentel, J. M. Papadimitriou, M. F. D'Antuono, and H. J. Dawkins (1998). Estrogen receptor-negative epithelial cells in mouse mammary gland development and growth. *Differentiation* **62**:221–226.

23. W. S. Shim, J. DiRenzo, J. A. DeCaprio, R. J. Santen, M. Brown, and M. H. Jeng (1999). Segregation of steroid receptor coactivator-1 from steroid receptors in mammary epithelium. *Proc. Natl. Acad. Sci. USA* **96**:208–213.

24. S. Z. Haslam and K. A. Nummy (1992). The ontogeny and cellular distribution of estrogen receptors in normal mouse mammary gland. *J. Steroid Biochem. Mol. Biol.* **42**:589–595.

25. J. F. Couse, J. Lindzey, K. Grandien, J. A. Gustafsson, and K. S. Korach (1997). Tissue distribution and quantitative analysis of estrogen receptor-alpha (ERalpha) and estrogen receptor-beta (ERbeta) messenger ribonucleic acid in the wild-type and ERalpha-knockout mouse. *Endocrinology* **138**:4613–4621.

26. C. Brisken, S. Park, T. Vass, J. P. Lydon, B. W. O'Malley, and R. A. Weinberg (1998). A paracrine role for the epithelial progesterone receptor in mammary gland development. *Proc. Natl. Acad. Sci. USA* **95**:5076–5081.

27. G. Shyamala, M. H. Barcellos-Hoff, D. Toft, and X. Yang (1997). *In situ* localization of progesterone receptors in normal mouse mammary glands: absence of receptors in the connective and adipose stroma and a heterogeneous distribution in the epithelium. *J. Steroid Biochem. Mol. Biol.* **63**:251–259.

28. M. Shirota, M. Kurohmaru, Y. Hayashi, K. Shirota, and P. A. Kelly (1995). Detection of *in situ* localization of long form prolactin receptor messenger RNA in lactating rats by biotin-labeled riboprobe. *Endocr. J.* **42**:69–76.

29. G. R. Cunha, P. Young, Y. K. Hom, P. S. Cooke, J. A. Taylor, and D. B. Lubahn (1997). Elucidation of a role of stromal steroid hormone receptors in mammary gland growth and development by tissue recombination experiments. *J. Mammary Gland Biol. Neoplasia* **2**:393–402.

30. P. Cooke, D. Buchanan, P. Young, T. Setiawan, J. Brody, K. Korach, J. Taylor, D. Lubahn, and G. Cunha (1997). Stromal estrogen receptors (ER) mediate mitogenic effects of estradiol on uterine epithelium. *Proc. Natl. Acad. Sci. USA* **94**:6535–6540.

31. D. L. Buchanan, T. Kurita, J. A. Taylor, D. L. Lubahn, G. R. Cunha, and P. S. Cooke (1998). Role of stromal and epithelial estrogen receptors in vaginal epithelial proliferation, stratification and cornification. *Endocrinology* **139**:4345–4352.

32. G. R. Cunha (1976). Stromal induction and specification of morphogenesis and cytodifferentiation of the epithelia of the Mullerian ducts and urogenital sinus during development of the uterus and vagina in mice. *J. Exp. Zool.* **196**:361–370.

33. E. L. Boutin, R. D. Sanderson, M. Bernfield, and G. R. Cunha (1991). Epithelial-mesenchymal interactions in uterus and vagina influence the expression of syndecan, a cell surface proteoglycan. *Dev. Biol.* **148:**63–74.

34. D. L. Buchanan, T. Setiawan, D. L. Lubahn, J. A. Taylor, T. Kurita, G. R. Cunha, and P. S. Cooke (1998). Tissue compartment-specific estrogen receptor participation in the mouse uterine epithelial secretory response. *Endocrinology* **140:**484–491.

35. T. Kurita, P. Young, J. Brody, J. P. Lydon, B. W. O'Malley, and G. R. Cunha (1998). Stromal progesterone receptors mediate the inhibitory effects of progesterone on estrogen-induced uterine epithelial cell (UtE) proliferation. *Endocrinology* **139:**4708–4713.

36. G. R. Cunha, E. Battle, P. Young, J. Brody, A. Donjacour, N. Hayashi, and H. Kinbara (1992). Role of epithelial-mesenchymal interactions in the differentiation and spatial organization of visceral smooth muscle. *Epithelial Cell Biol.* **1:**76–83.

37. A. Pavlova, E. Boutin, G. R. Cunha, and D. Sassoon (1994). *Msx1 (Hox-7.1)* in the mouse uterus: cellular interactions underlying regulation of expression. *Development* **120:**335–346.

Chapter 26

Rescue of Mammary Epithelium of Early Lethal Phenotypes by Embryonic Mammary Gland Transplantation as Exemplified with Insulin Receptor Null Mice

Gertraud W. Robinson, Domenico Accili, and Lothar Hennighausen

Abstract.   We describe a method to transplant embryonic mammary anlagen into the mammary fat pad of a virgin host whose endogenous mammary epithelium has been removed. The transplanted epithelium grows into the fat pad and is exposed to a physiological hormonal milieu of puberty and pregnancy when the host is mated. This technique allows studies on the developmental potential of mammary epithelia of mutants that result in lethality after embryonic day 13. Transplanted mammary epithelial cells derived from insulin-receptor-deficient mice show reduced size of alveoli at lactation and reduced expression of milk protein genes. These results underscore the importance of insulin receptor signaling in mammary epithelial development.

Abbreviations.   Dulbecco's modified Eagle's medium (DMEM); fetal calf serum (FCS); insulin-like growth factor (IGF); insulin receptor (IR); phosphate buffered saline (PBS); polymerase chain reaction (PCR).

INTRODUCTION

The development of techniques for the deletion of genes by homologous recombination permits studies on the role of defined proteins in mouse development. Although powerful, this technique has limitations. (I) If the absence of a gene results in embryonic lethality, developmental processes that occur at later stages cannot be studied. (II) If the absence of a gene has pleiotropic effects, it is difficult to distinguish between primary and direct, and secondary events. Different approaches can be used to circumvent these problems. In the case of lethality through gene deletion in the germ line, cell-specific gene deletion can be achieved through the use of site-specific recombinases whose expression is directed to one cell type by specific promoters (1). Alternatively, some questions can be studied by *in vitro* culture of

Gertraud W. Robinson and Lothar Hennighausen   Laboratory of Genetics and Physiology, National Institute of Diabetes, Digestive, and Kidney Diseases, National Institutes of Health, Bethesda, Maryland 20892.
Domenico Accili   Endocrinology Branch, National Institute of Child Health and Human Development, National Institutes of Health, Bethesda, Maryland 20892.

Methods in Mammary Gland Biology and Breast Cancer Research, edited by Ip and Asch. Kluwer Academic/Plenum Publishers, New York, 2000.

material recovered before the death of the embryo. Both these approaches alleviate the problem of indirect influences on the cell type of interest. However, the study of organogenesis in culture over extended periods of time cannot always be achieved. This applies in particular to the mammary gland. Development of this organ takes place almost exclusively in postnatal life and depends on multiple signals from the endocrine system and the interaction of parenchymal and stromal tissues (2). Presently there are no culture methods available to recapitulate *in vitro* all the steps of development of the gland.

In mice a primordium of the mammary gland starts to develop around day 12 of embryonic life, and it undergoes limited growth until puberty. With the onset of ovarian steroid secretion ductal growth commences, and the ductal tree expands and fills the entire mammary fat pad at 10 weeks of age. Functional differentiation of the gland occurs during pregnancy under the influence of lactogenic hormones, which activate the transcription of milk protein genes and lactation (3).

One family of proteins that appears to play a role in mammary gland development is insulin and the insulin-like growth factors (IGFs). In pioneering studies Topper and co-workers determined that insulin acts as a mitogen in mammary epithelial cells and that development and differentiation of mammary tissue derived from pregnant mice requires addition of the lactogenic hormones insulin, hydrocortisone, and prolactin to the culture medium (reviewed in Ref. 4). Insulin-like growth factors are also thought to act as local mediators of systemic hormones in the mammary gland. Local administration of IGF-I stimulates cell proliferation (5). Ectopic expression of IGF-I in mammary epithelium causes delayed involution and ductal hypertrophy (6, 7), and IGF-II increases the incidence of mammary adenocarcinoma (8). These molecules bind with varying affinity to the insulin receptor (IR) as well as to two types of insulin-like growth factor receptor (9). The availability of mice with a deletion of IR allowed us to study the role of IR signaling in the mammary gland. These mice are born but quickly succumb to severe hyperglycemia and die within a few days (10). This early lethality made it necessary to utilize transplants to investigate mammary epithelial development and differentiation in the absence of insulin receptor.

MATERIALS AND INSTRUMENTATION

- PBS
- DMEM
- Ham's F-12 medium
- FCS
- Trypan blue (0.4% in 0.85% saline)
- Stereomicroscope (approx. 6- to 20-fold magnification)
- Dissecting tools to remove embryos from the uterus
- Petri dishes (100 mm and 35 mm)
- 6-well dishes (optional)
- Organ culture dishes (Falcon Cat. No. 3037) can be substituted by a Nuclepore filter (Thomas Scientific Cat. No. 4625-V10) resting on stainless steel grids (cut from round filter grids—Thomas Cat. No. 3435881) in 35-mm dishes
- Dissecting knives (e.g., Biomedical Research Instruments Cat. No. 12-1170 or Roboz Cat. No. RS-6270)
- Microdissecting spring scissors (de Wecker) (e.g., Biomedical Research Instruments Cat. No. 11-1800 or Roboz Cat. No. RS-5802)

- Watchmaker's forceps (Biomedical Research Instruments Cat. No. 10-630 or Roboz Cat. No. RS-4976)
- 9-mm wound clips
- Transfer pipettes made from $5\frac{3}{4}$-inch Pasteur pipettes

METHODS

Reagents

- PBS for isolating embryos
- DMEM and 10% FCS for dissecting embryos
- DMEM–Ham's F-12 with 10% FCS, 2mM glutamine, and 1% penicillin–strepto-mycin for culture

Detailed Procedures

Mammary glands can be isolated from embryonic day 12 onwards, but mammary anlagen from E13.5 and 14.5 are easiest to collect. At this stage the five pairs of glands can be distinguished as bright dots surrounded by a slightly darker ring of mesenchyme (Figure 26-1). Their spacing and midventral position on the inside of the base of the limbs is the same as in the adult mouse with the three thoracic and two inguinal pairs separated by a larger gap.

ISOLATION OF MAMMARY GLANDS. All dissecting procedures are performed in petri dishes under a dissecting microscope (approx. 6- to 20-fold magnification) with sterile techniques. After sacrificing a pregnant mouse, remove the uterus and place into a 10-cm petri dish with

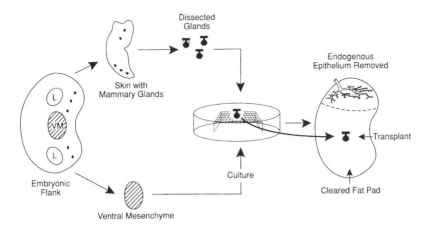

Figure 26-1. Outline of transplantation procedure. The skin is peeled from the embryonic flank and single mammary anlagen are dissected. They are combined with a piece of ventral mesenchyme (hatched area) and put in culture up to 36 h. At the time of transplantation the area between the nipple and the lymph node is surgically removed from a 3-week-old host and the embryonic mammary gland is trans-planted into the center of the cleared fat pad. L, stump of limbs; VM, ventral mesenchyme.

PBS. Carefully remove the embryos from the uterus and yolk sac with teethed forceps. Cut off the heads of the embryos with dissecting knives, and transfer the torsi to fresh PBS. When the mutant embryos can be distinguished by morphological features they can be pooled, otherwise each embryo has to be kept separate in a small petri dish (6-well plates make handling of larger numbers of embryos easier). Turn each embryo onto its belly and cut in half along the spinal cord with dissecting knives (Figure 26-2A). At this point, reserve a small amount of tissue for PCR genotyping, if required. Turn embryo half with skin side down, remove inner organs, and determine sex by the appearance of the gonads (Figure 26-2A). Male embryos are identified by the testis cords in the gonads (Figure 26-2B). Use only female embryos. Turn halved embryo skin side up and cut off the limbs. Peel off the skin starting from the back toward the belly. The glands now should be seen easily as small circles (Figure 26-2C). Collect mesenchyme from the flank by lifting the tissue overlying the rib cage and transfer it to a small petri dish with DMEM and 10% FCS. Transfer the skin pieces to another small petri dish with DMEM and 10% FCS for further dissection, and use dissecting knives to cut individual mammary glands from the skin pieces (Figure 26-3A). The developmental capacities of all the anlagen are identical.

CULTURE.   Since the individual mammary anlagen are too small to transplant, two to three glands are combined on a piece of mesenchyme, which serves as substrate for growth of the epithelia, and cultured overnight up to two days. The culture step serves two purposes. It yields larger aggregates of tissue that can be manipulated and transferred with forceps (Figure 26-3B). The culture period also allows time to perform PCR analysis in those cases in which the mutant embryos are not easily discerned by morphology. The cultures are placed on top of a piece of transparent filter (e.g., Nuclepore, which can be autoclaved) supported by a platform of stainless steel that touches the surface of the medium (Figure 26-3C). The medium contains 1:1 DMEM:Ham's F-12 with 10% FCS, 2 mM glutamine, and 1% penicillin–streptomycin. To assemble the cultures place a piece of mesenchyme on the filter and put two to three glands on the mesenchyme with a transfer pipette (these pipettes are produced by heating the tapered part of a Pasteur pipette and pulling it to a thinner pore size). Break the tip 1 inch from the taper by scoring with a diamond or vial file and bend the end to a 45° angle by holding it over a small flame. Keep the cultures in a humidified atmosphere of 5% CO_2 at 37°C.

HOST–GLAND PREPARATION.   "Clearing," i.e., removal of the endogenous mammary epithelium, is depicted in Figure 26-4. Briefly, at 3 weeks of age the area between the nipple and the lymph node of gland no. 4 is removed surgically. This leaves an epithelium-free fat pad into which the cultures are transplanted (Figure 26-1). A detailed description of the clearing procedure can be found in Ref. 11 and in Chapter 6 by Young *et al* in this volume (12). In general, clearing and transplantation are performed at the same time. However, since coordinating breeding of hosts and embryos at the same time can pose difficulties, mice whose fat pads have been cleared at 3 weeks of age can also be used at a later time point.

TRANSPLANTATION.   After a culture period of 16 to 36 h (determined by the time needed for genotyping), transplant the glands into the cleared fat pad of an appropriate host. For easier visualization during the tissue transfer the cultures can be stained by submerging the filters in trypan blue. After 3 to 5 min transfer the filters to PBS and carefully remove the cultures. Pick up the cultures with fine watchmaker's forceps and implant them into the center of a cleared fat pad. Each cleared fat pad receives one culture (two to three glands surrounded

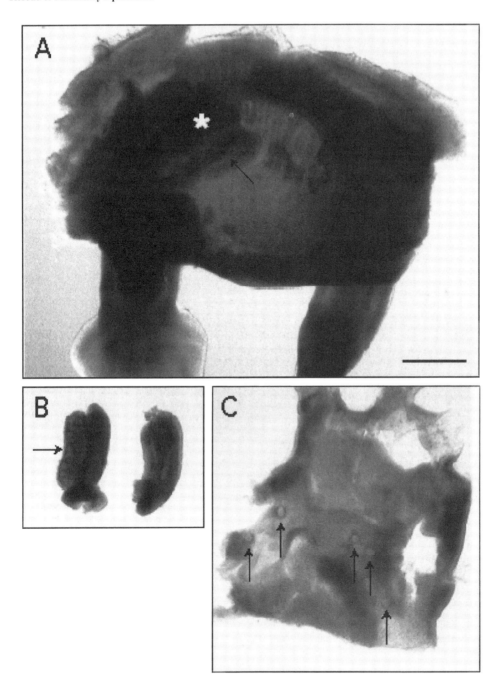

Figure 26-2. Dissection of embryos. (A) Dissected embryo half laying skin side down. All inner organs with exception of the gonad (arrow) and kidney (asterisk) are removed. Caudal is to the left. (B) Gonads of 13-day embryo. Testis cords (arrow) are visible in the testis on the left while the ovary on the right looks rather inconspicuous at this stage. (C) After peeling of the skin the five mammary anlagen (arrows) can be seen. Scale bar 1 mm.

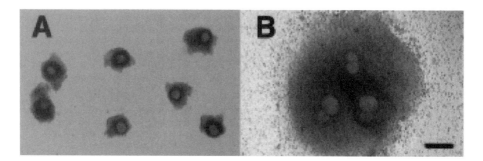

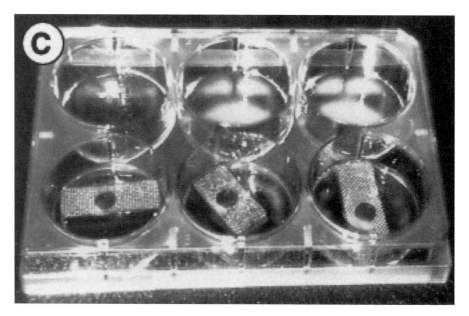

Figure 26-3. (A) Single mammary anlagen dissected from a 13-day-old embryo. (B) Three mammary glands grown for 24 h on a piece of ventral mesenchyme before transplantation. (C) Six-well dish with stainless steel grids used for culture of embryonic mammary tissues. Scale bar in (A) and (B) 200 μm.

by the ventral mesenchyme). For an internal control it is advisable to implant mutant glands on one side of the host and a control (wild type) gland on the contralateral side.

HARVEST.   Time and method of harvest of the transplanted tissues are determined by the experimental design. The fat pad containing the transplant is removed from the host in the same way as an endogenous gland through an incision along the midline in the ventral skin. In order to evaluate full ductal outgrowth transplants are harvested from virgin mice after 8 weeks. To assess epithelial development after pregnancy, we mate the hosts 8 weeks after the transplantation and harvest the transplants immediately after delivery (13, 14). Since the transplanted epithelium has no connection to a nipple, milk stasis will set in and induce the first stage of involution (15).

In each case it has to be ascertained that the transplant was successful. It is relatively easy to see the transplanted epithelium in the fully lactating state without aid, but it is harder to evaluate the epithelial content in the virgin animal. This is done most easily by reserving

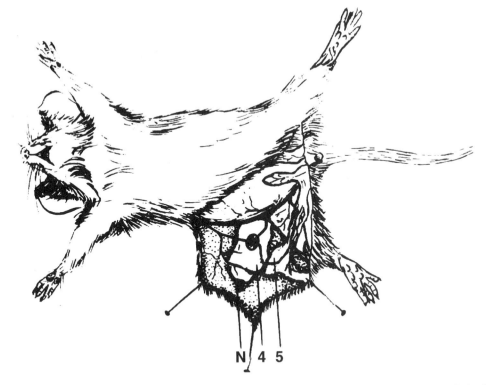

Figure 26-4. Clearing of mammary gland in 3-week-old mouse. N, nipple; 4, proximal part of gland no. 4 that is excised; 5, fat pad of gland no. 5. (Reproduced from Ref. 11 with kind permission from *Cancer Research*.)

a small piece of the fat pad on a glass slide, fixing and staining for whole mount examination (16). Depending on the amount of material needed, the glands can be divided into two or three parts that can be subject to different assays such as histology, RNA, or protein analysis in addition to the whole mount.

COMMENTS

Results Obtained Using the IR Knockout Mice

Inactivation of the IR results in perinatal lethality (10). To assess the role of IR signaling in mammary epithelial development, mammary anlagen were harvested from E14.5 C57BL/6 embryos derived by mating siblings heterozygous for a disrupted IR I gene (10) and cultured overnight as described. After genotyping of each embryo by PCR, tissues from IR deficient and wild-type embryos were transplanted into contralateral cleared fat pads of recipient hosts. Four hosts were harvested after 8 weeks and development of the transplants was assessed by whole mount analysis. No difference was observed in the extent of ductal development between control and mutant tissues (data not shown). Four hosts were mated and the transplanted tissues were harvested the morning after the delivery of pups. A small piece of tissue was reserved for whole mount analysis (16), and the rest of the transplanted

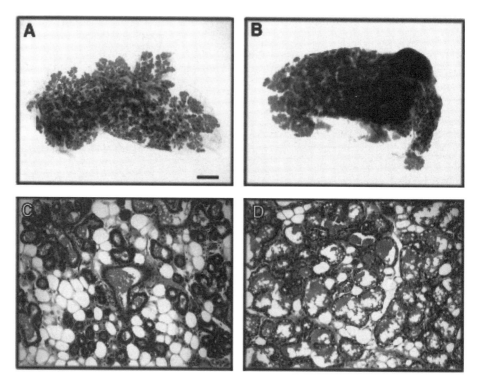

Figure 26-5. Transplanted IR-deficient mammary epithelium (A, C) and wild-type epithelium (B, D) harvested after parturition. The sparse development of the mutant epithelium is evident in the whole mounts (A, B) as well as in the histological sections (B, D). Scale bar 1 mm (A, B); 50 μm (C, D).

gland was processed for RNA extraction (17) and Northern analysis. After photographic documentation the whole-mounted tissue was embedded in paraffin, and 5-μm sections were prepared and stained with hematoxylin and eosin by standard methods.

Although the transplanted IR-null epithelium is able to form alveoli, the tissue harvested at the onset of lactation has a sparser appearance than the transplanted wild-type tissue harvested from the same host (Figure 26-5A, B). In the histological section a slight reduction in alveolar density and size is seen in IR-deficient mammary epithelium compared to the wild-type transplant. The alveolar cells show signs of secretory activity; however, they have a reduced number of lipid droplets in the cytoplasm (Figure 26-5C, D). The ducts are filled with secretory material. Milk protein synthesis as determined by the expression of β-casein and whey acidic protein is reduced in the gland containing an IR-deficient transplant compared to glands with a wild-type epithelial transplant (data not shown). This reflects the reduced epithelial contents and indicates that signaling through the epithelial IR receptor is required for alveolar growth.

Special Hints and Pitfalls

We describe here a method for transplantation of mammary anlagen of embryonic stages into prepubescent hosts. This permits evaluation of the developmental capacity of mammary tissues from mutants that do not survive to adulthood. The embryonic glands are originally cultured on a small piece of ventral mesenchyme. As in the embryo, the outgrowing primary sprout pushes through this layer of surrounding cells into the distal fat pad and thus becomes juxtaposed to the host's stroma. By transfer of the embryonic glands to the mammary fat pad of a prepubescent host whose mammary epithelium has been removed prior to transplantation the mammary epithelium is able to develop in a homotopic site. Under normal conditions the epithelium will branch and fully penetrate the host fad pad. Furthermore, the transplanted tissue will be exposed to the authentic hormonal milieu of pregnancy when the host is impregnated.

In order to prevent rejection of the graft by a host-versus-graft reaction the transplant should be made into isogenic hosts. If this is not possible immunocompromised hosts also can be used. We have successfully transplanted tissues from several mutants into nude mice. Recently the use of RAG1$^{-/-}$ hosts has been described (18).

In most cases, i.e., when the tissue is not damaged or lost during the procedure and the mutation does not affect mammary epithelial development, ducts will grow out and permeate the fat pad in about 5 to 7 weeks. Sometimes the transplant also may contain a small piece of epidermis, which will form a cyst with enclosed hair.

One source of problems derives from the incomplete removal of the endogenous gland from the recipient. This is crucial, particularly when the glands are harvested for RNA or protein preparation and not every transplant can be evaluated by whole mount or histology. It is important to use mice that are between 3 and 4 weeks of age (less than 13 g weight). At this stage the gland has not grown beyond the lymph node and will be removed entirely by the described clearing procedure. To validate complete removal of the host epithelium it is advisable to perform whole mount staining of the fragments removed in the clearing pocedure. Special care also has to be taken to sever the connection with the fat pad of the second inguinal (no. 5) gland, and one should determine that the fat pad of the transplanted gland is not connected to the fifth gland at the time of harvest. Finally, depending on the specific conditions, proof that the outgrowth is derived from the transplanted tissue can be obtained by PCR analysis or histochemistry or any other suitable test.

REFERENCES

1. K.-U. Wagner, E. B. Rucker III, and L. Hennighausen (2000). Adenoviral and transgenic approaches for the conditional deletion of genes from mammary tissue, Chapter 24 this volume.
2. C. W. Daniel and G. B. Silberstein (1987). Postnatal development of the rodent mammary gland. In M. C. Neville and C. W. Daniel (eds.), *The Mammary Gland. Development, Regulation, and Function*, Plenum Press, New York, pp. 3–36.
3. W. Imagawa, J. Yang, R. Guzman, and S. Nandi (1994). Control of mammary gland development. In E. Knobil and J. D. Neill (eds.), *The Physiology of Reproduction*, Second Edition, Raven Press, New York, pp. 1033–1059.
4. Y. J. Topper and C. S. Freeman (1980). Multiple hormone interactions in the developmental biology of the mammary gland. *Physiol. Rev.* **60**:1049–1056.
5. W. Ruan, V. Catanese, R. Wieczorek, M. Feldman, and D. L. Kleinberg (1995). Estradiol enhances the stimulatory effect of insulin-like growth factor-I (IGF-I) on mammary development and growth hormone-induced IGF-I messenger ribonucleic acid. *Endocrinology* **136**:1296–1302.
6. D. L. Hadsell, N. M. Greenberg, J. M. Fligger, C. R. Baumrucker, and J. M. Rosen (1996). Targeted expression of des(1–3) human insulin-like growth factor I in transgenic mice influences mammary gland development and IGF-binding protein expression. *Endocrinology* **137**:321–330.
7. S. Neuenschwander, A. Schwartz, T. L. Wood, C. T. Roberts, Jr., L. Henninghausen, and D. LeRoith (1996). Involution of the lactating mammary gland is inhibited by the IGF system in a transgenic mouse model. *J. Clin. Invest.* **97**:2225–2232.

8. P. Bates, R. Fisher, A. Ward, L. Richardson, D. J. Hill, and C. F. Graham (1995). Mammary cancer in transgenic mice expressing insulin-like growth factor II (IGF-II). *Br. J. Cancer* **72:**1189–1193.

9. D. Accili (1997). Insulin receptor knock-out mice. *Trends Endocrinol. Metab.* **8:**101–104.

10. D. Accili, J. Drago, E. J. Lee, M. D. Johnson, M. H. Cool, P. Salvatore, L. D. Asico, P. A. Jose, S. I. Taylor, and H. Westphal (1996). Early neonatal death in mice homozygous for a null allele of the insulin receptor gene. *Nat. Genet.* **12:**106–109.

11. K. B. DeOme, L. J. Faulkin, Jr., H. A. Bern, and P. E. Blair (1959). Development of mammary tumors from hyperplastic alveolar nodules transplanted into gland-free mammary fat pads of female C3H mice. *Cancer Res.* **19:**515–520.

12. L. J. T. Young (2000). The cleared mammary fat pad and the transplantation of mammary gland morphological structures and cells, Chapter 6 this volume.

13. G. W. Robinson and L. Hennighausen (1997). Inhibins and activins regulate mammary epithelial cell differentiation through mesenchymal-epithelial interactions. *Development* **124:**2701–2708.

14. G. W. Robinson, P. F. Johnson, L. Hennighausen, and E. Sterneck (1998). The C/EBPβ transcription factor regulates epithelial cell proliferation and differentiation in the mammary gland. *Genes Dev.* **12:**1907–1916.

15. M. Li, X. Liu, G. Robinson, U. Bar-Peled, K. U. Wagner, W. S. Young, L. Hennighausen, and P. A. Furth (1997). Mammary-derived signals activate programmed cell death during the first stage of mammary gland involution. *Proc. Natl. Acad. Sci. U.S.A.* **94:**3425–3430.

16. S. B. Rasmussen, L. J. T. Young, and G. H. Smith (2000). Preparing mammary gland whole mounts from mice, Chapter 7 this volume.

17. P. Chomczynski and N. Sacchi (1987). Single step method of RNA isolation by acid guanidinium thiocyanate-phenol-chloroform extraction. *Anal. Biochem.* **162:**156–159.

18. C. Brisken, S. Park, T. Vass, J. P. Lydon, and B. W. O'Malley (1998). A paracrine role for the epithelial progesterone receptor in mammary gland development. *Proc. Natl. Acad. Sci. U.S.A.* **95:**5076–5081.

Index